Teaching Atlas of Urologic Imaging

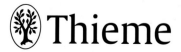

Teaching Atlas of Urologic Imaging

Robert A. Older, MD
Professor Emeritus, Department of Radiology
University of Virginia Health Sciences Center
University of Virginia
Charlottesville, Virginia
and
Director of Imaging
Virginia Urology Center
Richmond, Virginia

Matthew J. Bassignani, MD
Associate Professor, Department of Radiology
Section Chief, Genitourinary Imaging
Medical Director for Radiology Information Systems
Medical Director of the University of Virginia Imaging Center
University of Virginia Health Sciences Center
University of Virginia
Charlottesville, Virginia

Thieme
New York • Stuttgart

Thieme Medical Publishers, Inc.
333 Seventh Avenue
New York, NY 10001

Editor: Timothy Y. Hiscock
Editorial Assistant: David Price
Vice President, Production and Electronic Publishing: Anne T. Vinnicombe
Production Editor: Martha L. Wetherill
Vice President, International Sales and Marketing: Cornelia Schulze
Sales Director: Ross Lumpkin
Chief Financial Officer: Peter van Woerden
President: Brian D. Scanlan
Compositor: Macmillan Solutions
Printer: Everbest Printing Company Ltd.

Library of Congress Cataloging-in-Publication Data

Older, Robert A.
    Teaching atlas of urologic imaging / Robert A. Older, Matthew J. Bassignani.
        p. ; cm.
    Includes bibliographical references and index.
    ISBN 978-1-60406-016-4
    1. Urinary organs—Imaging—Atlases. I. Bassignani, Matthew J. II. Title.
    [DNLM: 1. Urologic Diseases—diagnosis—Atlases. 2. Urologic
Diseases—therapy—Atlases. 3. Diagnostic Imaging—methods—Atlases.
    4. Urology—methods—Atlases. WJ 17 O44t 2008]
    RC874.O43 2008
    616.6'075—dc22   2008028142

Important note: Medical knowledge is ever-changing. As new research and clinical experience broaden our knowledge, changes in treatment and drug therapy may be required. The authors and editors of the material herein have consulted sources believed to be reliable in their efforts to provide information that is complete and in accord with the standards accepted at the time of publication. However, in view of the possibility of human error by the authors, editors, or publisher of the work herein, or changes in medical knowledge, neither the authors, editors, or publisher, nor any other party who has been involved in the preparation of this work, warrants that the information contained herein is in every respect accurate or complete, and they are not responsible for any errors or omissions or for the results obtained from use of such information. Readers are encouraged to confirm the information contained herein with other sources. For example, readers are advised to check the product information sheet included in the package of each drug they plan to administer to be certain that the information contained in this publication is accurate and that changes have not been made in the recommended dose or in the contraindications for administration. This recommendation is of particular importance in connection with new or infrequently used drugs.

Some of the product names, patents, and registered designs referred to in this book are in fact registered trademarks or proprietary names even though specific reference to this fact is not always made in the text. Therefore, the appearance of a name without designation as proprietary is not to be construed as a representation by the publisher that it is in the public domain.

Printed in China
5 4 3 2 1

ISBN 978-1-60406-016-4

DEDICATIONS

To my wife, Linda, who has lovingly tolerated book chapters in progress covering much of the table and counter space of our home. Without her support, this book could not have been completed.

—Robert A. Older

To my partner, Alan Higgins, for his continued and unwavering support for all my academic pursuits. His continual encouragement challenges me to accomplish more than I ever thought that I could, and with that, it brings meaning and fulfillment to those pursuits.

—Matthew J. Bassignani

CONTENTS

PREFACE

Teaching Atlas of Urologic Imaging has been written by two radiologists specializing in urologic imaging. It is intended to create the equivalent of "viewbox" learning. Each case is initially presented as an image or series of images with a brief clinical history, much as would occur in clinical practice. The case can be initially viewed as an unknown. After viewing the images, the reader can then view the radiographic findings pertinent to the images presented. This is followed by the correct diagnosis. A brief differential diagnosis of other entities that might be considered given the imaging findings then follows. After the diagnosis is presented, clinical and pathologic data and treatment options are given where appropriate. The Imaging Findings section that follows is meant to do two things: to discuss the reasons the other choices in the differential diagnosis list are not the correct diagnosis and to discuss the role of imaging modalities other than the imaging study used for the initial case discussion. Sometimes this includes many modalities, but for other cases only limited modalities are appropriate. Diagnostic "pearls" are included as appropriate. At the end of each case, there is a list of suggested readings.

Urologic radiology has undergone dramatic changes. The intravenous pyelogram (IVP), for many years the mainstay of urologic imaging, has largely been replaced by abdominal computed tomography (CT) scans and ultrasound for many clinical indications. More recently, advances in CT instrumentation with multiplanar reconstruction have allowed the development of the CT-IVP, a study incorporating the basic principles of the IVP and the technology of CT. This study, which is now the basic means for evaluating hematuria and other urologic indications, has essentially replaced the IVP. It is important, however, to understand that the principles developed over many years to diagnose urologic diseases with the IVP need to be carried over to the interpretation of the CT-IVP. Experience with the CT-IVP is limited but growing rapidly. In this atlas we have selected cases to illustrate the imaging findings of many common and relatively common urologic abnormalities. We present not only the newer modalities of CT, CT-IVP, magnetic resonance imaging (MRI), and ultrasound, but also the traditional studies, such as KUB (kidneys, ureters, and bladder) abdominal radiography, IVP, voiding cystourethrogram (VCUG), cystogram, retrograde pyelogram, and retrograde urethrogram.

Teaching Atlas of Urologic Imaging is intended for radiologists and urologists in training, as well as for practicing board-certified physicians wanting to review the imaging findings of many common urologic diseases.

ACKNOWLEDGMENTS

The authors would like to acknowledge the editors of Thieme Medical Publishers for their help and support in this project, specifically David Price, Tim Hiscock, and Martha Wetherill, who have worked closely with us throughout the project and have made production of this book a smooth and pleasant process.

We would also like to thank and acknowledge Craig Luce who created the artwork in this atlas.

CASE 1

Clinical Presentation

A middle-aged female presented with a suspected right renal mass on an intravenous pyelogram (IVP).

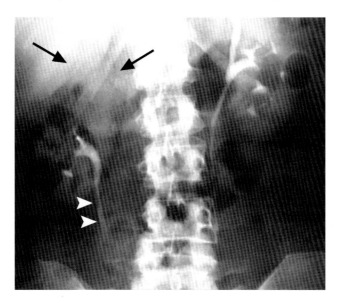

Fig. 1.1 Excretory phase of an intravenous pyelogram. The abdominal radiograph is coned to the kidneys.

Radiologic Findings

- In this patient with complete duplication, the IVP (**Fig. 1.1**) shows an ill-defined mass in the upper pole of the right kidney (*arrows*) deviating the remainder of the kidney's collecting system inferiorly. This represents an obstructed upper pole moiety. The lower moiety ureter is deviated laterally (*arrowheads*) by the dilated right upper ureter, which is not opacified.

Diagnosis

Complete duplication with obstructed upper moiety

Differential Diagnosis

- Renal mass
- Adrenal mass

Discussion

Background

Ureteral duplication occurs more commonly in females and is most often unilateral. Ectopic insertions in females may be below the external urethral sphincter, but in males, insertion is above the sphincter (most commonly into the posterior urethra). In females, most ectopic ureters are associated with duplications, whereas a single kidney and ureter are more commonly found in males with ectopic ureteral insertions.

Clinical Findings

Duplications are often discovered during the work-up of urinary tract infection (UTI) symptoms. Vesicoureteral reflux is a common complication of the lower moiety ureter. Obstruction is seen with the upper moiety ureter due to its abnormal insertion into the bladder (or due to ureterocele) presenting with pain or UTI.

In a young girl who should be old enough to be continent, the history of being continually wet should result in a work-up for an ectopic ureteral insertion below the external sphincter.

Pathology

Induction of the kidney parenchyma is believed to occur when the ureteric bud contacts the metanephric blastema. The bud originates from the mesonephric duct (precursor to the Gartner duct, located in the lateral vaginal wall, in women and the vas deferens, ejaculatory ducts, and seminal vesicles in men). In incomplete duplication, a bifid renal pelvis forms where upper and lower poles drain to separate collecting systems that fuse at the ureteropelvic junction (UPJ) level or lower to form one ureter that drains into the bladder. In complete duplication, two separate renal units (i.e., upper and lower moieties) will drain into separate ureters that have separate bladder insertions. Using the Weigert-Meyer rule, the upper moiety will drain into the bladder lower and medial when compared with the lower moiety. The upper moiety is prone to distal ureteral obstruction, whereas the lower moiety's ureter is prone to vesicoureteral reflux and UPJ obstruction. The upper moiety ureteral insertions may be ectopic and/or associated with ureterocele (**Fig. 1.2**).

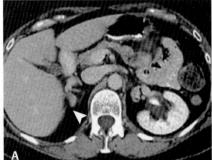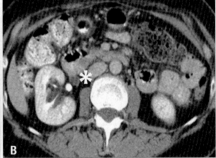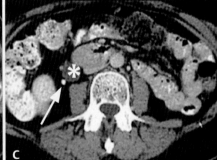

Fig. 1.2 Contrast-enhanced computed tomography (CT) from the patient in **Fig. 1.1**. **(A)** Obstructed atrophic upper moiety with cortical thinning (*arrowhead*). **(B)** CT at this level shows a normal lower moiety and the medially placed dilated upper moiety's ureter (*asterisk*). **(C)** CT at this level shows the dilated upper moiety's ureter (*asterisk*) displacing the lower moiety's ureter laterally (*arrow*).

Imaging Findings

RADIOGRAPHY

- An upper pole renal mass should enhance more than that seen in this case, and there should be some excretion from an upper pole renal mass.
- An adrenal mass may present with these findings; thus, cross-sectional imaging is indicated.
- Deviation of the lower moiety of a complete duplication is seen due to the mass effect from the obstructed upper moiety (see "drooping lily" in **Fig. 1.3**).
- As the upper moiety's ureter is dilated, it produces mass effect on the adjacent lower moiety's ureter, deviating it laterally (arrowheads in **Fig. 1.1** and arrows in **Fig. 1.3**).
- The complete duplication is not always apparent on the IVP; computed tomography (CT)-IVP should be performed even if the IVP is negative if symptoms, such as continual urine leak in a young female, suggest complete duplication.

The classic sign on IVP of a duplicated collecting system with obstruction is the "drooping lily" sign (**Fig. 1.3**). This results from the obstructed, poorly functioning upper moiety with mass effect on the lower moiety, which is normally functioning. Excretion into the lower moiety's collecting system shows the contrast-filled calyces to be bunched together and to resemble the drooping petals of a lily. Even though the obstructed upper moiety may not excrete, the nephrogram phase will show the kidney to be larger than what is being drained by the lower moiety's collecting system.

COMPUTED TOMOGRAPHY

- CT-IVP is an excellent modality to show all of the features associated with an obstructed duplicated kidney (**Fig. 1.4**).

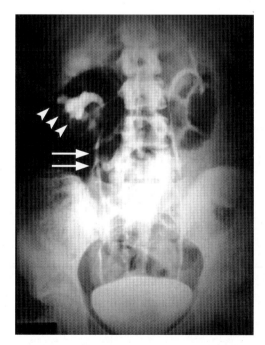

Fig. 1.3 Abdominal radiograph from the excretory phase of an intravenous pyelogram. Lower pole calyces (*arrowheads*) are displaced downward to form the "drooping lily" sign. Note the lateral displacement of the lower moiety's ureter (*arrows*). Courtesy of Theodore Keats, M.D.

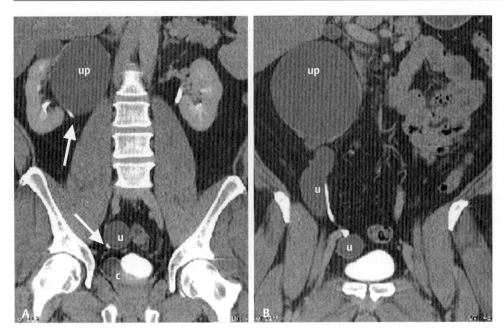

Fig. 1.4 Coronal reconstruction of a CT-IVP in the excretory phase at two levels **(A** and **B)**. **(A)** Right upper moiety hydronephrosis (up) with deviation of lower moiety's ureter laterally (*arrows*). C, distal ureter. **(B)** Upper moiety hydronephrosis (up) and hydroureter (u).

ULTRASOUND

- Observing hydronephrosis and hydroureter localized to an upper pole (as in **Fig. 1.5A**) should raise suspicion of a duplicated system with obstruction. This can, however, be confused with renal or parapelvic cysts.
- Evaluation of the bladder may show the dilated ureter near the expected trigone (**Fig. 1.5B**).
- An ectopic ureter may cause a fluid-filled bulge in the lateral bladder wall, or the ectopic ureter may end in a ureterocele (**Fig. 1.5B**).

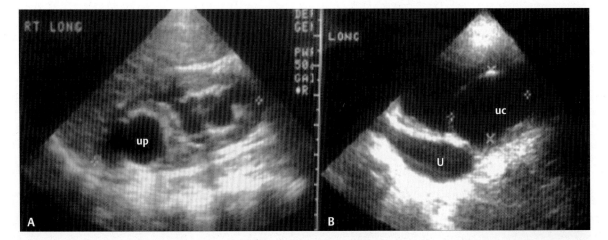

Fig. 1.5 Complete duplication on a renal sonogram. **(A)** Sagittal image of the right kidney shows the dilated upper collecting system (up) out of proportion to the lower collecting system. This mismatch suggests complete duplication with obstruction. The lower moiety collecting system is also somewhat prominent, most likely from reflux. **(B)** Sagittal bladder images show the dilated upper moiety's ureter (U) ending in a ureterocele (uc), the cause for the obstruction.

Treatment

- In symptomatic patients, if the renal function of both moieties is preserved, the ureters are reimplanted to prevent further damage from reflux or obstruction.
- In a long-standing obstruction, the upper moiety will be atrophic. If its function is minimal, the upper moiety will be resected along with its ureter.
- It is important to exclude bilateral duplicated systems (seen in up to 20% of cases) and to confirm which is the symptomatic system to avoid surgery on the wrong kidney.

Prognosis

- Good

PEARLS _____

- The difference in degree of dilatation of the upper and lower poles (**Fig. 1.5**) is an important clue to the diagnosis of complete duplication in these patients.

Suggested Readings

Berrocal T, Lopez-Pereira P, Arjonilla A, Gutierrez J. Anomalies of the distal ureter, bladder, and urethra in children: embryologic, radiologic, and pathologic features. Radiographics 2002;22(5):1139–1164.

Braverman RM, Lebowitz RL. Occult ectopic ureter in girls with urinary incontinence: diagnosis by using CT. AJR Am J Roentgenol 1991;156(2):365–366.

Decter RM. Renal duplication and fusion anomalies. Pediatr Clin North Am 1997;44(5):1323–1341.

Wein A, ed. Campbell-Walsh Urology. 9th ed. Philadelphia: Saunders; 2007.

Zissin R, Apter S, Yaffe D, et al. Renal duplication with associated complications in adults: CT findings in 26 cases. Clin Radiol 2001;56(1):58–63.

CASE 2

Clinical Presentation

A 35-year-old male presents with hematuria.

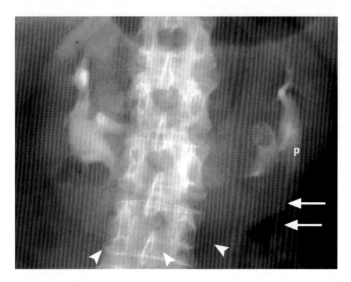

Fig. 2.1 Delayed film from an intravenous pyelogram.

Radiologic Findings

- Abnormal axis of both sides of the horseshoe kidney (lower poles directed medially)
- Midline fusion of the lower pole renal parenchyma (*arrowheads,* **Fig. 2.1**)
- Bilateral malrotation, with the renal pelvis directed laterally. Note the lateral position of the left ureter (*arrows,* **Fig. 2.1**) exiting an anteriorly and laterally placed renal pelvis (p).

Diagnosis

Horseshoe kidney

Differential Diagnosis

- Bilateral congenital renal malrotation without fusion
- Bilateral renal malrotation secondary to retroperitoneal mass
- Crossed fused renal ectopia

Discussion

Background

When it is discovered, horseshoe kidney is often incidentally detected, and as many as 90% of cases may be asymptomatic. Those discovered early are often found during the work-up for urinary tract infection or when a palpable abdominal mass is felt in a child. Horseshoe kidney occurs in ~1 in 400 to 500 live births, and males are affected more often than females. Many genetic syndromes are associated with horseshoe kidney (e.g., Turner syndrome).

6

Clinical Findings

Clinical presentation depends on secondary complications, such as stones, infection, or trauma.

Pathology

During renal development and ascent, it is believed that fusion of the metanephric blastema causes both developing kidneys to touch and fuse at their lower poles. This fusion anomaly causes the characteristic shape of the horseshoe kidney. The fused portion is termed the isthmus and can be composed of renal parenchyma (*arrowheads*, **Fig. 2.1**) or fibrous tissue. The isthmus rests just under the inferior mesenteric artery.

The ureters of horseshoe kidneys insert into an anteriorly placed renal pelvis (p, **Fig. 2.1**), which drapes over the anterior lip of the renal parenchyma and can result in impaired urine drainage. This configuration may result in urinary stasis, vesicoureteral reflux, stone formation, obstruction (**Figs. 2.2** and **2.3**), and/or infection. There also is an increased risk of transitional cell carcinoma in adults and Wilms tumor in children. The vascular supply is often complex, as the malformed renal tissue recruits its blood supply from the adjacent aorta and iliac vessels. The kidneys are at increased risk for blunt trauma, as they are no longer protected by the rib cage as are normally placed kidneys in the renal fossa. Rather, the isthmus lies just anterior to the spine, where it is quite easily injured from blunt abdominal trauma.

Imaging Findings

RADIOGRAPHY

- Visualizing the enhancing parenchymal isthmus excludes bilateral congenital renal malrotation without fusion and malrotation secondary to a retroperitoneal mass. If there were a fibrous isthmus, these diagnoses could be entertained.
- With renal units on either side of the spine, crossed fused renal ectopia is excluded.
- Malposition of the kidneys is seen, with both being lower than expected.
- Abnormal axis is seen, where the upper poles will be laterally oriented, and the lower poles are medially oriented.
- A parenchymal band of isthmus may be shown to enhance, whereas a fibrous band will not.

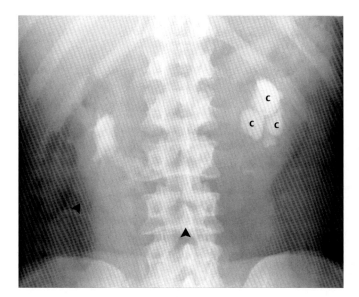

Fig. 2.2 Intravenous pyelogram film coned to the kidneys shows a curvilinear soft tissue density in the midabdomen (*arrowheads*) representing the outline of this patient's horseshoe kidney. There is a left-sided obstruction at the ureteropelvic junction. Note the dilated calyces (c).

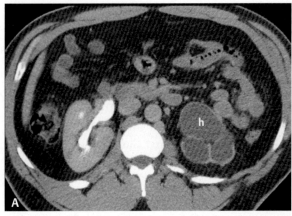 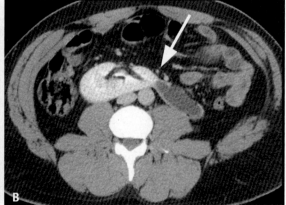

Fig. 2.3 Excretory phase of an enhanced computed tomography scan at two levels through a horseshoe kidney **(A** and **B)**. **(A)** There is a severely hydronephrotic left kidney with cortical thinning (h). **(B)** The left half of the horseshoe kidney has a ureteropelvic junction obstruction. Note the inferior mesenteric artery (*arrow*).

COMPUTED TOMOGRAPHY

- Malposition of the kidneys is seen on computed tomography (CT), with both kidneys being lower than expected.
- Abnormal axis is seen, where the upper poles are laterally oriented, and the lower poles are medially oriented.
- A parenchymal band of isthmus may be shown to enhance, whereas a fibrous band will not. Isthmus is seen at the L4–L5 level between the aorta and the inferior mesenteric artery.
- The renal pelvis and ureters are situated anteriorly.
- Multiple renal arteries may be seen.

ULTRASOUND

- Findings on ultrasound may be confusing. Because of the kidneys' slightly lower position and medial orientation, as well as midline bowel gas, the ultrasound technologist may not appreciate the fusion anomaly (**Fig. 2.4**). One kidney may not be appreciated, suggesting agenesis or ectopia.
- In the setting of renal ectopia, the sonographer should try to identify the second kidney in the contralateral renal fossa (e.g., crossed fused or crossed unfused ectopia) and anywhere along the path of renal ascent in the contralateral retroperitoneum or in the pelvis.

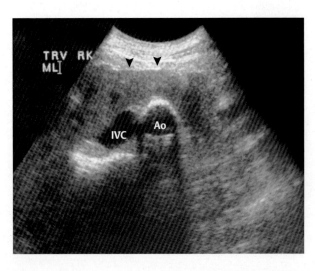

Fig. 2.4 Ultrasound showing an abnormal axis to both kidneys. The lower poles extend to the midline, where this isthmus of tissue (*arrowheads*) was demonstrated, consistent with a horseshoe kidney. Ao, aorta; IVC, inferior vena cava.

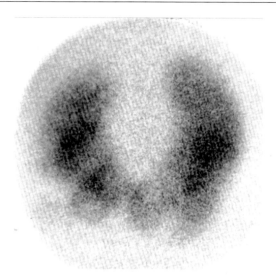

Fig. 2.5 Nuclear medicine renal scan. Anterior converging image obtained on the midabdomen shows a horseshoe kidney with tracer uptake in both renal units and in a prominent isthmus.

NUCLEAR MEDICINE

- A diuretic renal scan may be employed to evaluate obstruction and function of the kidney.
- Obstruction is determined by a delay in the excretion of 50% of the tracer from the collecting system beyond 20 minutes (i.e., prolonged T½).
- Differential renal function of each side of the horseshoe can be determined by relative tracer uptake (**Fig. 2.5**).

MAGNETIC RESONANCE IMAGING

- Findings are identical to CT (**Fig. 2.6**).

Treatment

- Based on associated complications/symptoms

Prognosis

- In the absence of complications, usually asymptomatic

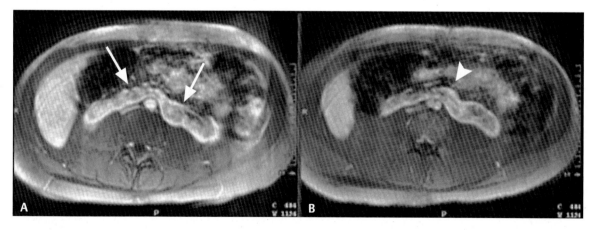

Fig. 2.6 (A,B) Postgadolinium T1-weighted gradient echo image at two levels through a horseshoe kidney shows a parenchymal band of tissue (*arrows* in **A**) just under the inferior mesenteric artery (*arrowhead* in **B**) consistent with a horseshoe kidney.

PEARLS

- A voiding cystourethrogram (VCUG) should be performed during work-up to exclude vesicoureteral reflux.

Suggested Readings

Boubaker A, Prior JO, Meuwly JY, Bischof-Delaloye A. Radionuclide investigations of the urinary tract in the era of multimodality imaging. J Nucl Med 2006;47(11):1819–1836.

Buntley D. Malignancy associated with horseshoe kidney. Urology 1976;8(2):146–148.

Decter RM. Renal duplication and fusion anomalies. Pediatr Clin North Am 1997;44(5):1323–1341.

Friedland GW, de Vries P. Renal ectopia and fusion: embryologic basis. Urology 1975;5(5):698–706.

Gleason PE, Kelalis PP, Husmann DA, Kramer SA. Hydronephrosis in renal ectopia: incidence, etiology and significance. J Urol 1994;151(6):1660–1661.

Grainger R, Murphy DM, Lane V. Horseshoe kidney: a review of the presentation, associated congenital anomalies and complications in 73 patients. Ir Med J 1983;76(7):315–317.

Pitts WRJr, Muecke EC. Horseshoe kidneys: a 40-year experience. J Urol 1975;113(6):743–746.

Walsh P, ed. Campbell's Urology. Philadelphia: Saunders; 2002.

CASE 3

Clinical Presentation

Urinary tract infections

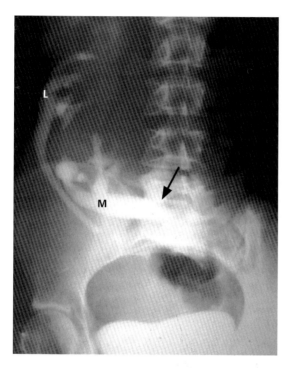

Fig. 3.1 KUB (kidneys, ureters, and bladder) examination from the excretory phase of an intravenous pyelogram. Demonstrated is the classic S-shaped configuration of the contrast-filled collecting systems and ureters in a patient with crossed fused ectopia.

Radiologic Findings

- Both kidneys are on one side of the spine (i.e., one kidney is crossed).
- The lower kidney's ureter crosses the midline (*arrow*, **Fig. 3.1**) and inserts into the orthotopic trigone.
- The upper kidney's ureter enters the ipsilateral trigone.
- Both kidneys show malrotation: the upper kidney's renal pelvis faces laterally (L, **Fig. 3.1**), and the lower kidney's renal pelvis faces medially (M, **Fig. 3.1**).
- The classic S-shaped configuration of the contrast-filled collecting systems and ureters is seen on excretory urography.

Diagnosis

Crossed fused ectopia

Differential Diagnosis

- Crossed nonfused kidneys
- Horseshoe kidney
- Pelvic kidney

Discussion

Background

Ectopic kidney is defined as a kidney not resting in its normal position in the renal fossa. Varieties include, from most common to least common, simple ectopia, crossed fused ectopia, crossed unfused ectopia, and pelvic kidney. Congenital absence of one (**Fig. 3.2**) or both kidneys is known as renal agenesis.

Clinical Findings

Most patients with renal ectopia are asymptomatic, but the ectopic kidney may show vesicoureteral reflux during a voiding cystourethrogram (VCUG). An abnormal ureteropelvic junction anatomy pre-disposes patients to urinary stasis and its attendant complications (e.g., stones and infection).

Pathology

A simple ectopic kidney can lie anywhere along the path of normal renal ascent, but not in the renal fossa. An ectopic kidney may assume a nonreniform shape, as the ectopic kidney conforms to the ectopic location; it may present as a mass. Blood supply is variable.

In fusion anomalies, the ectopic kidney commonly fuses its upper pole to the lower pole of the orthotopic kidney. The ectopic kidney can be identified as its ureter crosses midline at the pelvic brim (*arrow*, **Fig. 3.1**), showing a normal ureteral insertion into the bladder at the ipsilateral trigone (e.g., a crossed left kidney's ureter will insert, orthotopically, into the left trigone). The ureter often arises from an anteriorly facing renal pelvis.

Imaging Findings

RADIOGRAPHY

- The fusion anomaly may be difficult to determine without cross-sectional imaging.
- Horseshoe kidney would be centered in the midline.
- Pelvic kidney does not cross to the opposite side of the pelvis.
- The typical appearance of a crossed fused kidney during excretory urography is the S shape seen in **Fig. 3.1.** See findings above.
- Renal agenesis may mimic an ectopic configuration (**Fig. 3.2**).

COMPUTED TOMOGRAPHY

- Both kidneys are on one side of the spine (i.e., one kidney is crossed).
- The crossed kidney's ureter crosses midline and inserts into the orthotopic trigone, and the upper kidney's ureter enters the ipsilateral trigone.
- These findings may be difficult to sort out when the crossed fused ectopic kidneys are in the pelvis (**Fig. 3.3**).
- A pelvic ectopic kidney will show the absence of a normal kidney in the renal fossa that will be found in the ipsilateral pelvis (K, **Fig. 3.4**). The pelvic kidney's ureter will drain to the ipsilateral trigone.

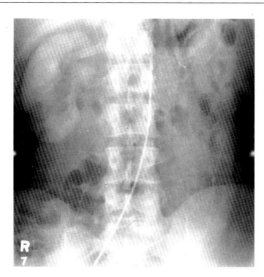

Fig. 3.2 KUB (kidneys, ureters, and bladder) examination from an aortogram shows a solitary enhancing right kidney and no enhancing renal parenchyma in the rest of the abdomen or pelvis (not shown), consistent with left renal agenesis.

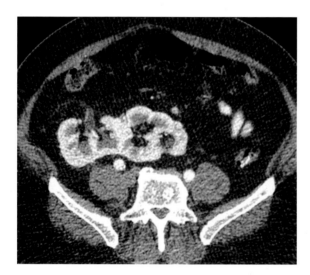

Fig. 3.3 Incidental finding. Enhanced computed tomography scan through the upper pelvis shows bilateral kidneys that are fused in the low abdomen/upper pelvis. This is consistent with crossed fused ectopia. This represents the so-called pancake kidney because of its flattened configuration.

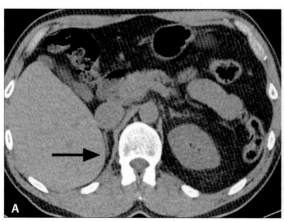
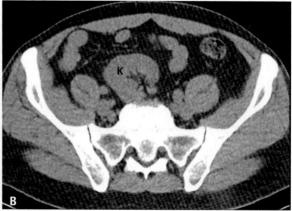

Fig. 3.4 Abdominal pain. Stone protocol computed tomography scan through the abdomen **(A)** and pelvis **(B)** shows the right renal fossa is empty (*arrow* in **A**), suggesting renal ectopia or agenesis. Pelvic kidney (K in **B**) represents the ectopic right kidney.

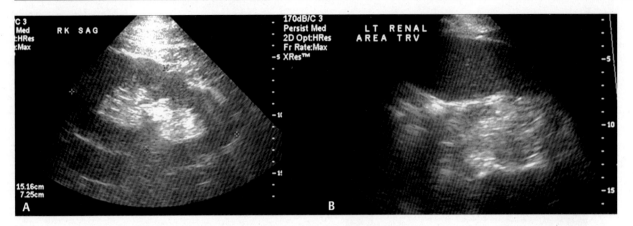

Fig. 3.5 Abdominal sonogram for pain. **(A)** Sagittal view of the right renal fossa shows a hypertrophied kidney (15.2 cm). **(B)** Sagittal view of the left renal fossa shows no left kidney identified here or anywhere along the tract of renal ascent down to the pelvis, suggesting left renal agenesis.

ULTRASOUND

- Sonograms may show a solitary, hypertrophied kidney with absence of a kidney in the contralateral renal fossa (**Fig. 3.5**). However, if an evaluation of the ipsilateral migratory pathway (i.e., pelvis to renal fossa) does not identify the contralateral kidney, a renal cortical scintigram is probably the single best test to identify contralateral functional renal tissue.

Treatment

- None is necessary except in symptomatic cases (e.g., vesicoureteral reflux, infection, or stones).

Prognosis

- Agenesis of both kidneys is incompatible with life.
- Unilateral agenesis is more common and found in 1 in 500 to 1000 live births, is usually asymptomatic, and results in no renal impairment.
- There is an association between abnormalities of the urinary tract and the genital system.
  - In males, seminal vesicle cysts may be found on the side of unilateral renal agenesis.
  - In females with urinary tract anomalies, müllerian anomalies should be considered, especially in those patients who cannot conceive.

PEARLS _____

- An ectopic kidney can "hide" over the spine on excretory urography, as the contrast-filled collecting structures blend in with the bone density of the spine. Obtain oblique abdominal radiographs during an intravenous pyelogram when only one kidney is seen.

Suggested Readings

Decter RM. Renal duplication and fusion anomalies. Pediatr Clin North Am 1997;44(5):1323–1341.

Friedland GW, de Vries P. Renal ectopia and fusion: embryologic basis. Urology 1975;5(5):698–706.

Wein A, ed. Campbell-Walsh Urology. 9th ed. Philadelphia: Saunders; 2007.

CASE 4

Clinical Presentation

A 31-year-old male presents with hematuria.

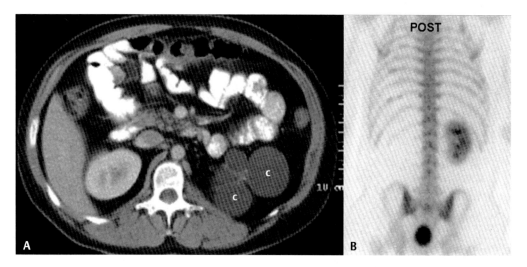

Fig. 4.1 (A) Enhanced computed tomography scan shows the left kidney replaced by cysts (c) of varying sizes. **(B)** The posterior view from a bone scan.

Radiologic Findings

- On a computed tomography (CT) scan, the left kidney is replaced by cysts (c, **Fig. 4.1**) of varying sizes.
- There is no significant left renal parenchyma.
- On a bone scan, a normal right kidney is seen, with no functioning left kidney.

Diagnosis

Multicystic dysplastic kidney

Differential Diagnosis

- Hydronephrosis
- Localized cystic disease of the kidney
- Multilocular cyst

Discussion

Background

Multicystic dysplastic kidney (MCDK) is one of the most common causes of a palpable mass in newborns. It is unilateral in ~1 in 3000 to 5000 live births. Bilateral MCDK is seen in ~1 in 10,000 live births, which is a serious finding, resulting in in utero oligohydramnios and its attendant malformations.

These lesions are almost never symptomatic and should be left alone. Over time, many will involute without a trace. There may be a slight increased risk of Wilms tumors in childhood in these patients; thus, ultrasound follow-up may be indicated to assess for worrisome changes, such as development of a mass in MCDK.

Associations include contralateral renal abnormality in up to half of patients with MCDK. Abnormalities of the contralateral kidney may include ureteropelvic junction obstruction, duplication abnormalities, vesicoureteral reflux, ectopia, or agenesis.

Clinical Findings

A palpable mass may be present in a newborn. It is usually asymptomatic in adults.

Pathology

MCDK is felt to result from abnormal interaction between the ureteric bud and the metanephric blastema. The derangement results in cysts and abnormal and nonfunctioning renal parenchyma in the involved kidney. The associated ureters are often atretic, and vascular supply is scant.

Imaging Findings

COMPUTED TOMOGRAPHY

- Hydronephrosis would connect to the collecting system, and these lesions are clearly individual cysts.
- Localized cystic disease may involve a portion of or an entire kidney, but the cysts are separated by normal-enhancing parenchyma, not seen in this case.
- Multilocular cysts arise from otherwise normal renal parenchyma, not seen in this case.
- MCDK will appear as a cystic mass in the renal fossa, with no normal renal tissue noted. Cysts may be calcified. The mass should not enhance significantly following intravenous contrast administration. If there is an enhancing component, a neoplasm must be considered. No function (i.e., contrast uptake or excretion) will be shown (**Fig. 4.1** and **Fig. 4.2**).

RADIOGRAPHY

- Abdominal radiography may show multiple calcified cysts (*arrow*, **Fig. 4.3**).

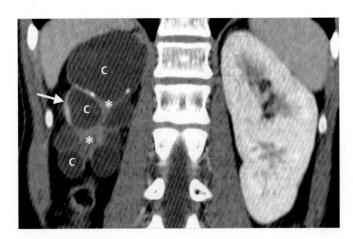

Fig. 4.2 Enhanced computed tomography three-dimensional coronal reconstruction shows multicystic dysplastic kidney on the right with multiple cysts (c), calcified cyst walls (*arrow*), and minimal abnormal renal parenchyma (*asterisks*). The cysts do not communicate to a renal pelvis. There is a normally enhancing left kidney.

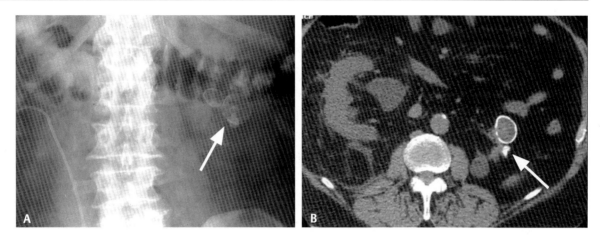

Fig. 4.3 **(A)** KUB during placement of a right double J nephroureteral stent for right-sided ureteropelvic junction obstruction. Disorganized cystic structures in the left upper quadrant with eggshell calcifications (*arrow*) are noted, suggesting multicystic dysplastic kidney. **(B)** A noncontrast computed tomography scan confirms atretic cystic structures in the left upper quadrant with little normal parenchyma (*arrow*).

ULTRASOUND

- On prenatal or antenatal sonography:
  - The sparse renal parenchyma is echogenic (**Fig. 4.4**).
  - The renal outline will be distorted and not reniform (**Fig. 4.4**).
  - MCDK is characterized as renal replacement by innumerable nonconnecting fluid-filled cysts (**Fig. 4.5**). Cysts are commonly large.
  - Little flow is seen in the residual parenchyma on color imaging.
  - No renal pelvis or ureter is identified.
  - The contralateral kidney may show signs of compensatory hypertrophy if it is otherwise unaffected.

Treatment

- Unilateral MCDK is now left untreated if asymptomatic (in most cases).
- In bilateral disease, renal transplantation may be entertained when the newborn is large enough and if lung development can support the child through the newborn period.

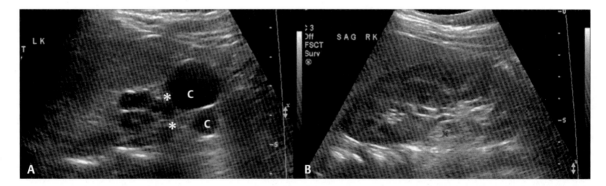

Fig. 4.4 **(A)** Renal sonogram for chronic renal insufficiency shows multiple noncommunicating cysts (c) in the left renal fossa with no normal parenchyma (*asterisks*) and no hydronephrosis. **(B)** The contralateral kidney shows hypertrophy.

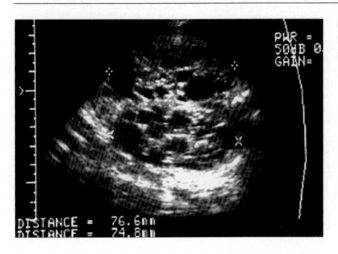

Fig. 4.5 Bilateral multicystic kidneys in utero, with both kidneys marked by cursors. This was incompatible with life.

Prognosis

• In unilateral cases, prognosis is generally good. Associated anomalies in the other kidney will result in added morbidities (e.g., early renal failure, hypertension).

PEARLS

• Although the affected kidney is large in the newborn, MCDK is usually smaller in an adult due to atrophy.

Suggested Readings

Glassberg K. Renal dysgenesis and cystic disease of the kidney. In: Wein A, ed. Campbell-Walsh Urology. 9th ed. Philadelphia: Saunders Elsevier; 2007:3334–3339.

Winyard P, Chitty L. Dysplastic and polycystic kidneys: diagnosis, associations and management. Prenat Diagn 2001;21(11):924–935.

CASE 5

Clinical Presentation

A 51-year-old female presents with a urinary tract infection (UTI).

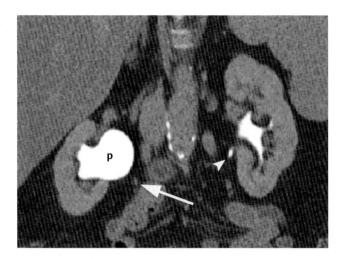

Fig. 5.1 Coronal reconstruction from a CT-IVP. Mild right ureteropelvic junction obstruction with dilated renal pelvis (p) and mild hydronephrosis are seen. The right ureter is of normal size, but it does not contain contrast (*arrow*). Normal contrast filled left ureter (*arrowhead*).

Radiologic Findings

- With an intravenous pyelogram (IVP) or computed tomography (CT)-IVP, the typical features of ureteropelvic junction (UPJ) obstruction are varying degrees of hydronephrosis in association with a dilated renal pelvis and nondilated ureter.
- The degree of hydronephrosis and parenchymal loss will depend on the severity of the obstruction and the length of time the obstruction has been present, which in turn is related to the age of the patient, as this condition is usually congenital.

Diagnosis

Congenital ureteropelvic junction obstruction

Differential Diagnosis

- Obstructing ureteral stone
- Obstructing neoplasm
- Vesicoureteral reflux

Discussion

Background

UPJ obstruction in the neonatal period is common. It presents as the most common cause of a palpable abdominal mass in a newborn. However, with the widespread use of prenatal imaging, hydronephrosis is more commonly diagnosed today during fetal sonography. Following birth, a work-up ensues after the first few days of birth, allowing the newborn to be adequately hydrated, thus negating any masking of hydronephrosis from the normal oliguric newborn. If hydronephrosis is still present, it can be staged using the Society of Fetal Urology classification, on a scale of I through IV (**Table 5.1**).

Table 5.1   Society of Fetal Urology Classification

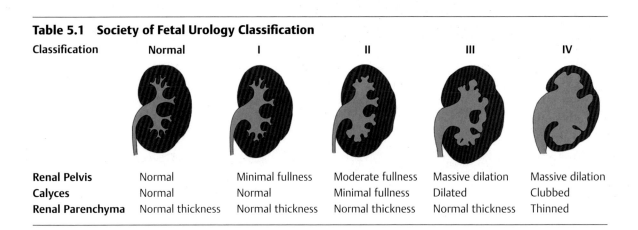

Classification	Normal	I	II	III	IV
Renal Pelvis	Normal	Minimal fullness	Moderate fullness	Massive dilation	Massive dilation
Calyces	Normal	Normal	Minimal fullness	Dilated	Clubbed
Renal Parenchyma	Normal thickness	Normal thickness	Normal thickness	Normal thickness	Thinned

Clinical Findings

A palpable mass is often present in infants representing the dilated collecting system. UTI, failure to thrive, or renal failure may occur.

Pathology

Congenital unilateral UPJ obstruction is a result of several factors resulting in the mechanical obstruction to urine flow. It is likely that causes include both an anatomical and a functional explanation. Anatomically, the area of the UPJ is narrowed, possibly limiting the movement of normal urine bolus into the proximal ureter. Some patients with UPJ obstruction have a decreased number of smooth muscle fibers at the UPJ, which may result in ineffective peristalsis and poor urine clearing from the collecting system. Crossing renal vessels, though rare, may play a part in UPJ obstruction, or they may simply be near the dilated renal pelvis as it approximates normal vessels. Finally, insertion of the pelvis into the ureter may not form a normal funnel shape or may not empty into the most dependent portion of the ureter.

Imaging Findings

WORK-UP FOR UPJ OBSTRUCTION IN THE NEWBORN

The work-up includes a voiding cystourethrogram to discount reflux, although unlikely, as the cause of unilateral collecting system distension. Renal ultrasound can confirm and can follow the collecting system dilation. IVP may be performed to determine function and anatomy. Nuclear medicine is the most commonly applied test (see below).

RADIOGRAPHY

- An obstructing ureteral stone resulting in a UPJ obstruction would present with typical clinical symptoms of renal colic, not present in this case.
- Obstructing neoplasm at the UPJ is a possibility, requiring further evaluation with cross-sectional imaging such as CT or magnetic resonance imaging (MRI). None was seen in this case.
- Nonvisualization of the ureter makes vesicoureteral reflux an unlikely diagnosis.
- Typical findings in cases of UPJ obstruction include varying degrees of hydronephrosis in association with a dilated renal pelvis and nondilated ureter (**Fig. 5.2**).

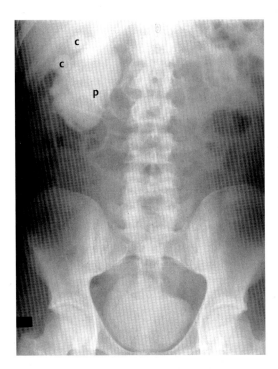

Fig. 5.2 KUB from an adult intravenous pyelogram shows a high-grade obstruction of the right collecting system with caliectasis (c) and a dilated renal pelvis (p) in this patient with left renal agenesis and a ureteropelvic junction obstruction on the right.

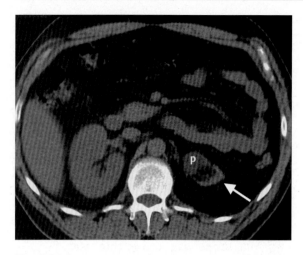

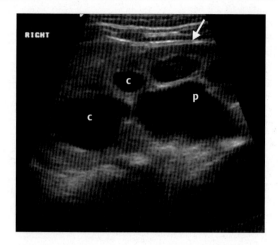

Fig. 5.3 Chronic ureteropelvic junction (UPJ) obstruction on the left in an adult. Stone protocol computed tomography without oral or intravenous contrast shows compensatory hypertrophy, seen on the right, and left cortical atrophy (*arrow*) and dilated renal pelvis (p) from a high-grade left UPJ obstruction. The left ureter (not shown) was of normal caliber.

Fig. 5.4 Sonogram of a child with a ureteropelvic junction obstruction shows hydronephrosis with dilated calyces (c) and a prominent renal pelvis (p). Parenchymal thinning is present (*arrow*), and no stones are identified.

COMPUTED TOMOGRAPHY

- Varying degrees of hydronephrosis in association with a dilated renal pelvis and nondilated ureter is seen. The degree of hydronephrosis and parenchymal loss will depend on the severity of the obstruction and the length of time it has been present, which in turn is related to the age of the patient, as this is usually congenital (**Fig. 5.3**).

ULTRASOUND

- Caliectasis (c, **Fig. 5.4**)
- Pyelectasis (p, **Fig. 5.4**)
- Cortical thinning in severe cases (*arrow*, **Fig. 5.4**)
- Dilated ureter not identified
- Serial sonography may be used to follow the progression/resolution of hydronephrosis when managing patients expectantly. Sonography is also useful to reassess patients following surgical treatment.

NUCLEAR MEDICINE

- Nuclear medicine renal scan with furosemide, also known as diuretic renogram (DR), is the most commonly employed exam to determine the significance of the obstruction.
- The time for 50% of the tracer to empty from the collecting system (T½) is calculated, with normal being < 10 minutes and obstruction being > 20 minutes (**Fig. 5.5**). The in-between range is considered "equivocal."
- DR will allow for calculation of split renal function (normal is 45–50% for each kidney).

MAGNETIC RESONANCE IMAGING

- MR urography with heavily T2-weighted and postgadolinium T1-weighted images with fat saturation are used to assess obstructive uropathy.

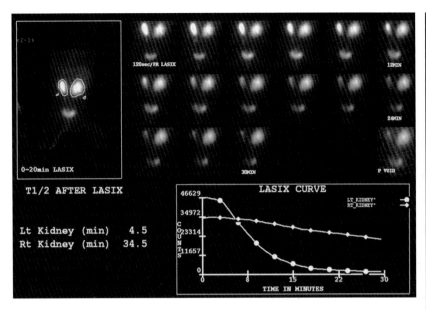

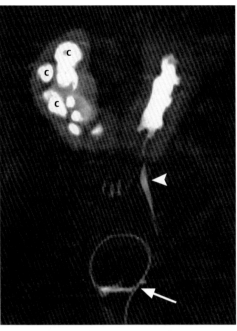

Fig. 5.5 Diuretic renogram in a 5-month-old with horseshoe kidney and right-sided ureteropelvic junction obstruction. T½ for the left is normal (< 10 minutes) and markedly abnormal on the right (34.5 minutes), consistent with a high-grade obstruction.

Fig. 5.6 Known left ureteropelvic junction obstruction in a 1-year-old. Magnetic resonance urogram using coronal postgadolinium T1-weighted gradient echo sequence, in the same patient with a horseshoe kidney (**Fig. 5.5**), shows normal excretion into the left ureter (*arrowhead*) at 10 minutes postcontrast; there is marked caliectasis (c) but no ureteral filling on the right. The arrow indicates the bladder catheter.

- UPJ obstruction presents with varying degrees of hydronephrosis in association with a dilated renal pelvis and nondilated ureter.
- Quantitiative techniques similar to a DR may be used to quantify the severity of the obstruction (**Fig. 5.6**).

Treatment

- Dismembered pyeloplasty is the procedure of choice where the narrowed UPJ is resected, the renal pelvis will be reshaped into a funnel, and the ureter and reformed pelvis are anastomosed. Indications include
  - Sufficient function in the hydronephrotic kidney, but the obstruction is deemed significant
  - If the patient's renal function declines between screening intervals
  - If symptoms develop between screening intervals

Prognosis

- With prompt recognition and treatment, prognosis is generally good for preservation of overall renal function.

PEARLS _____

- Multicystic dysplastic kidney (MCDK) can present and appear similar to a hydronephrotic kidney in an infant or young child. An important differentiating feature is communication of the fluid-filled spaces, seen in hydronephrosis but not with MCDK. MCDK replaces most of the renal parenchyma with cysts.

Suggested Readings

Gonzalez R, Schimke CM. Ureteropelvic junction obstruction in infants and children. Pediatr Clin North Am 2001;48(6):1505–1518.

McDaniel BB, Jones RA, Scherz H, Kirsch AJ, Little SB, Grattan-Smith JD. Dynamic contrast-enhanced MR urography in the evaluation of pediatric hydronephrosis, II: Anatomic and functional assessment of uteropelvic junction obstruction. AJR Am J Roentgenol 2005;185(6):1608–1614.

Mercado-Deane MG, Beeson JE, John SD. US of renal insufficiency in neonates. Radiographics 2002;22(6):1429–1438.

Park JM, Bloom DA. The pathophysiology of UPJ obstruction: current concepts. Urol Clin North Am 1998;25(2):161–169.

CASE 6

Clinical Presentation

Hematuria

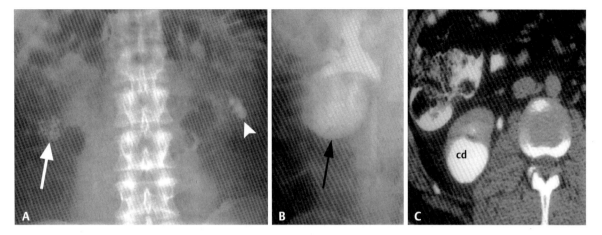

Fig. 6.1 **(A)** An abdominal radiograph coned to the kidneys. **(B)** An abdominal radiograph coned to the kidneys during the excretory phase of an intravenous pyelogram. **(C)** A late phase enhanced computed tomography scan.

Radiologic Findings

- On an intravenous pyelogram (IVP), clustered stones in a calyceal diverticulum (*arrow,* **Fig. 6.1A**) are seen. This finding could be confused with gallstones. A left renal stone is also present (*arrowhead,* **Fig. 6.1A**).
- Excretory phase from an IVP shows the diverticulum fills with contrast, with stones barely visible (*black arrow,* **Fig. 6.1B**).
- On computed tomography (CT), a large calyceal diverticulum (cd, **Fig. 6.1C**) filled with contrast-obscuring stones (stones were seen on the unenhanced portion of the CT study) is seen.

Diagnosis

Calyceal diverticulum

Differential Diagnosis

See **Table 6.1** for a breakout of differential diagnoses with and without stones.

Table 6.1 Differential Diagnosis of Calyceal Diverticulum

Without Stones	With Stones
• Renal cyst	• Gallstones
• Parapelvic cyst	• Renal stones
• Papillary necrosis	• Milk of calcium

25

Discussion

Background

A 1971 study of 16,000 IVPs found an incidence of 3.3 per 1000 in the pediatric population and 4.5 per 1000 in adults for calyceal diverticula. The differences were believed to be due to increased numbers of IVPs performed in adults. The calyceal diverticulum is urine containing and is lined by urothelium. The narrow neck predisposes to stasis with stone formation and, occasionally, infection.

Clinical Findings

Most patients do not have symptoms from their calyceal diverticulum, but stones and infection can occur. Most cases of calyceal diverticulum are incidentally detected on imaging studies for other reasons. About 40% will contain stones, and approximately one quarter may become infected.

Pathology

Similar incidences in children and adults point to the likelihood that these lesions are congenital and probably result from abnormal budding of the ureteric bud, with subsequent lack of parenchymal induction and resultant cystic cavity formation. A narrow connection from the cyst to the pyelocalyceal system remains. Calyceal diverticulum occurs more commonly in the upper poles.

Imaging Findings

RADIOGRAPHY

With conventional abdominal radiography:

- Without stones:
  - Calyceal diverticulum would not be detectable on abdominal films.
- With stones:
  - Renal calculi, gallstones, and milk of calcium cysts could not be differentiated.
  - Clustered stones in the right upper quadrant typically suggest gallstones, but clustered stones often occur in calyceal diverticula. These clustered stones often have faceted margins.
  - A renal stone can appear fragmented, but it would not be made up of multiple uniform calcifications, as in this case (**Fig. 6.1A**).
  - Milk of calcium would appear as uniform high density without discrete calcifications.
  - With decubitus positioning, the calculi will fall to the dependent portion of the cyst, forming a meniscus, which is highly suggestive of the diagnosis of calyceal diverticulum.

INTRAVENOUS PYELOGRAM

- Without stones, filling of the calyceal diverticulum on delayed IVP (**Fig. 6.1B**) excludes renal and parapelvic cysts, gallstones, renal parenchymal calcifications, and milk of calcium cysts. Papillary necrosis may still be a consideration, but the adjacent calyx should be normal in calyceal diverticulum, excluding papillary necrosis.
- With stones, the cystic cavity becomes progressively opacified, giving the appearance that the stones are growing. This is referred to as the "growing calculus" sign.
- Calyceal diverticulum opacifies late because it fills, not from excretion into the collecting tubules, but rather in a retrograde fashion from the opacifying collecting system. Occasionally, the diverticulum will not fill on an IVP.
- Calyceal diverticula and their narrow connection to the collecting system are better demonstrated on retrograde pyelography due to increased pyelocalyceal distension.

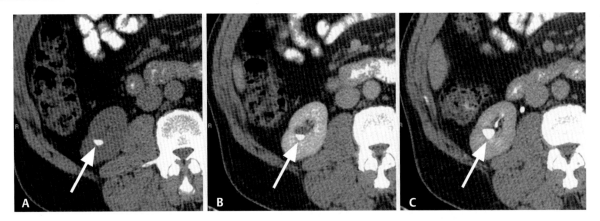

Fig. 6.2 CT-IVP for hematuria. **(A)** The unenhanced CT scan shows curvilinear calcification in the right midpole cortex (*arrow*). **(B)** During the nephrogram phase, stones are seen layering in a cystic cavity (*arrow*). **(C)**. The delayed pyelogram phase shows increasing density in the cystic cavity analogous to the "growing calculus" sign on intravenous urography, confirming the lesion's connection to the adjacent collecting system.

COMPUTED TOMOGRAPHY

- Nontailored CT scans may not reveal the true nature of these "cystic" lesions. Calyceal diverticula will be fluid density on unenhanced CT scans. Enhanced scans may show simply fluid-containing structures, resulting in misdiagnosis as a simple cyst. It is on delayed images (e.g., in a renal neoplasm protocol CT or CT-IVP) that sufficient delay time may permit the diverticulum to fill in a retrograde fashion from the opacifying collecting system (**Fig. 6.1C**).
- With stones in the calyceal diverticulum, the diagnosis is straightforward. The diverticulum will be fluid density with layering stone material on unenhanced CT scans (*arrow,* **Fig. 6.2A**). Enhanced scans reveal the stones contained within a cystic cavity (*arrow,* **Fig. 6.2B**). Delayed images will show the growing calculus sign, confirming a connection to the adjacent collecting system (*arrow,* **Fig. 6.2C**).

ULTRASOUND

- Calyceal diverticula may be indistinguishable from other renal cysts. They will be anechoic, rounded structures in the renal cortex with imperceptibly thin walls, with increased sound through transmission.
- Layering echogenic material may be detected representing stone material (**Fig. 6.3**). Stones will move with changes in positioning, often forming a meniscus or crescent.

MAGNETIC RESONANCE IMAGING

- As with CT and ultrasound, lesions on MRI may be indistinguishable from other renal cysts.
- On MRI, a calyceal diverticulum should follow the signal of simple fluid on all sequences (i.e., low signal intensity on T1-weighted images and high signal intensity on T2-weighted images).
- Delayed images may show excreted gadolinium layering in the cavity, confirming its true nature.

Treatment

- No specific treatment is required for an asymptomatic calyceal diverticulum.
- Surgical treatment for symptomatic lesions is geared toward obliterating the cyst cavity and/or its connection to the collecting system. Indications for surgical treatment include recurrent stone formation, recurrent urinary tract infections, pain, or evidence of ongoing renal damage.

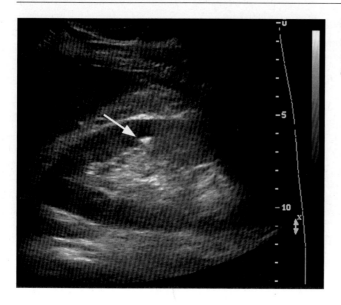

Fig. 6.3 An ultrasound image of the right kidney shows a cystic lesion containing layered echogenic material in a crescent or meniscus shape (*arrow*), consistent with a calyceal diverticulum.

Prognosis

- Treatment of symptomatic lesions is 80% effective in relieving recurrent problems.

PEARLS

- It is possible that slow retrograde filling of a calyceal diverticulum on a renal neoplasm protocol CT scan could mimic a slowly enhancing renal mass. Thus, adequate delay should be built into renal neoplasm protocol CT and CT-IVP studies to allow for filling of the diverticulum.

Suggested Readings

Hewitt MJ, Older RA. Calyceal calculi simulating gallstones. AJR Am J Roentgenol 1980;134(3):507–509.

Middleton AW Jr, Pfister RC. Stone-containing pyelocaliceal diverticulum: embryogenic, anatomic, radiologic and clinical characteristics. J Urol 1974;111(1):2–6.

Rathaus V, Konen O, Werner M, Shapiro Feinberg M, Grunebaum M, Zissin R. Pyelocalyceal diverticulum: the imaging spectrum with emphasis on the ultrasound features. Br J Radiol 2001;74(883):595–601.

Timmons JW Jr, Malek RS, Hattery RR, Deweerd JH. Caliceal diverticulum. J Urol 1975;114(1):6–9.

CASE 7

Clinical Presentation

Infant with urinary tract infections (UTIs)

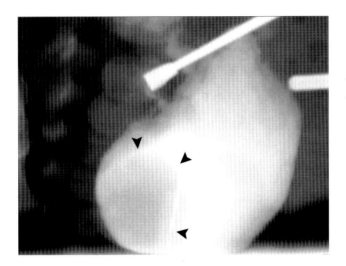

Fig. 7.1 Oblique image of the bladder from voiding cystoure-throgram (VCUG) in infant with urinary tract infection.

Radiologic Findings

- A large, well-circumscribed, right-sided bladder-filling defect is seen during a voiding cystoure-throgram (VCUG) (*arrowheads,* **Fig. 7.1**), representing a simple or orthotopic ureterocele. This was confirmed with ultrasound.

Diagnosis

Orthotopic ureterocele

Differential Diagnosis

- Ectopic ureterocele
- Pseudo-ureterocele
- Sarcoma botryoides

Discussion

Background

Ureteroceles are most likely congenital, although some can be acquired. A ureterocele is defined as a cystic outpouching of the distal ureter. Two varieties exist: orthotopic ureterocele (OU), where the cystic dilatation occurs at the trigone at the normally located ureteral orifice, and ectopic uretero-cele (EU), which inserts low and medial to the normal trigone as far inferior as the bladder neck or urethra (**Fig. 7.2**).

29

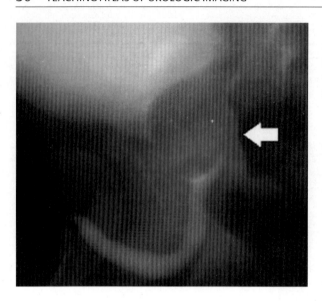

Fig. 7.2 Voiding cystourethrogram in an infant male. A large filling defect at the bladder neck obstructing the proximal urethra (*arrow*) represents an ectopic ureterocele associated with complete duplication of collecting structures (not shown).

OU is found incidentally in adults and often is asymptomatic. Women demonstrate this anomaly more commonly than men. EU is most commonly associated with duplication of the kidney and ureter, where the EU arises from the upper pole renal moiety and inserts low and medial (below the trigone). This is the Weigert-Meyer rule for duplicated systems. With EU, the upper moiety of a duplicated system is frequently hydronephrotic. The lower pole moiety will frequently show reflux.

Clinical Findings

The EU may cause bladder outlet obstruction due to its low insertion into the bladder or urethra, as seen in **Fig. 7.2**. EUs are more commonly found in children, usually because they are symptomatic with UTI from obstruction or reflux. EU can also be associated with continual urine leak in a female past the age of continence because the ureter inserts below the external sphincter.

Pathology

OU represents an outpouching of the ureteral mucosa that invaginates into the bladder, bringing along with it mucosa and muscular layers of the bladder wall and forming a balloon-like dilatation at the trigone, the so-called cobra head deformity. The ureterocele and the ureteral orifice are located in the bladder. EU dilatation is seen within the wall of the bladder, with some part extending into the bladder neck or urethra and most often presenting as a filling defect on VCUG or intravenous pyelogram (IVP) (**Fig. 7.2**).

A mimicking abnormality is known as a "pseudo-ureterocele" and includes a stone, stricture, or mass-causing distal ureteral obstruction, with the dilated ureteral segment bulging into the bladder.

Imaging Findings
RADIOGRAPHY

- OU is seen on IVP as the classic cobra head deformity in the later part of the IVP, when the dilated ureterocele is filled with contrast and it bulges into the contrast-filled bladder. The thin mucosal wall of the ureterocele forms the outline of the cobra's head. The intramural component to the dilated EU will present as a filling defect in the bladder or urethra on contrast-filled images,

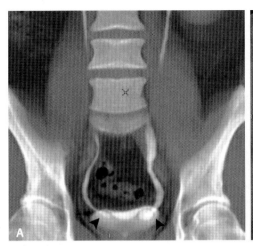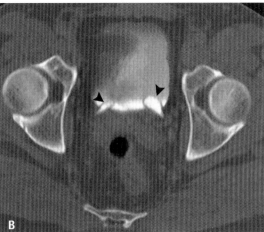

Fig. 7.3 CT-IVP with **(A)** three-dimensional reconstruction and **(B)** axial images in bone windows. Bilateral cobra head deformities (*arrowheads*) are seen at the bladder trigones in this patient with bilateral simple (orthotopic) ureteroceles.

as seen in **Fig. 7.2.** Either type of ureterocele may obstruct the bladder outlet. In the setting of obstruction, delayed imaging may be required to show contrast in the ballooned ureterocele.

COMPUTED TOMOGRAPHY

- OU may be seen on unenhanced CT as a cystic structure with a thin wall at the ureteral trigone.
- The classic cobra head deformity of OU will be most apparent in the excretory phase of a CT-IVP when the dilated ureterocele is filled with contrast and it bulges into the contrast-filled bladder. The thin mucosal wall of the ureterocele forms the outline of the cobra's head (**Fig. 7.3**).
- The intramural component to the dilated EU will present as a cystic structure in the bladder or urethra that may fill with contrast on the delayed images from a CT-IVP.

ULTRASOUND

- A cystic anechoic fluid collection surrounded by a thin wall will be seen at the trigone (OU) or in the wall of the bladder (EU). It may change size over the observation time as urine enters and exits, depending on the degree of obstruction (**Fig. 7.4**).

NUCLEAR MEDICINE

- Split function assessment of the kidneys is often performed in patients with symptomatic EU to determine if there is significant function in the associated renal moiety. If there is little function, the symptomatic moiety can be resected with little adverse impact on renal function.

Treatment

- Symptomatic ureteroceles are treated with transurethral fenestration to temporize.
- In long-term symptomatic patients, if the ureterocele is associated with a poorly functioning upper moiety, resection of the upper moiety and its ureter will be performed.
- If there is good renal function in the upper moiety, ureteral reimplantation of both ureters will be undertaken.

Prognosis

- Most symptomatic patients, when treated early as above, respond favorably.

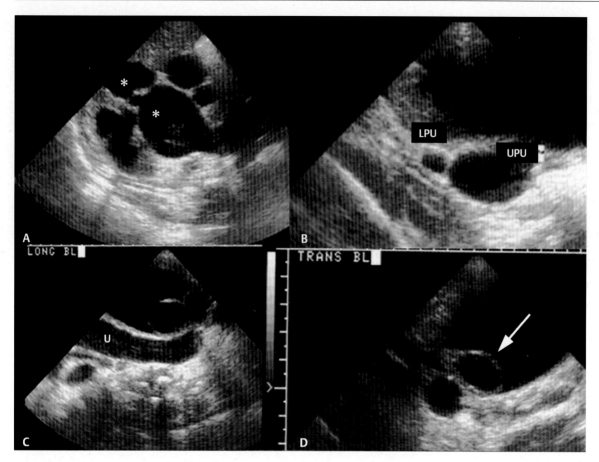

Fig. 7.4 Postnatal ultrasound in the same patient as in **Fig. 7.2. (A)** Transverse right kidney with dilated upper moiety to a duplex kidney (*asterisks*). **(B)** Transverse of the ureters in the midabdomen. Two ureters are identified in the retroperitoneum draining the separate renal units. LPU, lower pole ureter; UPU, dilated upper pole ureter. **(C)** Sagittal view of the ureterocele showing the dilated right upper moiety ureter (U) behind the bladder. **(D)** Transverse view of a right-sided ureterocele (*arrow*) in the bladder.

Suggested Readings

Chavhan GB. The cobra head sign. Radiology 2002;225(3):781–782.

Decter RM. Renal duplication and fusion anomalies. Pediatr Clin North Am 1997;44(5):1323–1341.

CASE 8

Clinical Presentation

A 50-year-old male presents with abdominal pain. The patient is alert but has a blood pressure of 90/60.

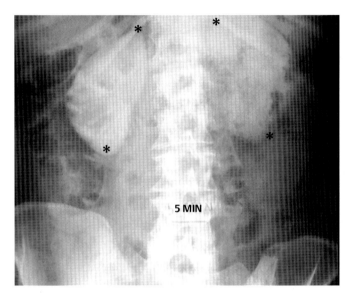

Fig. 8.1 A 5-minute radiograph from intravenous urography coned to the kidneys (*asterisks*).

Radiologic Findings

- Bilateral persistent nephrogram (*asterisks*, **Fig. 8.1**).
- No calyceal filling bilaterally

Diagnosis

Hypotensive contrast reaction

Differential Diagnosis

- Contrast-induced nephrotoxicity
- Preexisting acute tubular necrosis
- Bilateral ureteral obstruction

Discussion

Background

Mild to moderate reactions to the injection of iodinated contrast media (ICM) occur in 7 to 12% of patients. Hypotension is considered a moderately severe reaction. Nearly all clinically important reactions occur within 20 minutes of injection. Most reactions cannot be predicted. Hypotension with bradycardia represents a vasovagal reaction. Anxiety plays a part in this event. Hypotension with tachycardia is thought to be related, at least in part, to the hypertonicity of the ICM.

Clinical Findings

Identifying the response to hypotension is essential in the characterization of the type of reaction the patient is experiencing and the subsequent treatment thereof. With hypotension, the correct response is tachycardia, as the body attempts to correct for decreased blood pressure by increasing cardiac output. Treatment is geared to supporting blood pressure with fluid boluses and elevation of the lower extremities. A vasovagal reaction represents an inappropriate response to hypotension, and the treatment is geared toward diminishing vagal activity [e.g., with intravenous (IV) atropine] and supporting blood pressure.

Pathology

Vasovagal reaction is mediated by the autonomic nervous system, where excessive vagal activity results in hypotension and bradycardia. In a nonvasovagal reaction, hypotension is mediated by the release of vasoactive substances, histamines, and other factors in a complex immunologic response, and tachycardia is the body's response in an attempt to support blood flow.

Imaging Findings
RADIOGRAPHY

- A persistent nephrogram at 5 minutes with no calyceal filling must raise immediate suspicion for a hypotensive contrast reaction, with urgent evaluation of the patient to include an immediate blood pressure measurement.
- The patient may be alert and not complaining of specific symptoms.
- Contrast-induced nephrotoxicity (CIN) can have an identical radiographic appearance to an acute hypotensive reaction, and if hypotension is excluded, CIN becomes the primary diagnosis. CIN does not require immediate therapy, whereas a hypotensive reaction does. Hypotension should always be excluded before making the diagnosis of CIN.
- Preexisting acute tubular necrosis can cause a persistent nephrogram without calyceal filling, but preexisting renal insufficiency should be detected using standard clinical and laboratory screening prior to injection of contrast media.
- Bilateral persistent nephrograms due to acute obstruction are very unlikely.

COMPUTED TOMOGRAPHY

- Similar findings are noted on a computed tomography (CT) scan as are noted with an intravenous pyelogram (IVP).
- Bilateral persistent nephrograms with absent calyceal filling seen soon after contrast injection should raise the suspicion of acute hypotension, with immediate evaluation and support of the patient given.

Treatment

For a detailed summary of the management of acute contrast reactions, see Section B in Appendix.

HYPOTENSION WITH TACHYCARDIA

- Legs should be elevated 60 degrees or more.
- Administer bolus IV of large volumes of isotonic Ringer lactate or normal saline. If patient is unresponsive to fluid resuscitation, administer epinephrine subcutaneously or intramuscularly (1:1000) 0.1 to 0.3 mL. Repeat as needed up to a maximum of 1 mg.
- Activate the advanced cardiac life support (ACLS) team for assistance.

HYPOTENSION WITH BRADYCARDIA (VAGAL REACTION)

- Legs should be elevated 60 degrees or more.
- Administer bolus IV of large volumes of isotonic Ringer lactate or normal saline. If patient is unresponsive to fluid resuscitation, administer atropine 0.6 to 1 mg IV slowly.
- Repeat atropine up to a total dose of 0.04 mg/kg (2–3 mg) in adults.
- Activate the ACLS team for assistance.

Prognosis

- With early recognition and timely treatment, prognosis for return to normotension is excellent.

PEARLS

- Remember "O_2, IV, and monitor" from basic life support. These maneuvers should be performed on every patient you are called to evaluate for potential life-threatening contrast reaction until assessment shows these interventions are not needed.
- Administer O_2 6 to 10 L per minute via face mask.
- Maintain adequate IV access, preferably with an 18-gauge antecubital angiocatheter.
- Attach monitor for O_2 saturation, blood pressure, and heart rate.

Suggested Readings

American College of Radiology. ACR Manual on Contrast Media. 5th ed. Reston, VA: American College of Radiology; 2004.

Friedenberg R, Harris R. Excretory urography. In: Pollack H., McClennan B., eds. Clinical Urography. Vol 1. 2nd ed. Philadelphia: WB Saunders; 2000:147–257.

Saunders HS, Dyer RB, Shifrin RY, Scharling ES, Bechtold RE, Zagoria RJ. The CT nephrogram: implications for evaluation of urinary tract disease. Radiographics 1995;15(5):1069–1085, discussion 1086–1068.

CASE 9

Clinical Presentation

A 35-year-old male presented with lymphoma.

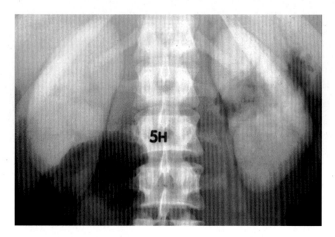

Fig. 9.1 Five-hour abdominal radiograph following an intravenous pyelogram (IVP). The IVP study was normal. Source: Resnick, Older, Diagnosis of Genitourinary Disease, New York: Thieme, 1997: 53. Reprinted by permission.

Radiologic Findings

- Bilateral persistent nephrogram
- No calyceal filling

Diagnosis

Contrast-induced renal failure

Differential Diagnosis

- Bilateral ureteral obstruction
- Contrast reaction with hypotension
- Preexistent acute tubular necrosis (ATN)

Discussion

Background

Acute renal failure (ARF) is defined as an absolute increase in serum creatinine of 0.5 mg/dL or a 25% increase from baseline. Contrast-induced nephrotoxicity (CIN) in association with intra-arterial iodinated contrast media (ICM) administration is ~8% in patients with normal renal function and no diabetes. Data regarding intravenous ICM administration and the risk of CIN are limited. ARF has been reported to occur in anywhere from 1 to 30% of patients in clinical trials of various contrast agents, many receiving intra-arterial injection for cardiac studies. In the outpatient setting, any ARF is short-lived and reversible. However, ICM has been implicated as the third-leading cause of ARF in hospitalized patients, with an associated mortality of 14%: nearly 50% of these cases were related to cardiac catheterizations, and slightly over 33% were related to diagnostic computed tomography (CT) examinations. Keep in mind that concomitant medical conditions could have been contributors to these deaths.

Clinical Findings

The most common cause of contrast-induced renal failure is preexistent decreased renal function, especially in diabetics, which is not present in this case.

Pathology

Contrast induced renal failure results from ATN, which is an ischemic (reduced blood flow) or toxic insult to the tubular epithelial cells. Resultant cell death causes tubular dysfunction with failure of the kidney to adequately concentrate urine. Urinary sediment findings suggesting ATN include muddy brown granular casts and tubular epithelial and epithelial casts.

Imaging Findings

RADIOGRAPHY

- Acute ureteral obstruction produces a dense, persistent nephrogram, but it would be highly unlikely to be bilateral.
- Hypotension secondary to a contrast reaction is a possibility but unlikely at 5 hours without clinical findings of hypotension. Always check the patient's blood pressure when a bilateral persistent nephrogram is seen.
- Preexistent ATN would have produced an immediate abnormal nephrogram, and the history indicates initial normal appearance to the intravenous pyelogram (IVP).
- A persistent nephrogram can be seen on abdominal radiographic exams days following a contrast load in patients who develop acute renal insufficiency.

COMPUTED TOMOGRAPHY

- Bilateral persistent nephrograms can be seen with no calyceal filling (as in **Fig. 9.2**).
- Vicarious excretion of contrast into the gallbladder also may be present.

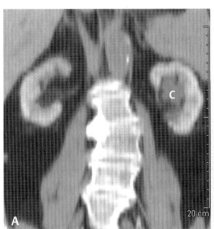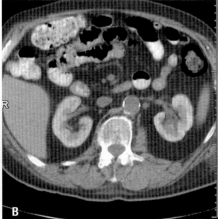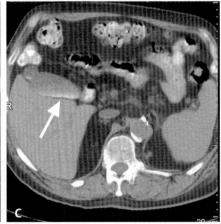

Fig. 9.2 Non-contrast-enhanced computed tomography scan following cardiac catheterization to evaluate for a source of dropping hematocrit. **(A)** A reconstructed coronal image through the kidneys and **(B)** an axial view show bilaterally persistent nephrograms with no calyceal filling. c, parapelvic cyst. **(C)** High-density material layering in the gallbladder (*arrow*) is consistent with vicarious excretion, another finding that can be seen with contrast-induced renal failure.

Treatment

- Treatment options are limited once ARF ensues.
- Treatment is supportive with most patients' renal function improving spontaneously days to weeks after the insult.
- The best treatment for ATN is prevention by reducing the patient's risks for contrast-induced nephrotoxicity: initiate hydration, discontinue use of nephrotoxic drugs, limit contrast dose, use low osmolar contrast agents, and consider free radical scavenger administration (e.g., sodium bicarbonate or *N*-acetylcysteine).

Prognosis

- Most cases of contrast-induced renal failure resolve spontaneously within days to weeks.
- Patients with no underlying acute medical condition will have a 7 to 23% mortality rate.
- Intensive care unit patients with ARF have a 50 to 80% mortality rate.

PEARLS

- Always check blood pressure when bilateral persistent nephrograms are noted, as this may be due to hypotension that requires immediate therapy.
- If a persistent nephrogram is seen following a contrast-enhanced study and does not represent an acute hypotensive event, notification to the ordering clinician of potential acute renal failure is important so that supportive measures (restrict further contrast loads, discontinue nephrotoxic drugs, maintenance of renal perfusion) can be instituted.

Suggested Readings

Barrett BJ, Parfrey PS. Clinical practice: preventing nephropathy induced by contrast medium. N Engl J Med 2006;354(4):379–386.

Gill N, Nally JV Jr, Fatica RA. Renal failure secondary to acute tubular necrosis: epidemiology, diagnosis, and management. Chest 2005;128(4):2847–2863.

Nash K, Hafeez A, Hou S. Hospital-acquired renal insufficiency. Am J Kidney Dis 2002;39(5):930–936.

Rudnick MR, Goldfarb S, Wexler L, et al. Nephrotoxicity of ionic and nonionic contrast media in 1196 patients: a randomized trial. The Iohexol Cooperative Study. Kidney Int 1995;47(1):254–261.

Saunders HS, Dyer RB, Shifrin RY, Scharling ES, Bechtold RE, Zagoria RJ. The CT nephrogram: implications for evaluation of urinary tract disease. Radiographics 1995;15(5):1069–1085, discussion 1086–1068.

CASE 10

Clinical Presentation

A 40-year-old female with chronic renal insufficiency who underwent magnetic resonance imaging (MRI) with gadolinium several weeks before presenting with skin thickening and redness.

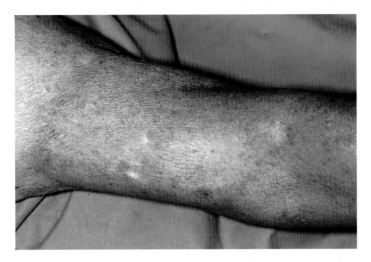

Fig. 10.1 Photograph of the left elbow shows dermatologic changes of nephrogenic systemic fibrosis, including plaquelike induration involving the limbs. With thanks to Julie Padgett, M.D., and Kenneth Greer, M.D.

Dermatologic Findings

- Skin thickening and induration in the left upper extremity (**Fig. 10.1**)

Pathologic Findings

- Biopsy shows exuberant fibrotic tissues, increased cellularity, myxoid background stroma (*arrow,* **Fig. 10.2**), and innumerable fibroblasts that are positive for factor XIIIa and CD34 (*arrowhead,* **Fig. 10.2**).

Diagnosis

Nephrogenic systemic fibrosis (NSF)

Differential Diagnosis

- Other rashes for which dermatology consultation and biopsy would be required

Discussion

Background

Cases of NSF in association with gadolinium have been reported since 1997. All patients diagnosed with NSF have at least one exposure to gadolinium administration, generally within 2 weeks to 3

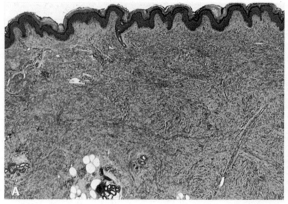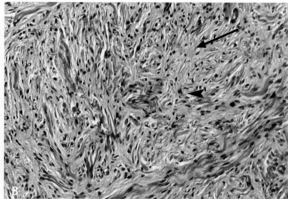

Fig. 10.2 **(A)** Low-power and **(B)** high-power photomicrograph of skin biopsy from a patient with nephrogenic systemic fibrosis. The highpower image shows fibroblasts (*arrowhead*) and exuberant fibrotic (myxoid) stroma (*arrow*). With thanks to James W. Patterson, M.D.

months of the onset of NSF. At least one researcher has found free, unbound gadolinium in biopsy specimens of NSF skin lesions. These findings do not prove a cause-and-effect relationship, but they are pieces of evidence that have led the U.S. Food and Drug Administration (FDA) to issue a strong recommendation to avoid gadolinium agents in patients with renal insufficiency and/or who are on dialysis. Approximately 3 to 5% of patients with stage 4 or 5 chronic kidney disease (glomerular filtration rate [GFR] < 30 mL/min) develop NSF. A dose-dependent response also seems likely, as all patients in the study by Broome et al. received "double-dose" gadolinium (i.e., 0.2 mmol/kg). Omniscan (gadodiamide, GE Healthcare, Buckinghamshire, UK) has been the agent reported in nearly 90% of NSF cases to date compared with other gadolinium chelates.

Clinical Findings

NSF represents a systemic response resulting in fibrotic lesions in the skin and also in parenchymal organs. This progressive disease can be a painful and debilitating illness that can lead to death. No definite age, sex, or racial predilection is documented.

Pathology

NSF is a systemic fibrosing process that involves primarily the skin, with skin thickening and tightening occurring. Patients usually present with acute plaquelike induration involving the lower and upper limbs or torso. The face is spared. Lesions are often painful or pruritic. Severity and rapid progression correlate with poorer prognosis. Fibrosis may involve skeletal muscle and heart as well as other organ systems.

Imaging Findings

• None

Treatment

• There is no specific treatment for NSF except for prevention. The FDA recommends that patients with compromised renal function (GFR < 30 mL/min) and patients in any degree of acute renal insufficiency should not be given gadolinium for contrast-enhanced studies. Kanal et al (2007) recommend withholding gadolinium administration in patients with GFR < 60 mL/min and avoiding Omniscan at any level of renal insufficiency. If a contrast-enhanced study is indicated (e.g., in life-threatening situations), a contrast-enhanced computed tomography scan may be considered if the potential benefits of using contrast outweigh the risks of contrast-induced renal failure.

Prognosis

- NSF is painful and may be a rapidly progressive, debilitating condition. Organ involvement can occur. Severe cases can be fatal.

Suggested Readings

Broome DR, Girguis MS, Baron PW, Cottrell AC, Kjellin I, Kirk GA. Gadodiamide-associated nephrogenic systemic fibrosis: why radiologists should be concerned. AJR Am J Roentgenol 2007;188(2):586–592.

Grobner T, Prischl FC. Gadolinium and nephrogenic systemic fibrosis. Kidney Int 2007;72(3):260–264.

Jamboti J. A timely reminder about an evolving clinical entity: nephrogenic systemic fibrosis and gadolinium use in CKD. Nephrology (Carlton) 2007;12(3):316.

Kanal E, Barkovich AJ, Bell C, et al. ACR guidance document for safe MR practices: 2007. AJR Am J Roentgenol 2007;188(6):1447–1474.

Karlik SJ. Gadodiamide-associated nephrogenic systemic fibrosis. AJR Am J Roentgenol 2007;188(6):584.

Kuo PH, Kanal E, Abu-Alfa AK, Cowper SE. Gadolinium-based MR contrast agents and nephrogenic systemic fibrosis. Radiology 2007;242(3):647–649.

Leiner T, Herborn CU, Goyen M. Nephrogenic systemic fibrosis is not exclusively associated with gadodiamide. Eur Radiol 2007;17(8):1921–1923.

Partain CL. On the potential causal relationship between gadolinium-containing MRI agents and nephrogenic systemic fibrosis. J Magn Reson Imaging 2007;25(5):879–880.

Pedersen M. Safety update on the possible causal relationship between gadolinium-containing MRI agents and nephrogenic systemic fibrosis. J Magn Reson Imaging 2007;25(5):881–883.

Thomsen HS, Morcos SK. Nephrogenic systemic fibrosis and nonionic linear chelates. AJR Am J Roentgenol 2007;188(6):580.

CASE 11

Clinical Presentation

A 43-year-old female presents with a metabolic abnormality.

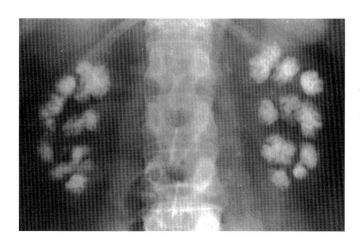

Fig. 11.1   Abdominal radiograph coned to the kidneys. Source: CRITICAL REVIEWS IN DIAGNOSTIC IMAGING by Older RA, Moore AV and McClelland R. Copyright 1981 by Taylor & Francis Informa UK Ltd — Journals. Reproduced with permission of Taylor & Francis Informa UK Ltd — Journals in the format Textbook via Copyright Clearance Center.

Radiologic Findings

- Bilateral calcifications throughout medullary pyramids
- "Popcorn"-type calcifications

Diagnosis

Medullary nephrocalcinosis

Differential Diagnosis

- Staghorn calculi
- Cortical nephrocalcinosis
- Medullary sponge kidney

Discussion

Background

Nephrocalcinosis (increased calcium deposition within the renal parenchyma) results from metabolic disease caused by hypercalcemia due to primary hyperparathyroidism, distal-type renal tubular acidosis, milk alkali syndrome, or medullary sponge kidney.

Clinical Findings

Aside from clinical findings related to the metabolic derangement, patients may present with typical signs and symptoms of renal colic when any of the innumerable renal calculi move into the collecting system and cause obstruction.

43

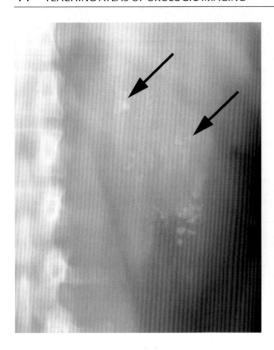

Fig. 11.2 A tomogram from intravenous urography in a patient with hematuria shows extensive medullary calcifications (*arrows*).

Pathology

Increased calcium deposition is seen in the medullary regions of the kidney.

Imaging Findings

RADIOGRAPHY

- Staghorn calculi fill the collecting system as if forming a cast of the collecting system. Although it would be impossible to exclude some stones in the collecting structures on the abdominal film shown, the overall pattern is predominantly medullary calcification.
- Cortical nephrocalcinosis produces bandlike calcification of the cortex; there is no cortical calcification in this case.
- Medullary sponge kidney with calcifications in dilated tubules can be a cause of medullary nephrocalcinosis, but it cannot be diagnosed on an abdominal film. Diagnosis is based on a contrast-enhanced study revealing globular collections of contrast within the dilated tubules.
- Multiple bilateral, peripherally located calcifications in the distribution of the renal medullary pyramids with a "popcorn" appearance (**Fig. 11.1**) represent medullary nephrocalcinosis.
- This patient's medullary nephrocalcinosis was secondary to hyperparathyroidism (**Fig. 11.2**).

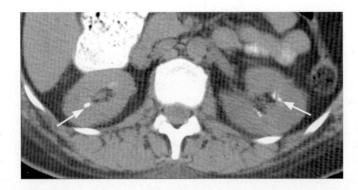

Fig. 11.3 An unenhanced computed tomography scan shows bilateral medullary calcifications (*arrows*) in this patient with hyperparathyroidism.

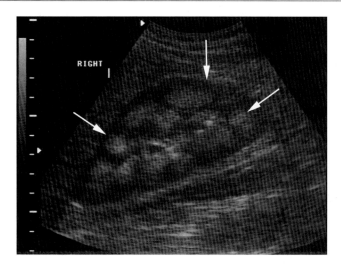

Fig. 11.4 A renal sonogram shows extensive echogenic renal medullary pyramids (*arrows*) with mild shadowing (seen best during real-time sonographic imaging) in a patient with medullary nephrocalcinosis secondary to a metabolic disorder.

CT

- Highly accurate for renal calculi detection; nearly all calculi are dense on CT.
- Calcifications are localized to the renal medullary pyramids (**Fig. 11.3**).

ULTRASOUND

- Echogenic renal pyramids (*arrows*, **Fig. 11.4**)
- Mild acoustic shadowing is seen intermittently, but it is less than that which would be seen with actual stones.
- Ultrasound is more sensitive than abdominal radiography for mild nephrocalcinosis.

Treatment

- Treatment is directed at the underlying cause of hypercalcemia.
- In patients with hyperparathyroidism, only ~20% will become symptomatic and form stones. Those patients will benefit from removal of hyperplastic or adenomatous functional parathyroid tissue.

Prognosis

- Prognosis depends on the underlying cause of hypercalcemia. Following removal of hyperplastic or adenomatous parathyroid tissue, calcium levels return to normal.

Suggested Readings

Glazer GM, Callen PW, Filly RA. Medullary nephrocalcinosis: sonographic evaluation. AJR Am J Roentgenol 1982;138(1):55–57.

Ramshandani P. Radiologic evaluation of renal calculus disease. In: Pollack H, McClennan B, eds. Clinical Urography. 2nd ed. Philadelphia: WB Saunders; 2000:2147–2199.

CASE 12

Clinical Presentation

A 37-year-old male presents with chronic renal disease.

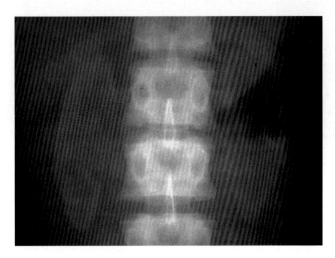

Fig. 12.1 Coned radiograph of the upper abdomen. Source: CRITICAL REVIEWS IN DIAGNOSTIC IMAGING by Older RA, Moore AV and McClelland R. Copyright 1981 by Taylor & Francis Informa UK Ltd — Journals. Reproduced with permission of Taylor & Francis Informa UK Ltd — Journals in the format Textbook via Copyright Clearance Center.

Radiologic Findings

- Bilateral cortical calcification. Kidneys should not be this apparent on a noncontrast abdominal radiograph.
- Small kidneys

Diagnosis

Cortical nephrocalcinosis secondary to chronic glomerulonephritis

Differential Diagnosis

- Acute cortical necrosis
- Hyperparathyroidism
- Medullary sponge kidney

Discussion

Background

Cortical nephrocalcinosis (CNC) is a rare condition with calcification deposited in the renal cortical parenchyma. A wide array of pathologic entities can result in CNC, but the most common are chronic glomerulonephritis and acute cortical necrosis. Sepsis, toxemia of pregnancy, chronic pyelonephritis, drugs, and other entities have been implicated.

Clinical Findings

Initially, CNC may be asymptomatic, with renal dysfunction ensuing weeks to months after the original insult. Clinical findings depend on the severity of the original insult, but most patients will develop chronic renal insufficiency.

Pathology

Deposition of calcium in the renal cortex is the primary finding.

Imaging Findings

RADIOGRAPHY

- Acute cortical necrosis produces CNC, but it is usually due to pregnancy-related hemorrhage or sepsis.
- Hyperparathyroidism causes medullary nephrocalcinosis, not CNC.
- Medullary sponge kidney also produces medullary nephrocalcinosis, not CNC.
- A combination of bilateral cortical calcification and small kidneys (**Fig. 12.1**) indicates a chronic process such as chronic glomerulonephritis.

COMPUTED TOMOGRAPHY

- A band or bands of linear calcification or diffuse punctate calcifications are located in the renal cortex with medullary sparing.

ULTRASOUND

- Increased echogenicity of the renal cortex
- Occasional shadowing from the cortical echogenicities

Treatment

- There is usually little that can be done for this chronic process to mitigate the preexisting renal damage.

Prognosis

- Most cases progress to renal failure.

Suggested Readings

Dyer RB, Chen MY, Zagoria RJ. Abnormal calcifications in the urinary tract. Radiographics 1998;18(6):1405–1424.

Schepens D, Verswijvel G, Kuypers D, Vanrenterghem Y. Images in nephrology: renal cortical nephrocalcinosis. Nephrol Dial Transplant 2000;15(7):1080–1082.

CASE 13

Clinical Presentation

Hematuria

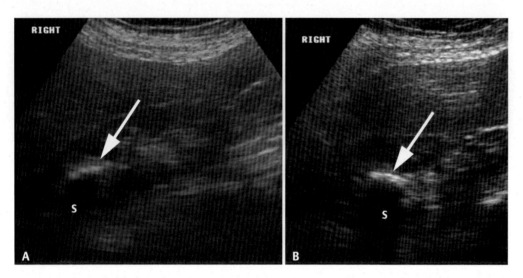

Fig. 13.1 Renal sonogram. **(A)** Longitudinal and **(B)** transverse views of the right kidney.

Radiologic Findings

- Hyperechoic foci in the upper pole (*arrows*, **Fig. 13.1**)
- Clean acoustic shadowing (S, **Fig. 13.1**) presenting as a black band posterior to echogenic foci

Diagnosis

Renal stones

Differential Diagnosis

- Angiomyolipoma
- Medullary nephrocalcinosis
- High-density cyst

Discussion

Background

The prevalence of urinary calculi is increasing, with several factors implicated in their genesis, including hot, sunny environments. Renal colic is a disease that will recur within 5 to 10 years in 50% of patients having already experienced one episode. Subsequent to that, additional bouts will become more frequent. Family history, infection, or an underlying metabolic condition (e.g., hyperparathyroidism) predisposes to renal calculi.

Renal stone analysis can identify specific stone types. Urinary pH analysis can also suggest particular stone types. Causes for renal stone formation are complex and include

- Decreased urine volume is believed to cause supersaturated urine, resulting in the precipitation of crystals.
- Hypercalciuria is the most important factor in calcium stone formation (the most common type of stone being calcium oxalate or calcium phosphate).
- Urinary tract infection with urease-splitting organisms (*Klebsiella* and *Proteus* species) predisposes to stone formation (e.g., staghorn calculi).

Clinical Findings

Many renal calculi are now detected incidentally with increased use of diagnostic imaging. Some degree of urinary obstruction is required to cause renal colic. Fifty percent of incidentally detected calculi will at some point become symptomatic (i.e., will obstruct the collecting system) within 5 years of their discovery. Symptomatic renal calculi present with classic abrupt onset of severe flank pain (renal colic) that may migrate toward the groin as the stone travels down the ureter. Pain is unrelieved by positional changes. Gross hematuria is found in 80 to 100% of cases.

Pathology

Some calculi are believed to form on a calcium substrate found in the renal medulla, which protrudes into the collecting system; these are referred to as Randall's plaques. Exposure of Randall's plaques to urine results in precipitation of stone-forming material on this nidus.

Imaging Findings

ULTRASOUND

- Angiomyolipoma (AML) is a hyperechoic lesion, but it is not as echogenic as the stones in this case. The prominent acoustic shadow of stones is more pronounced than that typically seen with AML. A position within the central echo complex (i.e., in the renal hilum) also indicates stones, not AML.
- Medullary nephrocalcinosis typically produces multiple hyperechoic areas within the medulla. These typically are not as echogenic as the well-formed stone seen in this case.
- A high-density cyst is not hyperechoic. Generally, a cyst is hypoechoic or anechoic and shows increased sound through transmission and not shadowing.
- Ultrasound is ~80% sensitive for renal stone detection but is of limited value for detection of ureteral stones (only 20%), as ureters are not well seen with sonography. It is quite sensitive for detecting hydronephrosis but less sensitive for determining the cause.
- Renal stones less than 5 mm may be difficult to detect with sonography.

RADIOGRAPHY

- Approximately 85% of urinary tract stones contain enough calcium to be detectable on abdominal radiographs, but only ~50% in fact are detected. The reasons for the poor detection of calculi include the small size of the stone and the position over areas where stones can be obscured (bone structures, bowel).

COMPUTED TOMOGRAPHY

- Stone protocol computed tomography without oral or intravenous contrast is the gold standard for detection of renal, ureteral, and bladder calculi, with nearly 100% sensitivity and specificity for urinary tract stones. Very few calculi are nonopaque on CT, with the exception of protein matrix calculi and calculi resulting from treatment with protease inhibitors such as Indinavir.

- Even in the setting of nonopaque calculi, a secondary finding such as hydronephrosis or hydroureter, together with perirenal and/or periureteric stranding, has a 92% positive predictive value for ureteral obstruction.

MAGNETIC RESONANCE IMAGING

- MR urography can demonstrate a dilated, fluid-filled collecting system with heavily T2-weighted imaging (**Fig. 13.2A,B**). In nondilated systems, the collecting system can be demonstrated on dynamic postcontrast T1-weighted imaging (**Fig. 13.2C**) with Furosemide administration.
- MRI is a useful second-line test in patients who should avoid ionizing radiation (e.g., pregnant females). Sensitivity for detecting hydronephrosis (H, **Fig. 13.2B**) and hydroureter (u, **Fig. 13.2B**) is similar to that for an intravenous pyelogram (IVP) with normal renal function and surpasses IVP in patients with renal failure.
- Renal calculi may not be visualized due to MRI's inability to adequately detect calcification (*arrowhead*, **Fig. 13.2B**); however, an obstructed collecting system is easily visualized.

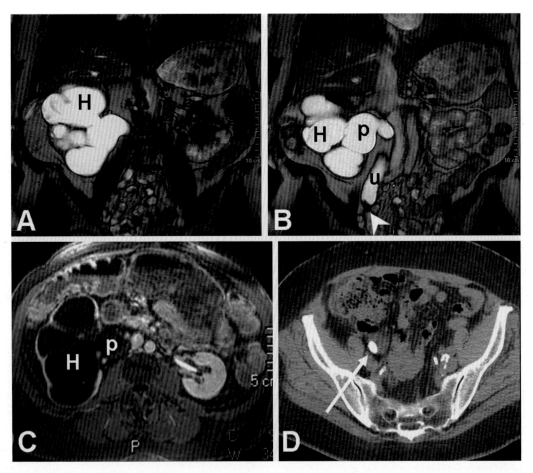

Fig. 13.2 Magnetic resonance urogram using **(A,B)** T2-weighted coronal images showing massive right hydronephrosis (H), dilation of the renal pelvis (p), and upper half of the right ureter (u). Hydronephrosis terminates at the signal void (*arrowhead*), representing a large stone in the lower right ureter. **(C)** Contrast-enhanced axial T1-weighted image showing massive hydronephrosis (H) and dilated renal pelvis (p). **(D)** Corresponding stone protocol computed tomography scan confirming a large obstructing stone (*arrow*) in the distal right ureter.

Treatment

- Diagnosis is directed at identifying the specific type of stone (and therefore its cause). Underlying factors leading to stone formation, such as dehydration, specific causes of hypercalciuria, and urinary tract infection, are sought and treated.
- Immediate treatment is directed at relieving the obstruction. Stones < 5 mm will most likely pass spontaneously, so supportive measures include pain relief with analgesics and hydration. For stones that do not pass spontaneously, lithotripsy or ureteroscopic extraction is pursued.

Prognosis

- Recurrent stone disease is expected in up to 50% of patients.

Suggested Readings

Fowler KA, Locken JA, Duchesne JH, Williamson MR. US for detecting renal calculi with nonenhanced CT as a reference standard. Radiology 2002;222(1):109–113.

Lingeman J, Matlaga B, Evan A. Surgical management of upper urinary tract calculi. In: Wein A, ed. Campbell-Walsh Urology. 9th ed. Philadelphia: Saunders Elsevier; 2007.

Moe OW. Kidney stones: pathophysiology and medical management. Lancet 2006;367(9507):333–344.

Roy C, Saussine C, Guth S, et al. MR urography in the evaluation of urinary tract obstruction. Abdom Imaging 1998;23(1):27–34.

CASE 14

Clinical Presentation

A 47-year-old male presents with chronic urinary tract infections (UTIs).

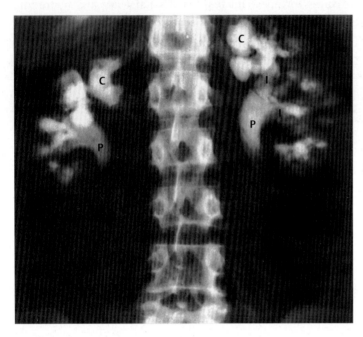

Fig. 14.1 Abdominal radiograph coned to the kidneys. Source: Resnick, Older, Diagnosis of Genitourinary Disease, New York: Thieme, 1997: 40. Reprinted by permission.

Radiologic Findings

- Bilateral calculi fill the collecting system, creating a cast of the calyces (c), infundibuli (i), and renal pelvis (p) in **Fig. 14.1**.

Diagnosis

Bilateral staghorn calculi

Differential Diagnosis

- Medullary nephrocalcinosis
- Bilateral ureteral obstruction
- Cortical calcinosis

Discussion

Background

Staghorn calculi are those calculi that fill the renal pelvis, the adjacent infundibuli, and calyces. These stones form as the result of infectious agents that produce urease (urea-splitting enzyme). Women are more commonly affected than men because women develop UTIs more often.

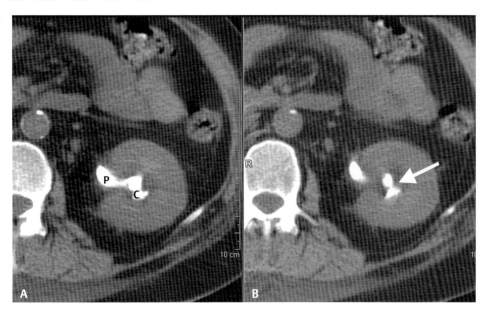

Fig. 14.2   An unenhanced computed tomography scan at two levels through the left kidney. **(A)** Calcifications form a cast involving the renal pelvis (p) and calyx (c). **(B)** Calcification involving the infundibulum (*arrow*).

Clinical Findings

Symptoms may be referral to UTI, an obstructing stone, or both. Some patients may be entirely asymptomatic despite the stone's occupation of the entire collecting system.

Pathology

Staghorn calculi are usually struvite (magnesium ammonium phosphate) crystallized with carbonate apatite. These stones develop in response to UTI with urease-splitting organisms such as *Proteus* and *Klebsiella* species.

Imaging Findings

RADIOGRAPHY

- Medullary nephrocalcinosis could look similar to the peripheral portions of the staghorn calculi, but medullary nephrocalcinosis would not fill the central portions of the collecting system.
- Ureteral obstruction would be a consideration if contrast had been given, but the patient's history in this case indicates abdominal radiograph only.
- Cortical calcinosis does not fit the diagnosis, as calcification does not involve the cortex.

COMPUTED TOMOGRAPHY

- Large stones filling and forming a cast of the collecting system is classic (**Fig. 14.2**).

ULTRASOUND

- Calcifications should be quite apparent as echoic interfaces, although determining the extent to which the stones fill the collecting system may be difficult.
- Posterior acoustic shadowing will be seen, as in **Fig. 14.3**.

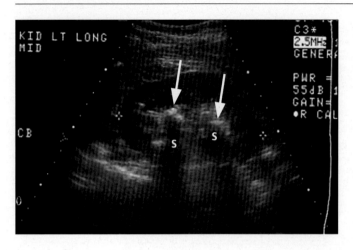

Fig. 14.3 Left renal sonogram in a patient with staghorn calculi. Calcification forms a cast of the collecting system (*arrows*) with posterior acoustic shadowing (S).

Treatment

- Treatment is directed at (1) treating the underlying infection and (2) removing all the stone material from the collecting system so that it does not serve as a nidus for new stone crystallization.
- Percutaneous stone removal without or with combination shock wave lithotripsy and surgical removal are therapeutic options.

Prognosis

- Stone-free rates following stone removal without or with lithotripsy reach 80 to 87%; surgical removal achieves a near 100% stone-free rate.

Suggested Readings

Dyer RB, Chen MY, Zagoria RJ. Classic signs in uroradiology. Radiographics 2004;24(Suppl 1):S247–S280.

Segura JW. Staghorn calculi. Urol Clin North Am 1997;24(1):71–80.

CASE 15

Clinical Presentation

A 22-year-old female presents with right flank pain.

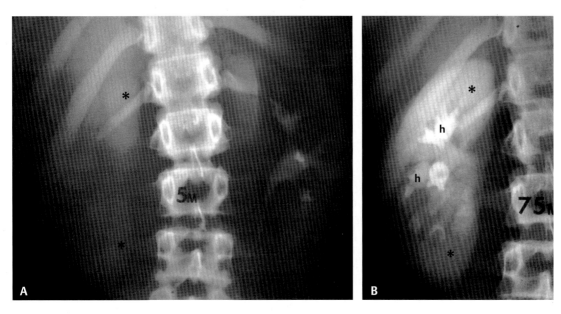

Fig. 15.1 Two images from an intravenous pyelogram: **(A)** at 5 minutes and **(B)** at 75 minutes.

Radiologic Findings

- Progressively increasing right nephrogram (*asterisks,* **Fig. 15.1**)
- Delayed filling of right collecting system (**Fig. 15.1A**)
- Mild dilatation of right collecting system (h, **Fig. 15.1B**)
- Normal left kidney

Diagnosis

Acute right ureteral obstruction on intravenous pyelogram (IVP) secondary to distal right ureteral stone (not shown)

Differential Diagnosis

- Renal vein thrombosis
- Renal artery stenosis
- Contrast-induced renal failure

Discussion

BACKGROUND

Up to 12% of the U.S. population will experience at least one bout of renal colic; 50% of those patients will suffer at least one recurrence. Caucasian patients are affected more often than African-American patients and males more often than females.

Clinical Findings

Renal colicky pain is classic, with flank pain migrating to the groin as the stone travels down the ureter. Stones in the distal ureter may cause pain at the tip of the urethra or into the groin, together with dysuria, urgency, and frequency. Patients will writhe in pain and cannot find a comfortable position to alleviate the discomfort. Ninety percent of patients will have gross or microscopic hematuria. Nausea and vomiting may be present because of splanchnic innervation of the renal capsule.

Pathology

Etiologies associated with stone formation include hypercalciuria, acidic urine (seen with uric acid stones), and infection, especially with urease-producing bacteria.

Imaging Findings

RADIOGRAPHY

- Renal vein thrombosis can produce a similar delayed nephrogram, but it is very uncommon and would not produce the dilated calyces present in this case (*asterisks,* **Fig. 15.1B**).
- Renal artery stenosis can produce a delayed nephrogram, but the kidney would be small and smooth, and calyces would not be dilated.
- Contrast-induced renal failure produces a bilateral, not unilateral, persistent nephrogram.
- This case shows the classic IVP appearance of acute ureteral obstruction—the "lightbulb" nephrogram, meaning the nephrogram continually gets brighter or stays bright. With this IVP appearance in the setting of flank pain, acute ureteral obstruction is by far the most likely diagnosis.

Treatment

- In the absence of infection, renal failure, or intractable vomiting, management is expectant with observation until the stone passes, together with pain management.
- Stones remaining in the ureter longer than 4 weeks require intervention (e.g., ureteroscopic retrieval, lithotripsy).

Prognosis

- Stones < 5 mm (longest axis) are likely to pass spontaneously within 4 weeks.
- Recurrent renal colic in 50% of patients.

PEARLS _____

- Following IV injection of contrast, the osmotic diuresis caused by the contrast agent may result in an initial increase in the patient's flank pain as the obstructed system becomes more distended. Further distension may result in a fornical rupture, an extravasation of contrast, and, paradoxically, a resolution of the patient's pain and resolved persistent nephrogram. Fornical ruptures can be managed conservatively as long as the ureteral obstruction is ultimately removed.

Suggested Readings

Dyer RB, Chen MY, Zagoria RJ. Intravenous urography: technique and interpretation. Radiographics 2001;21(4):799–821, discussion 822–794.

Teichman JM. Clinical practice: acute renal colic from ureteral calculus. N Engl J Med 2004;350(7):684–693.

CASE 16

Clinical Presentation

A 27-year-old female presents with pyuria and left flank pain.

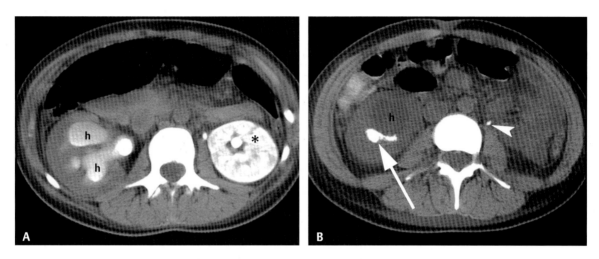

Fig. 16.1 CT-IVP **(A)** at 15 minutes postcontrast and **(B)** at 12 hours postcontrast at a slightly lower level.

Radiologic Findings

- Dense, persistent left nephrogram (*asterisk,* **Fig. 16.1A**)
- Small stone in the left proximal ureter (*arrowhead,* **Fig. 16.1B**)
- Right renal stones (*arrow,* **Fig. 16.1B**)
- Moderate right hydronephrosis (h, **Fig. 16.1A,B**)

Diagnosis

Acute left ureteral obstruction

Differential Diagnosis

- Acute right ureteral obstruction
- Left acute pyelonephritis
- Left renal vein thrombosis

Discussion

Background

Up to 12% of the U.S. population will experience at least one bout of renal colic; 50% of those patients will suffer at least one recurrence. Caucasian patients are affected more often than African-American patients and males more often than females.

Clinical Findings

Renal colicky pain is classic, with flank pain migrating to the groin as the stone travels down the ureter. Stones in the distal ureter may cause pain at the tip of the urethra or into the groin, together with dysuria, urgency, and frequency. Patients will writhe in pain and cannot find a comfortable position to alleviate the discomfort. Ninety percent of patients will have gross or microscopic hematuria. Nausea and vomiting may be present because of splanchnic innervation of the renal capsule.

Pathology

Etiologies associated with stone formation include hypercalciuria, acidic urine (seen with uric acid stones), and infection.

Imaging Findings

COMPUTED TOMOGRAPHY

- Right hydronephrosis indicates a chronic or prior obstructive process on the right (h, **Fig. 16.1A,B**), but the lack of a persistent nephrogram and the relatively prompt filling of the collecting system on the right exclude an acute right obstruction.
- Acute pyelonephritis produces a striated nephrogram but not a dense, persistent nephrogram (*asterisk,* **Fig. 16.1A**). That is the hallmark of acute obstruction.
- Renal vein thrombosis, which is rare, can produce a dense, persistent nephrogram. This is very unlikely, especially in view of the ureteral stone seen on the 12-hour delayed set of images after all contrast has cleared (*arrowhead,* **Fig. 16.1B**).

Treatment

- In the absence of infection, renal failure, or intractable vomiting, management is expectant with observation until the stone passes, together with adequate pain management.
- Stones remaining in the ureter longer than 4 weeks require intervention (e.g., ureteroscopic retrieval, lithotripsy).

Prognosis

- Stones < 5 mm (longest axis) are likely to pass spontaneously within 4 weeks.
- Recurrent renal colic in 50% of patients

PEARLS

- A unilateral dense, persistent nephrogram is almost always due to acute ureteral obstruction.

Suggested Readings

Abramson S, Walders N, Applegate KE, Gilkeson RC, Robbin MR. Impact in the emergency department of unenhanced CT on diagnostic confidence and therapeutic efficacy in patients with suspected renal colic: a prospective survey. 2000 ARRS President's Award, American Roentgen Ray Society. AJR Am J Roentgenol 2000;175(6):1689–1695.

Boridy IC, Kawashima A, Goldman SM, Sandler CM. Acute ureterolithiasis: nonenhanced helical CT findings of perinephric edema for prediction of degree of ureteral obstruction. Radiology 1999;213(3):663–667.

Boulay I, Holtz P, Foley WD, White B, Begun FP. Ureteral calculi: diagnostic efficacy of helical CT and implications for treatment of patients. AJR Am J Roentgenol 1999;172(6):1485–1490.

Kimme-Smith C, Perrella RR, Kaveggia LP, Cochran S, Grant EG. Detection of renal stones with real-time sonography: effect of transducers and scanning parameters. AJR Am J Roentgenol 1991;157(5):975–980.

Levine JA, Neitlich J, Verga M, Dalrymple N, Smith RC. Ureteral calculi in patients with flank pain: correlation of plain radiography with unenhanced helical CT. Radiology 1997;204(1):27–31.

Saunders HS, Dyer RB, Shifrin RY, Scharling ES, Bechtold RE, Zagoria RJ. The CT nephrogram: implications for evaluation of urinary tract disease. Radiographics 1995;15(5):1069–1085, discussion 1086–1088.

Smith RC, Verga M, McCarthy S, Rosenfield AT. Diagnosis of acute flank pain: value of unenhanced helical CT. AJR Am J Roentgenol 1996;166(1):97–101.

Teichman JM. Clinical practice: acute renal colic from ureteral calculus. N Engl J Med 2004;350(7):684–693.

CASE 17

Clinical Presentation

A 60-year-old male presents with right flank pain, hematuria, and a history of leukemia.

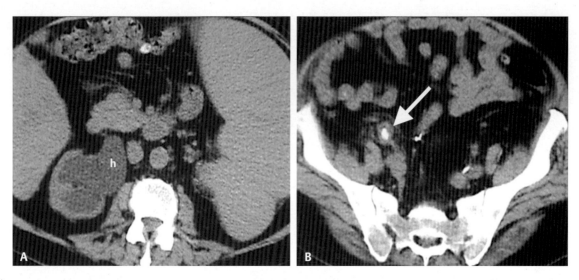

Fig. 17.1 Noncontrast computed tomography at two levels: **(A)** right kidney and **(B)** right midureter.

Radiologic Findings

- Hydronephrosis and hydroureter (h, **Fig. 17.1A**)
- Ureteral stone, periureteric stranding, and the "rim" sign produced by edematous ureter (*arrow,* **Fig. 17.1B**)
- Splenomegaly, incidentally noted (**Fig. 17.1A**)

Diagnosis

Obstructing ureteral stone on the right

Differential Diagnosis

- Nonobstructing ureteral stone
- Ureteral clot
- Ureteral tumor

Discussion

Background

Up to 12% of the U.S. population will experience at least one bout of renal colic; 50% of those patients will suffer at least one recurrence. Caucasian patients are affected more often than African-American patients and males more often than females.

Clinical Findings

Renal colicky pain is classic, with flank pain migrating to the groin as the stone travels down the ureter. Stones in the distal ureter may cause pain at the tip of the urethra or into the groin, together with dysuria, urgency, and frequency. Patients will writhe in pain and cannot find a comfortable position to alleviate the discomfort. Ninety percent of patients will have gross or microscopic hematuria. Nausea and vomiting may be present because of splanchnic innervation of the renal capsule.

Pathology

Etiologies associated with stone formation include hypercalciuria, acidic urine (seen with uric acid stones), and infection.

Imaging Findings
COMPUTED TOMOGRAPHY

- A nonobstructing stone would not produce hydronephrosis or hydroureter.
- A tumor or clot can produce secondary signs of obstruction but will lack the presence of a hyperdense stone.
- The noncontrast CT stone protocol has become the study of choice for suspected ureteral stones. Diagnosis of an obstructing ureteral stone with the CT protocol is based on primary and secondary signs:
  - Primary signs of obstructing ureteral stone include visualization of the stone within the ureter. The soft tissue "rim" sign represents visualization of the edematous ureter around the stone. Both of these signs are present on **Fig. 17.1B** in this case.
  - Secondary signs of hydronephrosis, hydroureter, perinephric stranding, and nephromegaly are > 90% accurate for obstructing ureteral stone. Hydronephrosis and hydroureter are present in this case (h, **Fig. 17.1A**).

RADIOGRAPHY

- Depending on stone composition, stones may be opaque or lucent on abdominal radiography.
- Visualization of opaque stones will vary depending on stone size, position, body habitus, and overlying structures, such as bowel gas or bony structures. Although ~85% of renal calculi are dense enough to be seen on conventional radiography, only ~50% are, in fact, detected.
- Opaque stones include
  - Calcium stones (calcium oxylate, calcium phosphate): ~80% of all stones
  - Struvite (magnesium ammonium phosphate bound to apatite): ~10% of all stones
- Lucent stones include
  - Uric acid: ~5 to 10% of all stones
  - Protein matrix and stones arising from protease inhibitors, such as Indinavir (these rare stones are also lucent on computed tomography (CT); therefore, secondary findings become important in diagnosing the obstructing stone)

INTRAVENOUS PYELOGRAM

- Scout film may show the obstructing calculus (*arrow,* **Fig. 17.2A**).
- Uptake and excretion of contrast by the obstructed kidney may be delayed depending on the severity of the obstruction and its detrimental effects on renal function.
- With excretion, hydroureteronephrosis should become apparent (h, **Fig. 17.2B**). Contrast may be diluted as it is excreted into the hydronephrotic volume.

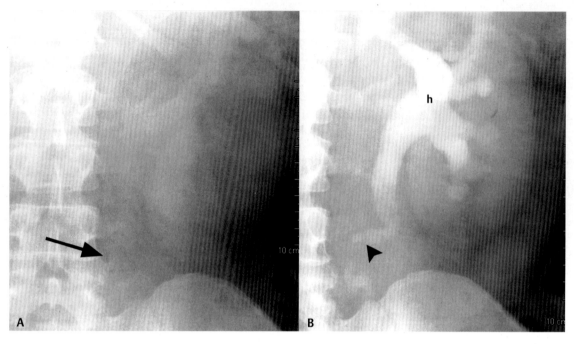

Fig. 17.2   Intravenous pyelogram. **(A)** Radiograph scout film coned to kidneys shows calcification in the location of the left ureteropelvic junction. **(B)** A delayed excretory phase image shows hydronephrosis (h) and hydroureter to the level of the obstructing stone (*arrowhead*).

- With continued delayed imaging, the level of the obstruction should become apparent as the contrast column will arrest at the level of the obstructing stone (*arrowhead*, **Fig. 17.2B**).

ULTRASOUND

- Most renal calculi present with an echogenic interface and clean posterior acoustic shadowing.
- Sensitivity for detecting renal calculi ranges from 60 to 91%.
- Sensitivity for detecting ureteral calculi is < 20%.

Treatment

- In the absence of infection, renal failure, or intractable vomiting, management is expectant with observation until the stone passes, together with adequate pain management.
- Stones < 5 mm (longest axis) are likely to pass spontaneously within 4 weeks.
- Stones remaining in the ureter longer than 4 weeks require intervention (e.g., basket retrieval, lithotripsy).

Prognosis

- Recurrent renal colic in 50% of patients

PEARLS

- Noncontrast spiral CT is the study of choice for acute renal colic pain and suspected acute ureteral obstructing stone, but it is not the study of choice for painless hematuria (i.e., painless hematuria requires CT-IVP).

Suggested Readings

Abramson S, Walders N, Applegate KE, Gilkeson RC, Robbin MR. Impact in the emergency department of unenhanced CT on diagnostic confidence and therapeutic efficacy in patients with suspected renal colic: a prospective survey. 2000 ARRS President's Award, American Roentgen Ray Society. AJR Am J Roentgenol 2000;175(6):1689–1695.

Boridy IC, Kawashima A, Goldman SM, Sandler CM. Acute ureterolithiasis: nonenhanced helical CT findings of perinephric edema for prediction of degree of ureteral obstruction. Radiology 1999;213(3):663–667.

Kimme-Smith C, Perrella RR, Kaveggia LP, Cochran S, Grant EG. Detection of renal stones with real-time sonography: effect of transducers and scanning parameters. AJR Am J Roentgenol 1991;157(5):975–980.

Smith RC, Verga M, McCarthy S, Rosenfield AT. Diagnosis of acute flank pain: value of unenhanced helical CT. AJR Am J Roentgenol 1996;166(1):97–101.

Teichman JM. Clinical practice: acute renal colic from ureteral calculus. N Engl J Med 2004;350(7):684–693.

CASE 18

Clinical Presentation

A 50-year-old male presents with intermittent right flank pain.

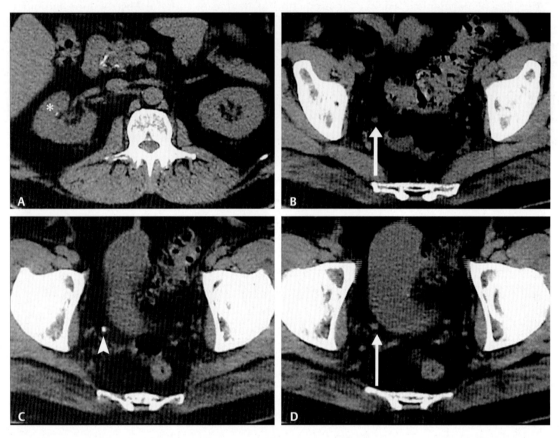

Fig. 18.1 Noncontrast computed tomography scans at four levels: **(A)** right kidney, **(B)** right ureter proximal to stone (*arrow*), **(C)** right ureteral stone (*arrowhead*), and **(D)** right ureter distal to stone (*arrow*).

Radiologic Findings

- Right renal stone (*asterisk*, **Fig. 18.1A**)
- No hydronephrosis or hydroureter (*arrow*, **Fig. 18.1B,D**)
- Distal right ureteral stone (*arrowhead*, **Fig. 18.1C**)
- No rim sign
- Distal ureter below stone is same size as ureter above stone (*arrow*, **Fig. 18.1D**)

Diagnosis

Nonobstructing distal right ureteral stone

Differential Diagnosis

- Obstructing ureteral stone
- Appendicitis
- Pyelonephritis

Discussion

Background

Up to 12% of the U.S. population will experience at least one bout of renal colic; 50% of those patients will suffer a recurrence. Caucasian patients are affected more often than African-American patients and males more often than females.

Clinical Findings

Flank pain and hematuria are the most common symptoms, but they can be variable with nonobstructing stones.

Pathology

Most stones are calcium oxylate.

Imaging Findings

COMPUTED TOMOGRAPHY

- An obstructing stone is excluded by the lack of hydronephrosis or hydroureter.
- Appendicitis cannot be excluded on the images shown, but it becomes unlikely as the cause of pain with identification of the ureteral stone.
- Noncontrast CT is not diagnostic for pyelonephritis.
- The noncontrast CT stone protocol has become the study of choice for suspected ureteral stones. Nearly 100% of renal calculi are dense and are detectable on CT.
- Diagnosis of a ureteral stone with the CT protocol is based on primary and secondary signs:
  - Primary sign of a stone within the ureter is present in this case and diagnostic (*arrowhead,* **Fig. 18.1C**).
  - Primary soft tissue "rim" sign, which represents the edematous soft tissue ureteral wall surrounding the stone, is absent in this case.
  - Secondary signs of obstruction are hydronephrosis, hydroureter, perinephric stranding, and nephromegaly. In the absence of a visualized ureteral stone, these findings result in > 90% positive predictive value for an obstructing ureteral stone, but secondary findings are absent in this case.

RADIOGRAPHY

- Depending on their composition, stones may be opaque or lucent on abdominal radiography.
- Visualization of even opaque stones will vary depending on stone size, position, body habitus, and overlying structures, such as bowel gas or bony structures. Although ~85% of renal calculi are dense enough to be seen on conventional radiography, only ~50% are, in fact, detected.
- Opaque stones include
  - Calcium stones (calcium oxylate, calcium phosphate): ~80% of all stones
  - Struvite (magnesium ammonium phosphate bound to apatite): ~10% of all stones
- Lucent stones include
  - Uric acid: ~5 to 10% of all stones
  - Protein matrix and stones arising from protease inhibitors, such as Indinavir (these rare stones are also lucent on computed tomography (CT); therefore, secondary findings become important in diagnosing the obstructing stone)

ULTRASOUND

- Although good for the detection of renal stones and hydronephrosis, ultrasound is not very useful for the detection of ureteral stones, especially nonobstructing ureteral stones.

Treatment

- Observation for stones < 4 to 5 mm
- Larger stones that do not pass after a period of observation require intervention (lithotripsy, basket stone removal).

Prognosis

- Good, as most small stones will pass spontaneously
- Once renal calculi have recurred, the number of recurrences and the rate of recurrences increase.

PEARLS _____

- The absence of secondary signs does not exclude a ureteral stone. Careful evaluation of the ureter on thin section images during a stone protocol CT is necessary to avoid overlooking a nonobstructing stone that could produce obstruction with slight changes in the position of the stone.

Suggested Readings

Abramson S, Walders N, Applegate KE, Gilkeson RC, Robbin MR. Impact in the emergency department of unenhanced CT on diagnostic confidence and therapeutic efficacy in patients with suspected renal colic: a prospective survey. 2000 ARRS President's Award, American Roentgen Ray Society. AJR Am J Roentgenol 2000;175(6):1689–1695.

Boulay I, Holtz P, Foley WD, White B, Begun FP. Ureteral calculi: diagnostic efficacy of helical CT and implications for treatment of patients. AJR Am J Roentgenol 1999;172(6):1485–1490.

Levine JA, Neitlich J, Verga M, Dalrymple N, Smith RC. Ureteral calculi in patients with flank pain: correlation of plain radiography with unenhanced helical CT. Radiology 1997;204(1):27–31.

Smith RC, Verga M, McCarthy S, Rosenfield AT. Diagnosis of acute flank pain: value of unenhanced helical CT. AJR Am J Roentgenol 1996;166(1):97–101.

CASE 19

Clinical Presentation

A 25-year-old male presents with right flank pain.

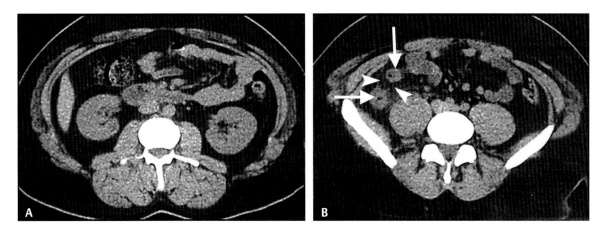

Fig. 19.1 Noncontrast stone protocol computed tomography through the level of the **(A)** kidneys and **(B)** upper pelvis.

Radiologic Findings

- No renal stones, hydronephrosis, and perirenal stranding are noted on images provided (**Fig. 19.1A**).
- Enlarged appendix with markedly thickened wall (*arrows,* **Fig. 19.1B**)
- Periappendiceal and pericecal stranding of fat (*arrowheads,* **Fig. 19.1B**)

Diagnosis

Acute appendicitis mimicking ureteral colic

Differential Diagnosis

- Ureteral stone
- Intestinal obstruction
- Diverticulitis
- Mesenteric adenitis

Discussion

Background

Appendicitis is the most common cause of acute abdominal pain and the most common indication for surgery in young children. It can be found rarely in extremely young and extremely old patients, but it often goes undiagnosed for some time.

Clinical Findings

Pain begins as vaguely nonlocalizing or epigastric, ultimately becoming periumbilical and progressively moving to the right lower quadrant. Anorexia is usually present. Fever or elevated white blood cell count may be minimal. Physical exam findings include pain localizing to McBurney point halfway between the anterosuperior iliac spine and the umbilicus in the right lower quadrant. Appendicitis and diverticulitis account for ~10 to 12% of alternative diagnoses on unenhanced computed tomography (CT) for suspected ureteral stones.

Pathology

Appendicitis results from appendiceal luminal obstruction from fecolith, external lymph nodes, or other factors. This obstruction results in appendiceal distension and poor blood flow to the appendiceal mucosa, with ischemic necrosis leading to infection of the appendiceal wall from gut organisms. If not treated during the acute inflammatory phase, perforation is likely with peritonitis and/or abscess formation, with resultant increased morbidity and mortality.

Imaging Findings

COMPUTED TOMOGRAPHY

- A ureteral stone is excluded, as no renal or ureteral stones and no hydronephrosis or hydroureter are identified on the images provided (**Fig. 19.1A**).
- No dilatation of the small or large intestine is seen to indicate intestinal obstruction.
- No diverticula are identified in this young patient to indicate diverticulitis.
- Mesenteric adenitis is a diagnosis of exclusion. However, a cause for the patient's pain is identified in this case.
- CT is highly accurate (94–98%) for appendicitis diagnosis.
- A normal appendix can measure anywhere from 6 to 10 mm measured from the outer wall to the outer wall with a thin wall. The measurements can vary compared with sonography because appendiceal compression is not applied with CT. The appendiceal lumen often contains gas. An appendicolith may be present but is not indicative of appendicitis as an isolated finding.
- An abnormal appendix includes
    - Fluid-filled appendix with transverse diameter > 7 mm measured from the outer wall to the outer wall is consistent with appendicitis.
- Ancillary findings that increase confidence in the diagnosis include
    - Appendiceal wall thickening > 3 mm
    - Appendiceal wall hyperemia
    - Appendiceal intramural gas
    - Periappendiceal inflammatory changes/stranding
    - Cecal apical wall thickening
- Abscess, extraluminal gas, or extraluminal fecolith is consistent with appendiceal perforation.

ULTRASOUND

- With graded compression sonography, a normal appendix should measure ≤ 6 mm from the outer wall to the outer wall. Often, a normal appendix is not identified.
- An abnormal appendix includes
    - Thickened transverse diameter > 6 mm measured from the outer wall to the outer wall on compression sonography (**Fig. 19.2**)
- Ancillary findings that increase confidence in the diagnosis include
    - Appendiceal wall hyperemia

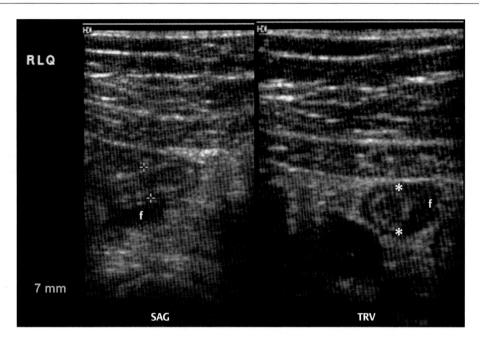

Fig. 19.2 Appendix sonogram in a patient with right lower quadrant pain. Sagittal images show a dilated blind-ending tubular structure in the region of the patient's pain. Plus calipers measure 7 mm on this compression sonogram. Transverse images show a similarly noncompressible appendix between the asterisks. f, periappendiceal fluid.

- Abscess, extraluminal gas, or extraluminal fecolith is consistent with appendiceal perforation.
- Nonvisualization of the appendix cannot exclude appendicitis.

MAGNETIC RESONANCE IMAGING

- Magnetic resonance imaging without gadolinium may be performed in pregnant females suspected of having appendicitis (**Fig. 19.3**).
- A normal appendix measures ≤ 6 mm and contains luminal air.
- An abnormal appendix includes
  - Thickened transverse diameter > 7 mm measured from the outer wall to the outer wall with a fluid-filled appendiceal lumen (**Fig. 19.3B,D**). Although not validated some normal appendices may measure up to 10 mm as has been found in the CT literature.
- Ancillary findings that increase confidence in the diagnosis include
  - Periappendiceal fluid seen as a high T2 signal
  - Obstructing appendicolith may be inconspicuous or may show a signal void (**Fig. 19.3A,C**) due to MRI's inability to demonstrate calcification.

Treatment

- Appendectomy in uncomplicated cases
- Cases with abscess formation usually require drainage and convalescence with antibiotics and bowel rest prior to subsequent surgical resection.

Prognosis

- When diagnosed early, excellent results

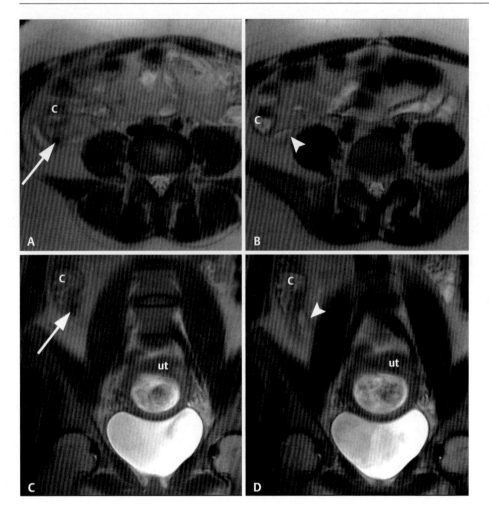

Fig. 19.3 Abdominal and pelvic magnetic resonance images in a pregnant female with right lower quadrant pain, heavily T2-weighted images in the axial **(A,B)** and coronal **(C,D)** planes. **(A)** Signal void in the base of the appendix (*arrow*) represents an appendicolith. **(B)** Dilated fluid-filled appendix (*arrowhead*) measures 10 mm, consistent with appendicitis. **(C)** Appendicolith (*arrow*). **(D)** Dilated fluid-filled appendix (*arrowhead*) beyond the obstructing appendicolith. Note gravid uterus (ut) impressing on the bladder in **C** and **D**. C, cecum.

- Delay in diagnosis results in increased risk for perforation, and with perforation comes increased morbidity and mortality.

PEARLS

- Appendicitis and diverticulitis account for ~10 to 12% of alternative diagnoses on unenhanced CT for suspected ureteral stones.

Suggested Readings

Jeffrey RB Jr, Laing FC, Townsend RR. Acute appendicitis: sonographic criteria based on 250 cases. Radiology 1988;167(2):327–329.

Pedrosa I, Levine D, Eyvazzadeh AD, et al. MR imaging evaluation of acute appendicitis in pregnancy. Radiology 2006;238(3):891–899.

Pinto Leite N, Pereira JM, Cunha R, Pinto P, Sirlin C. CT evaluation of appendicitis and its complications: imaging techniques and key diagnostic findings. AJR Am J Roentgenol 2005;185(2):406–417.

Rucker CM, Menias CO, Bhalla S. Mimics of renal colic: alternative diagnoses at unenhanced helical CT. Radiographics 2004;24(Suppl 1):S11–S28, discussion S28–S33.

CASE 20

Clinical Presentation

A 57-year-old female presents with hematuria.

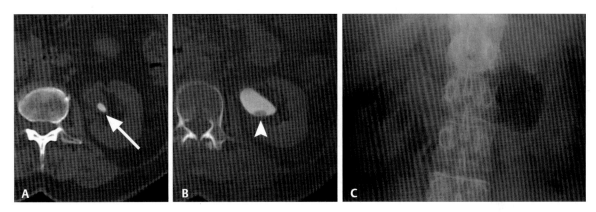

Fig. 20.1 **(A)** Noncontrast computed tomography (CT) scan, **(B)** delayed CT-IVP, and **(C)** abdominal radiograph coned to the kidneys.

Radiologic Findings

- High-density stone in the left renal pelvis on a noncontrast study measuring 400 Hounsfield units (HU). Region of interest measurement is not shown. (*arrow,* **Fig. 20.1A**).
- Filling defect in the left renal pelvis (*arrowhead,* **Fig. 20.1B**).
- No stone on abdominal film (**Fig. 20.1C**)

Diagnosis

Uric acid stone

Differential Diagnosis

- Blood clot
- Calcium stone
- Sloughed papilla
- Transitional cell carcinoma

Discussion

Background

Uric acid stones are the second most common type of renal calculi. An abnormally low urine pH, gout (and other causes of hyperuricemia), and obesity are implicated.

Clinical Findings

Many renal calculi are now detected incidentally with the increased use of diagnostic imaging. Some degree of urinary obstruction is required to cause symptoms. Fifty percent of incidentally detected calculi will become symptomatic (i.e., will obstruct the collecting system) within 5 years of discovery. Symptomatic renal calculi present with classic abrupt onset of severe flank pain (i.e., renal colic) that may migrate toward the groin, as the stone travels down the ureter. Pain is unrelieved by positional changes. Gross hematuria is found in 80 to 100% of patients with renal colic.

Pathology

An abnormally low urine pH of ~5.5 or increased uric acid in the urine, or both, results in the precipitation of uric acid stones.

Imaging Findings

COMPUTED TOMOGRAPHY

- A fresh blood clot can be high density compared with unenhanced abdominal soft tissue, but it is typically < 100 HU and not nearly as high as the 400 HU in this case.
- Densities range from around 400 to 500 HU for uric acid stones to well over 1000 HU for calcium stones. Calcium stones would likely be apparent on the abdominal film (**Fig. 20.1C**) and would measure > 400 HU on computed tomography (CT).
- Sloughed papilla would be soft tissue density (i.e., 50–70 HU) unless calcified, and no calcification is apparent on the abdominal radiograph.
- Transitional cell carcinoma (TCC) would not be high density on the noncontrast exam. TCC typically enhances only slightly on enhanced scans.
- Cysteine stones, not listed as a choice, could appear similar to the current case, as they are often not visible on routine abdominal radiographs, but they usually measure higher CT density than in this case.
- Virtually all calculi are detectable by unenhanced CT scan, and the CT density units can provide some indication of the composition of the stones.

RADIOGRAPHY

- Uric acid stones are generally not detectable on abdominal radiographs due to their low density.
- On intravenous urography, the stone would be detected as a nonspecific filling defect, which could represent uric acid stone, clot, sloughed papilla, or tumor. If it were shown to be mobile, all other entities except stones would be excluded.

ULTRASOUND

- Stones in the kidney or renal pelvis will be shown as hyperechoic foci with posterior acoustic shadowing.
- Stones in the ureter especially distally, are poorly demonstrated on sonography, although the associated hydronephrosis will be easily detected.

Treatment

- Increased fluid intake as with all stone diseases.
- Decrease uric acid stone precipitation in the urine:
  - Alkalinize the urine with oral potassium citrate.
  - Treat hyperuricemic states.
  - Diet with decreased purine intake.

Prognosis

- Alkalinization of the urine has an ~80% success rate in inhibiting uric acid stone formation.

Suggested Readings

Coe F, Favus M, Asplin J. Nephrolithiasis. In: Wein A, ed. Campbell-Walsh Urology. 9th ed. Philadelphia: Saunders Elsevier; 2007.

Moe OW. Kidney stones: pathophysiology and medical management. Lancet 2006;367(9507):333–344.

Mostafavi MR, Ernst RD, Saltzman B. Accurate determination of chemical composition of urinary calculi by spiral computerized tomography. J Urol 1998;159(3):673–675.

Saw KC, McAteer JA, Monga AG, et al. Helical CT of urinary calculi: effect of stone composition, stone size, and scan collimation. AJR Am J Roentgenol 2000;175(2):329–332.

Shekarriz B, Stoller ML. Uric acid nephrolithiasis: current concepts and controversies. J Urol 2002;168(4 Pt 1):1307–1314.

CASE 21

Clinical Presentation

A 27-year-old male presents with left flank pain and low-grade fever.

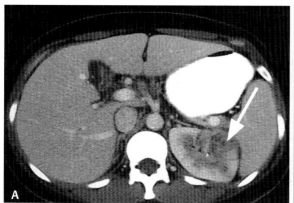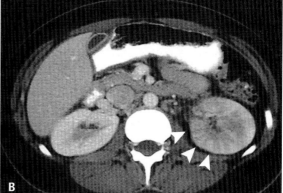

Fig. 21.1 **(A,B)** Enhanced computed tomography scans at two levels through the left kidney.

Radiologic Findings

- Focal hypodense area (*arrow*, **Fig. 21.1A**)
- Striated nephrogram (*arrowheads,* **Fig. 21.1B**)
- Slight nephrographic delay in function for the left kidney (**Fig. 21.1A,B**)

Diagnosis

Acute pyelonephritis (AP)

Differential Diagnosis

- Renal tumor
- Ureteral obstruction
- Contusion

Discussion

Background

Most AP results from an ascending urinary tract infection (UTI). The most common organism is *Escherichia coli* (80%) in adults. A minority of cases of AP are caused by hematogenous spread from distant sources (e.g., endocarditis, tooth abscess, intravenous drug abuse with septic thrombophlebitis). Most common hematogenously spread organisms are *Staphyloccus* and *Streptococcus* species.

Clinical Findings

Acute pyelonephritis is a clinical diagnosis consisting of flank pain, fever, and/or elevated white blood cell count, along with evidence for UTI on urinalysis. Renal imaging is required only if the

75

diagnosis is in doubt or if the patient is unresponsive to appropriate antibiotic coverage beyond 72 hours.

Pathology

In uncomplicated AP, imaging findings (i.e., poor enhancement, striated nephrogram) are attributed to interstitial edema and/or collecting tubules clogged with inflammatory cells, debris, or both.

Imaging Findings

COMPUTED TOMOGRAPHY

- Renal tumor is a consideration with a focal nephrographic defect, but it would not explain the diffuse left striated nephrogram also present (**Fig. 21.1B**).
- The striated nephrogram of obstruction is seen primarily during urography and consists of very fine striations and not the coarse striations present in this study (*arrowheads,* **Fig. 21.1B**). Obstruction also does not explain the hypodense area.
- Contusion can produce a striated nephrogram, but there was no history of trauma given.

RADIOGRAPHY

- Intravenous pyelogram (IVP) can show a swollen kidney, but IVP is normal in 75% of cases.

ULTRASOUND

- Ultrasound has poor sensitivity for AP compared with computed tomography (CT) but is used in the initial work-up to exclude hydronephrosis and obstruction as sources of infection.

NUCLEAR MEDICINE

- Cortical imaging with Technetium 99-m dimercaptosuccinic acid (DMSA) is used primarily in children.
- Focal areas of decreased uptake represent acute inflammation.

Treatment

- Uncomplicated AP responds well to antimicrobial therapy.

Prognosis

- In the absence of recurrent disease with scarring, the prognosis is excellent.

PEARLS _____

- All UTIs in male children and females < 5 years old require imaging to evaluate for vesicoureteral reflux and other predisposing conditions.

Suggested Readings

Kawashima A, LeRoy AJ. Radiologic evaluation of patients with renal infections. Infect Dis Clin North Am 2003;17(2):433–456.

Saunders HS, Dyer RB, Shifrin RY, et al. The CT nephrogram: implications for evaluation of urinary tract disease. Radiographics 1995;15(5):1069–1085, discussion 1086–1088.

Talner LB, Davidson AJ, Lebowitz RL, Dalla Palma L, Goldman SM. Acute pyelonephritis: can we agree on terminology? Radiology 1994;192(2):297–305.

CASE 22

Clinical Presentation

A 31-year-old presents with fever of unknown origin.

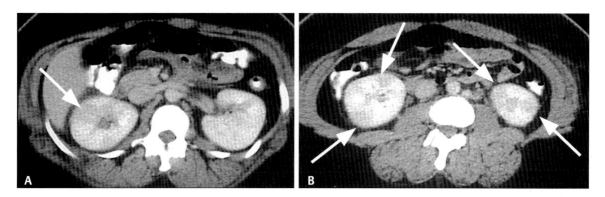

Fig. 22.1 **(A,B)** Enhanced computed tomography scans at two levels.

Radiologic Findings

- Bilateral focal hypodense areas (*arrows,* **Fig. 22.1**)
- No striated nephrogram

Diagnosis

Acute pyelonephritis (AP)

Differential Diagnosis

- Bilateral renal abscesses
- Lymphoma/leukemia
- von Hippel-Lindau disease with multiple renal cell carcinomas (RCCs)

Discussion

Background

Most AP results from an ascending urinary tract infection (UTI). The most common organism is *Escherichia coli* (80%) in adults. The minority of cases of AP are caused by hematogenous spread from distant sources (e.g., endocarditis, tooth abscess, intravenous drug abuse with septic thrombophlebitis). Most common hematogenously spread organisms are *Staphyloccus* and *Streptococcus* species.

Clinical Findings

Acute pyelonephritis is a clinical diagnosis consisting of flank pain, fever, and/or elevated white blood cell count, along with evidence of UTI on urinalysis. Renal imaging is required only if the diagnosis is in doubt or if the patient is unresponsive to appropriate antibiotic coverage beyond 72 hours. The presence of fever suggests an infectious process but does not exclude lymphoma, leukemia, or multifocal RCC.

Pathology

In uncomplicated AP, imaging findings (i.e., poor enhancement, striated nephrogram) are attributed to interstitial edema and/or collecting tubules clogged with inflammatory cells, debris, or both.

Imaging Findings

COMPUTED TOMOGRAPHY

- Renal abscess can appear on computed tomography (CT) as a relatively nondescript hypodense area (*arrows*, **Fig. 22.1**) or as a well-defined, low-density area surrounded by an enhancing rim.
- Although renal lymphoma or leukemia can present with multiple mass lesions, the lack of any abdominal adenopathy makes this diagnosis unlikely.
- Multiple renal tumors are a feature of von Hippel-Lindau disease, but the presenting complaint of fever makes this an unlikely diagnosis.
- The multiplicity of lesions is most consistent with AP despite the lack of a striated nephrogram. If any doubt exists to the certainty of the diagnosis, follow-up imaging is indicated following appropriate antibiotic therapy to ensure resolution of the lesions.

Treatment

- Confirmation of AP as the cause of these bilateral hypodense lesions can be obtained by image-guided percutaneous aspiration and culture versus follow-up CT scan in approximately 6 weeks to show improvement or resolution of the lesions following antibiotic therapy.

Prognosis

- In the absence of recurrent disease with scarring, the prognosis is excellent.

PEARLS _____

- The absence of a striated nephrogram does not exclude the diagnosis of AP.

Suggested Readings

Kawashima A, LeRoy AJ. Radiologic evaluation of patients with renal infections. Infect Dis Clin North Am 2003;17(2):433–456.

Saunders HS, Dyer RB, Shifrin RY, et al. The CT nephrogram: implications for evaluation of urinary tract disease. Radiographics 1995;15(5):1069–1085, discussion 1086–1088.

Sheeran SR, Sussman SK. Renal lymphoma: spectrum of CT findings and potential mimics. AJR Am J Roentgenol 1998;171(4):1067–1072.

Talner LB, Davidson AJ, Lebowitz RL, Dalla Palma L, Goldman SM. Acute pyelonephritis: can we agree on terminology? Radiology 1994;192(2):297–305.

Urban BA, Fishman EK. Tailored helical CT evaluation of acute abdomen. Radiographics 2000;20(3):725–749.

CASE 23

Clinical Presentation

A 25-year-old, on antibiotics for a urinary tract infection (UTI), presents with continued flank pain and fever.

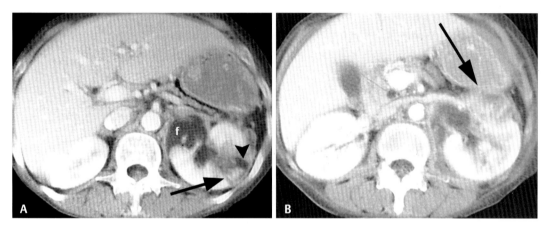

Fig. 23.1 **(A,B)** Enhanced computed tomography scans at two levels through the left kidney.

Radiologic Findings

- Striated nephrogram (*arrows*, **Fig. 23.1A,B**)
- Focal hypodense areas (*arrowhead*, **Fig. 23.1A**)
- Fluid density lesion medially (f, **Fig. 23.1A**)

Diagnosis

Acute pyelonephritis with intrarenal abscess

Differential Diagnosis

- Renal infarct
- Infected cyst
- Obstructed ureter
- Fractured kidney

Discussion

Background

Intrarenal abscess develops as a consequence of the patient's immune response to renal infection. The abscess may remain localized or may spread to the perirenal or pararenal spaces. Extrarenal processes may secondarily involve the genitourinary system (e.g., abscesses from appendicitis or diverticulitis). Diabetic patients and immunocompromised and transplant patients, as well as patients with septic emboli, urinary reflux or obstruction, are at increased risk for renal and perirenal abscess.

Clinical Findings

Flank pain and fever suggest pyelonephritis as opposed to flank pain and hematuria, which suggest ureteral stones with obstruction. This patient in **Fig. 23.1** received imaging because there was no clinical improvement following initiation of antibiotics.

Pathology

Renal abscesses usually develop as a complication of acute pyelonephritis. Common organisms are similar to those resulting in pyelonephritis, such as *Escherichia coli* and enterococci, but also *Klebsiella* and *Proteus*. Hematogenous spread of infection (e.g., from tooth abscess) is usually caused by *Staphylococcus* and *Streptococcus* species (**Fig. 23.2**).

Imaging Findings

COMPUTED TOMOGRAPHY

- Infected cyst may appear the same and would be treated similarly.
- Renal infarcts are usually well demarcated, follow vascular distribution, and often have a rim sign due to intact capsular flow, features not present in this case.
- Ureteral obstruction produces a generalized delayed nephrogram, not present in this case.
- A fractured kidney with disruption of the collecting structures might produce a nephrographic abnormality and fluid collection similar to the current case, but it is excluded by the history, which does not indicate trauma.
- Acute pyelonephritis produces a striated nephrogram (*black arrows,* **Fig. 23.1A,B**) due to delayed transit of contrast through areas of edematous parenchyma. An alternate pattern is multifocal hypodense areas representing focal inflammatory lesions (*arrowhead,* **Fig. 23.1A**). With inadequate treatment, an abscess may result (f, **Fig. 23.1A**).

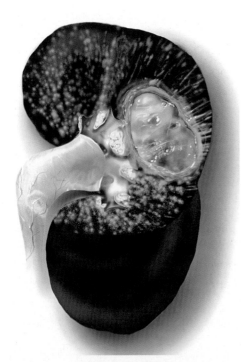

Fig. 23.2 Diffuse acute pyelonephritis with both microabscesses and large abscess formation.

- Computed tomography (CT) is the most accurate modality to assess for renal abscess. If present, CT assists in planning percutaneous or surgical drainage procedures. Additional findings on CT for intrarenal abscess include
  - Well-defined, low-density lesion
  - Liquefied material centrally that does not enhance with contrast
  - Thick, irregular wall that may enhance with contrast
  - Gas within the perinephric fluid collection suggests an infected abscess. Gas is usually caused by *E. coli,* which can ferment tissue glucose. These types of infections are most commonly encountered in poorly controlled diabetics.

Treatment

- Intravenous antibiotics and surgical or image-guided percutaneous drainage is required.

Prognosis

- Generally good

Suggested Readings

Kawashima A, LeRoy AJ. Radiologic evaluation of patients with renal infections. Infect Dis Clin North Am 2003;17(2):433–456.

Talner LB, Davidson AJ, Lebowitz RL, Dalla Palma L, Goldman SM. Acute pyelonephritis: can we agree on terminology? Radiology 1994;192(2):297–305.

CASE 24

Clinical Presentation

A 45-year-old female presents with recurrent urinary tract infections (UTIs).

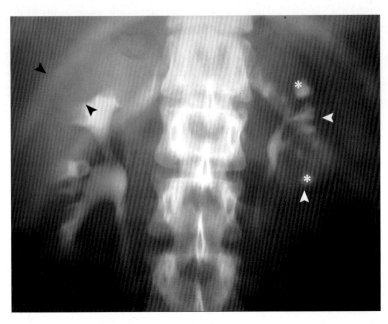

Fig. 24.1 A 5-minute radiograph coned to the kidneys from an intravenous pyelogram in the excretory phase.

Radiologic Findings

- Small, irregularly scarred left kidney (**Fig. 24.1**)
- Multiple clubbed calyces (*asterisks*) associated with parenchymal tissue loss/scars (*white arrowheads*)
- Normal to slightly hypertrophied contralateral renal cortex (*between black arrowheads*)

Diagnosis

Chronic pyelonephritis

Differential Diagnosis

- Postobstructive atrophy
- Renal artery stenosis
- Congenital hypoplastic kidney

Discussion

Background

Chronic pyelonephritis is synonymous with chronic reflux nephropathy. Damage to the renal parenchyma and collecting systems is due to repeated bouts of upper tract reflux of infected urine with associated recurrent renal infection and tissue loss.

Clinical Findings

A history of vesicoureteral reflux and/or recurrent UTI (e.g., intermittent fever, elevated white blood cell count, dysuria, positive urine cultures) may be elicited. There are no symptoms referable to chronic pyelonephritis until it produces renal failure and/or hypertension.

Pathology

The ascending UTI extends to the medullary pyramids. Subsequent inflammatory infiltration destroys the medulla and overlying parenchyma, resulting in a dilated calyx and overlying renal cortical loss/scar (*white arrowheads,* **Fig. 24.1**). See the drawing of chronic pyelonephritis in **Fig. 24.2**. Renal infection alone does not usually cause significant scarring unless recurrent bouts are related to functional or structural urinary tract abnormalities.

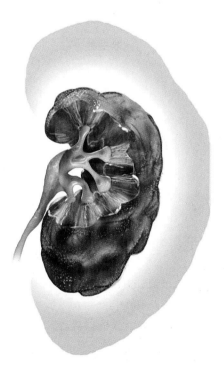

Fig. 24.2 Schematic drawing of chronic pyelonephritis showing a "peanut kidney" in the shadow of a normal parenchymal outline.

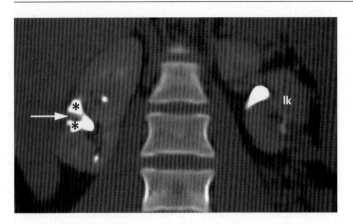

Fig. 24.3 Delayed image from a contrast-enhanced computed tomography scan show right lower pole clubbing (*asterisks*) and associated cortical thinning (*arrow*) from reflux nephropathy in a complete duplicated system on the right. Upper pole parenchyma appears normal. The left kidney is normal, although not well visualized on this image.

Imaging Findings

This case centers on the differential diagnosis of the unilateral small kidney.

RADIOGRAPHY/INTRAVENOUS PYELOGRAM

- Postobstructive atrophy produces global parenchymal loss with a smooth outline and no deep scars. There is usually some caliectasis.
- Renal artery stenosis produces a small, smooth kidney with normal collecting structures (no caliectasis).
- Congenital hypoplastic kidney may have a poorly developed collecting system but not deep scars or clubbed calyces.

COMPUTED TOMOGRAPHY

- The hallmark of chronic pyelonephritis on computed tomography is a small, scarred kidney. Cortical thinning will be seen in association with caliectasis (**Fig. 24.3**).

Treatment

- Early recognition and treatment of reflux is essential. In children, prophylactic antibiotics are administered and close monitoring is performed as reflux may resolve spontaneously. If the patient continues to develop urinary infections despite antibiotics, treatment may require ureteral reimplantation.

Prognosis

- Renal scarring may lead to early onset of hypertension and/or renal insufficiency, so the primary focus is to identify and treat the cause of recurrent infection as early as possible.

Suggested Readings

Dyer RB, Chen MY, Zagoria RJ. Intravenous urography: technique and interpretation. Radiographics 2001;21(4):799–821, discussion 822–794.

Kawashima A, LeRoy AJ. Radiologic evaluation of patients with renal infections. Infect Dis Clin North Am 2003;17(2):433–456.

Kenny P. Chronic inflammation. In: Pollack H, McClennan B, eds. Clinical Urography. Vol 1. 2nd ed. Philadelphia: WB Saunders; 2000:947–975.

CASE 25

Clinical Presentation

A 60-year-old diabetic female presents with a high fever.

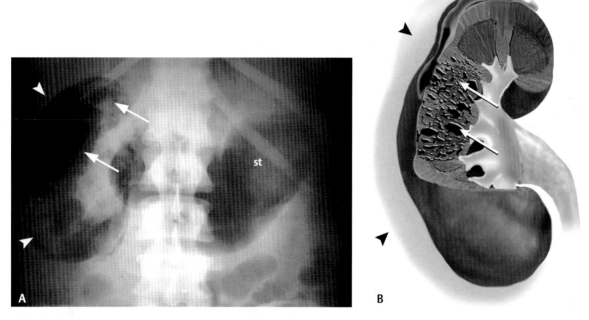

Fig. 25.1 **(A)** Conventional radiograph coned to the kidney region. **(B)** Schematic drawing illustrating gas locules infiltrating the renal parenchyma as in **Fig. 25.1A**. Source of **Fig. 25.1A**: CRITICAL REVIEWS IN DIAGNOSTIC IMAGING by Older RA, Moore AV and McClelland R. Copyright 1981 by Taylor & Francis Informa UK Ltd — Journals. Reproduced with permission of Taylor & Francis Informa UK Ltd — Journals in the format Textbook via Copyright Clearance Center.)

Radiologic Findings

- Gas in the perinephric space (*arrowheads,* **Fig. 25.1A,B**)
- Gas dissecting throughout the right kidney (*arrows,* **Fig. 25.1A,B**)
- Left-sided gas is in stomach (*st,* **Fig. 25.1A**)

Diagnosis

Emphysematous pyelonephritis

Differential Diagnosis

- Perinephric abscess
- Renal abscess
- Emphysematous pyelitis

Discussion

Background

Emphysematous pyelonephritis is an acute necrotizing renal parenchymal infection from gas-forming organisms. The most common bacteria are *Escherichia col*, *Klebsiella*, and *Proteus* species. Most patients are poorly controlled diabetics.

Clinical Findings

Patients present with severe acute pyelonephritis, urosepsis, or shock. Symptoms may include fever, vomiting, and flank pain. A history of poorly controlled blood glucose levels in a diabetic is also a factor. A urinary tract obstruction may be a predisposing factor.

Pathology

Emphysematous pyelonephritis is believed to be a consequence of severe pyelonephritis. Renal bacterial infection with gas-forming organisms results in parenchymal destruction due to the acute inflammatory process and is furthered by an inadequate host immune response and/or obstructive uropathy. Gas formation is thought to occur because of fermentation of tissue glucose by the organisms.

Imaging Findings

RADIOGRAPHY

- Perinephric abscess would have gas around the kidney but not within the kidney.
- Intrarenal abscess could contain gas within the kidney, but it would be localized to the abscess cavity (better prognosis) and not throughout the parenchyma (worse prognosis).
- Emphysematous pyelitis refers to an infection with gas only within the collecting system and not in the parenchyma (**Fig. 25.2**).
- Gas throughout the renal parenchyma is the distinguishing feature of emphysematous pyelonephritis (**Fig. 25.1**).

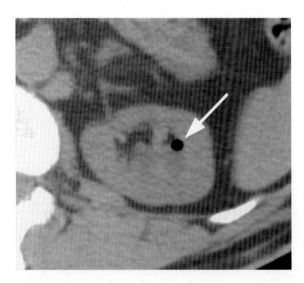

Fig. 25.2 Unenhanced computed tomography scan through the left kidney in a patient with flank pain and urinary symptoms shows a small collection of gas in the nondependent portion of the collecting system (*arrow*), consistent with emphysematous pyelitis.

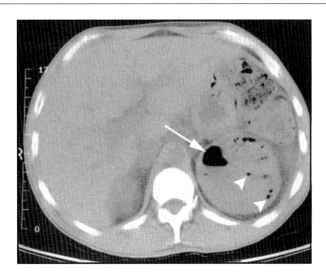

Fig. 25.3 Unenhanced computed tomography scan through the left kidney in a patient with symptoms of urosepsis shows a large air-fluid level in an intrarenal abscess (*arrow*), as well as gas scattered throughout the renal parenchyma (*arrowheads*), consistent with emphysematous pyelonephritis.

COMPUTED TOMOGRAPHY

- Computed tomography (CT) is the modality of choice for confirming gas in the renal parenchyma versus the collecting system (pyelitis) or perinephric space.
- CT is accurate for the diagnosis of parenchymal gas (worse prognosis) versus gas localized to a fluid-filled cavity (better prognosis).
- CT assists in planning surgical or percutaneous drainage procedures (**Fig. 25.3**).

Treatment

- In septic patients, emergent nephrectomy is indicated.
- In stable patients, a trial of medical therapy may be attempted.
- In the setting of urinary obstruction, emergent drainage is indicated.

Prognosis

- Gas in a localized abscess has ~20% mortality.
- Gas infiltrating the renal parenchyma has a high mortality of up to 60%.

PEARLS _____

- Be sure to clearly define the location of the gas collection (i.e., inside a fluid-containing cavity/abscess vs within the nonliquefied renal parenchyma), as these two findings have different severities and prognoses.

Suggested Readings

Grayson DE, Abbott RM, Levy AD, Sherman PM. Emphysematous infections of the abdomen and pelvis: a pictorial review. Radiographics 2002;22(3):543–561.

Kawashima A, LeRoy AJ. Radiologic evaluation of patients with renal infections. Infect Dis Clin North Am 2003;17(2):433–456

Schaeffer A, Schaeffer E. Infections of the urinary tract. In: Wein A, ed. Campbell-Walsh Urology. 9th ed. Philadelphia: Saunders Elsevier; 2007.

CASE 26

Clinical Presentation

A 50-year-old female presents with chronic urinary tract infections (UTIs) and a nonfunctioning kidney on an intravenous pyelogram (IVP) (not shown).

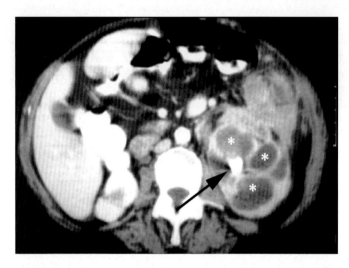

Fig. 26.1 Enhanced computed tomography scan at the level of the middle left kidney.

Radiologic Findings

- Enlarged left kidney
- Large left renal pelvis stone (*arrow*, **Fig. 26.1**)
- Multiple hypodense areas (*asterisks*, **Fig. 26.1**) in the left renal parenchyma with a "bear paw" appearance on contrast-enhanced computed tomography.

Diagnosis

Xanthogranulomatous pyelonephritis

Differential Diagnosis

- Pyonephrosis
- Cystic renal cell carcinoma
- Lymphoma

Discussion

Background

Xanthogranulomatous pyelonephritis is a form of chronic pyelonephritis. It is a rare inflammatory disorder associated with renal calculi (80%), often staghorn type, in the setting of chronic obstruction and infection. A history of chronic infection is important in the diagnosis.

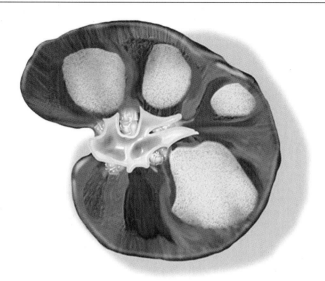

Fig. 26.2 Drawing of xanthogranulomatous pyelone-phritis showing the "bear paw" sign.

Clinical Findings

Patients often present with flank pain, fever, and chills, and about half show signs of UTI on urinalysis. Diabetics are at increased risk, as are women and patients in the 5th to 7th decade.

Pathology

Chronic inflammation and obstruction result in the replacement of renal cortical tissue by lipid-laden macrophages (xanthoma cells), leading to nonfunctional kidney. Infection may spread beyond the Gerota fascia. Diffuse and focal forms are seen. It is nearly always unilateral (**Fig. 26.2**).

Imaging Findings

COMPUTED TOMOGRAPHY

- Pyonephrosis may present with a very similar appearance and can be indistinguishable from xanthogranulomatous pyelonephritis. The classic "bear paw" sign in this case helps with the diagnosis.
- The presence of the central stone and the history make a cystic renal tumor unlikely. There is usually no function with xanthogranulomatous pyelonephritis (i.e., no enhancement), also making tumor unlikely.
- Lymphoma can produce multifocal hypodense lesions, but the stone, history, and lack of visible adenopathy make this diagnosis unlikely.
- The classic appearance includes poor renal function, nephromegaly, and renal calculi.
- Hypodense areas are arranged within the kidney as in hydronephrosis. These low density areas mimic the appearance of the pads on a bear's paw.

RADIOGRAPHY/INTRAVENOUS PYELOGRAM

- A large nonfunctioning kidney with central stone(s)

ULTRASOUND

- Enlarged kidney with central echogenic focus, representing stones, is seen, but this is nonspecific.

Treatment

- Long-term antibiotic therapy may be attempted. Alternatively, renal resection is indicated in septic patients.

Prognosis

- Good following resection

Suggested Readings

Kenny P. Chronic inflammation. In: Pollack H, McClennan B, eds. Clinical Urography. Vol 1. 2nd ed. Philadelphia: WB Saunders; 2000:947–975.

Kim JC. US and CT findings of xanthogranulomatous pyelonephritis. Clin Imaging 2001;25(2):118–121.

Pickhardt PJ, Lonergan GJ, Davis CJ Jr, Kashitani N, Wagner BJ. From the archives of the AFIP: infiltrative renal lesions: radiologic-pathologic correlation. Armed Forces Institute of Pathology. Radiographics 2000;20(1):215–243.

Schaeffer A, Schaeffer E. Infections of the urinary tract. In: Wein A, ed. Campbell-Walsh Urology. 9th ed. Philadelphia: Saunders Elsevier; 2007:223–302.

CASE 27

Clinical Presentation

A 54-year-old presents with pyuria, fever, and negative cytology and negative plain film.

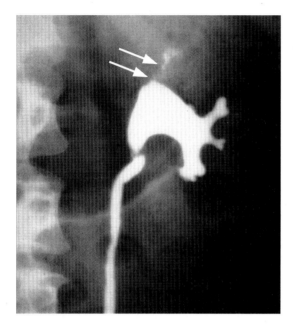

Fig. 27.1 Left retrograde pyelogram.

Radiologic Findings

- Amputated left upper pole calyx (*arrows,* **Fig. 27.1**)

Diagnosis

Tuberculosis (TB)

Differential Diagnosis

- Transitional cell carcinoma (TCC)
- Infundibular stone
- Infundibular clot

Discussion

Background

Renal TB infection occurs at the time of pulmonary infection. The organism will be controlled until the host's immune system becomes inadequate, at which point reactivation occurs in the renal parenchyma. Renal TB accounts for slightly over 1% of TB cases, so it is rare.

Clinical Findings

There may be long-standing urinary symptoms (e.g., frequent painless urination), but no cause isolated. Sterile pyuria is common. Hematuria is seen in 50% of cases.

Pathology

Caseating necrosis from tuberculous infection with granuloma formation occurs in the renal parenchyma and results in fibrosis and calcification with healing. Collecting system extension of the above process causes the classic multifocal urothelial stricturing seen with TB.

Imaging Findings

RADIOGRAPHY

- Transitional cell carcinoma can have an identical appearance on retrograde pyelogram or intravenous pyelogram, with irregularity and amputation of the calyx. Clinical features and urine findings are critical to the diagnosis. Ureteroscopy/biopsy may be required for definitive diagnosis.
- Stone and edema could appear similar, but negative scout film makes a stone unlikely, as in this case.
- The infundibular appearance in this case is more irregular than is typical for a clot.

Treatment

- As in any TB infection, multidrug antituberculous antibiotics are administered to decrease the time needed for treatment and decrease the possibility of drug-resistant organisms developing.
- Therapy may last from 6 to 9 months.
- Focal abscesses may require image-guided drainage.
- Nephrectomy may be required in cases unresponsive to standard medical therapy.

Prognosis

- Most compliant patients respond well to therapy, as above, with negative urine cultures 2 weeks after initiating treatment.
- Multidrug-resistant TB has become a problem in the last decade, requiring individualized treatment plans based on consultation with infectious disease specialists.

PEARLS

- This radiographic appearance (**Fig. 27.1**) necessitates work-up to rule out both TB and TCC.

Suggested Readings

Gibson MS, Puckett ML, Shelly ME. Renal tuberculosis. Radiographics 2004;24(1):251–256.

Kawashima A, LeRoy AJ. Radiologic evaluation of patients with renal infections. Infect Dis Clin North Am 2003;17(2):433–456.

McAleer S, Johnson C, Johnson W. Tuberculosis and parasitic and fungal infections of the genitourinary system. In: Wein A, ed. Campbell-Walsh Urology. 9th ed. Philadelphia: Saunders Elsevier; 2007:436–477.

CASE 28

Clinical Presentation

A 60-year-old diabetic female

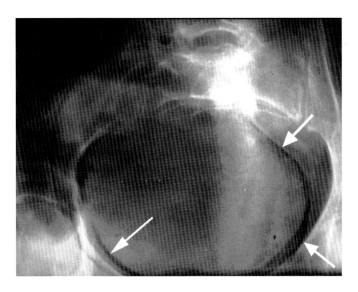

Fig. 28.1 Conventional radiograph coned to the pelvis. Source: Resnick, Older, Diagnosis of Genitourinary Disease, New York: Thieme, 1997: 43. Reprinted by permission.

Radiologic Findings

- Gas in the bladder wall (*arrows,* **Fig. 28.1**), allowing clear visualization of the bladder on noncontrast radiograph

Diagnosis

Emphysematous cystitis

Differential Diagnosis

- Colovesicle fistula
- Bladder stone
- Recent instrumentation of bladder

Discussion

Background

Gas forming infection in the bladder is seen commonly in diabetics (50% of cases). Women are affected more than men. Frequent urinary tract infections (UTIs), bladder outlet obstruction, and neurogenic bladder are associated with this condition.

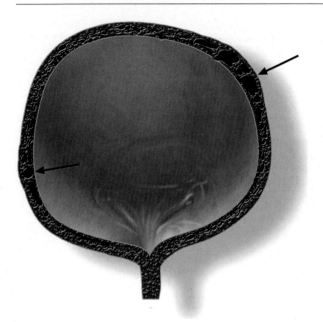

Fig. 28.2 Drawing of emphysematous cystitis demonstrating gas (*arrows*) in the bladder wall.

Clinical Findings

Common: dysuria, urinary frequency, and hematuria. Rare: pneumaturia, which represents gas in the urine stream, is a more specific finding.

Pathology

Emphysematous cystitis is a severe infection occurring in diabetic patients and is caused by *Escherichia coli* (and, rarely, other organisms). Gas in the bladder wall is produced when tissue glucose is fermented by the infecting organism (**Fig. 28.2**).

Imaging Findings

RADIOGRAPHY

- Colovesicle fistula will produce bladder gas, but it will be in the bladder lumen and not the wall, as in this case.
- Bladder stone would be dense, not lucent, as in this case.
- Recent bladder instrumentation will produce gas in the bladder lumen but not the bladder wall.
- Emphysematous cystitis begins with gas in the bladder wall, which can also extend into the bladder lumen. It is the gas in the bladder wall that is the diagnostic feature of emphysematous cystitis. Clear visualization of the bladder wall is usually not seen on a noncontrast radiograph. The bladder wall visualization in this case is not due to high density within the bladder, such as with a stone, but rather was due to low-density gas outlining the bladder wall.

COMPUTED TOMOGRAPHY

- Findings may mimic an enterovesical fistula, where gas may be seen within the bladder lumen, but the fistula will not produce gas within the bladder wall. The presence of gas in both the bladder lumen and the bladder wall indicates primary production of gas within the wall, as occurs in emphysematous cystitis (**Fig. 28.3**).
- Recent instrumentation of the bladder will often lead to gas in the bladder lumen but not in the bladder wall.

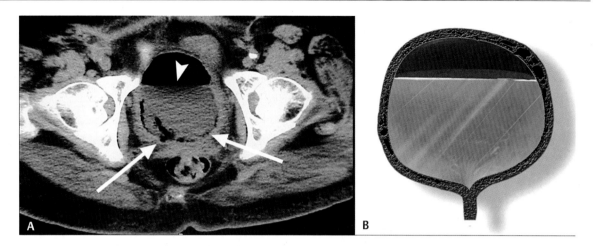

Fig. 28.3 **(A)** Computed tomography without intravenous contrast through the pelvis shows the gas urine level in the bladder (*arrowhead*) and gas in the nondependent portions of the bladder within the bladder wall (*arrows*). **(B)** Drawing of emphysematous cystitis with gas urine level and gas in the bladder wall.

Treatment

- Treat the bladder drainage problem (i.e., catheter drainage), in addition to broad-spectrum antibiotics, until the infecting organism is isolated, at which point antimicrobial coverage can be tailored.
- Maintain euglycemia.

Prognosis

- Most patients respond to appropriate antibiotic coverage.

Suggested Readings

Grayson DE, Abbott RM, Levy AD, Sherman PM. Emphysematous infections of the abdomen and pelvis: a pictorial review. Radiographics 2002;22(3):543–561.

CASE 29

Clinical Presentation

A 53-year-old male presents with recent onset of pneumaturia.

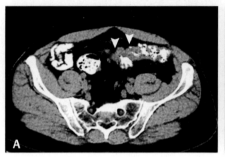 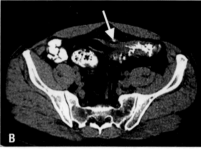 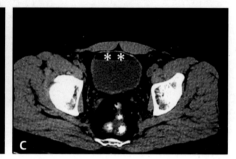

Fig. 29.1 Enhanced computed tomography scans at three levels: **(A)** just above the bladder, **(B)** at the bladder dome, and **(C)** mid-bladder.

Radiologic Findings

- Colonic diverticuli with surrounding inflammatory change immediately adjacent to the bladder wall (*arrowheads,* **Fig. 29.1A**)
- Probable fistulous tract between the inflamed colon and the bladder containing gas (*arrow,* **Fig. 29.1B**)
- Gas in the bladder lumen (*asterisks,* **Fig. 29.1C**)
- No gas in the bladder wall

Diagnosis

Colovesical fistula secondary to diverticulitis

Differential Diagnosis

- Emphysematous cystitis
- Recent instrumentation of the bladder
- Vesicoileal fistula secondary to regional enteritis

Discussion

Background

The most common causes for colovesical fistula are diverticulitis and colon cancer with fistulization to the bladder. Rarer causes include bladder cancer and pelvic radiation.

Clinical Findings

Pneumaturia is found in the majority of patients. A history of diverticulitis is common. Urinary tract infections, frequency, and dysuria occur in ~50% of cases.

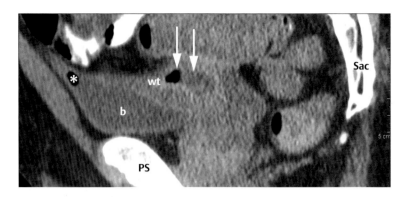

Fig. 29.2 Sagittal reconstructed computed tomography scan with intravenous and oral contrast shows the bladder (b) with gas in it (*asterisk*), bladder wall thickening (wt), and an adjacent diverticular abscess containing gas and fluid (*arrows*). PS, pubic symphysis; Sac, sacrum.

Pathology

Abnormal connection between the adjacent colon and the bladder is due to inflammatory adhesive process (e.g., serositis) and tissue breakdown between the two structures.

Imaging Findings

COMPUTED TOMOGRAPHY

- Emphysematous cystitis begins as gas in the bladder wall; there may be gas in the lumen as well. The absence of gas in the bladder wall excludes emphysematous cystitis.
- The patient's history gives no indication of prior instrumentation.
- The bladder is adherent to a loop of abnormal colon with evidence of diverticulitis; there is no evidence of small bowel abnormality to suggest regional enteritis.
- Computed tomography (CT) is the most accurate test compared with barium enema and cystography.
- With CT to evaluate for fistula, obtain a pelvic scan prior to contrast administration, then administer rectal or bladder contrast (but not both) and rescan. Contrast filling from one structure to the other confirms fistula. Obtain postvoid images as well, as the work of straining may force open the fistula, allowing contrast to pass through it and demonstrate the fistula to better effect (**Fig. 29.2**).

Treatment

- Surgical resection of the fistula and the diseased segment of the colon with fecal diversion and/or a multistaged procedure may be required. Repair the bladder wall.

Prognosis

- Following surgery, recurrence is unlikely, although complications may occur in up to 45% of patients.

PEARLS

- Whenever gas is present in the bladder, recent instrumentation or catheterization should be excluded, as these are common causes of bladder gas.

Suggested Readings

Grayson DE, Abbott RM, Levy AD, Sherman PM. Emphysematous infections of the abdomen and pelvis: a pictorial review. Radiographics 2002;22(3):543–561.

Najjar SF, Jamal MK, Savas JF, Miller TA. The spectrum of colovesical fistula and diagnostic paradigm. Am J Surg 2004;188(5):617–621.

CASE 30

Clinical Presentation

Incidental finding on intravenous urography (IVU) performed for urinary tract infection (UTI)

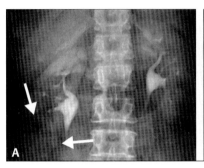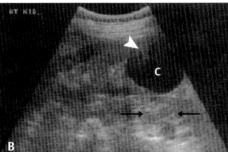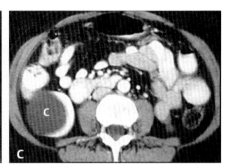

Fig. 30.1   **(A)** Intravenous urography, **(B)** ultrasound, and **(C)** computed tomography images of a right renal mass noted on intravenous pyelogram.

Radiologic Findings

- IVU shows a right lower pole mass effect with splaying of the right lower calyces (*arrows*, **Fig. 30.1A**).
- Ultrasound demonstrates an anechoic lesion (c, **Fig. 30.1B**) with features including
  - Round structure
  - Anechoic
  - Smooth, imperceptibly thin wall
  - Increased sound through-transmission posterior to the lesion (black arrows, **Fig. 30.1B**)
  - Reverberation artifact at near wall (*arrowhead*, **Fig. 30.1B**)
- Computed tomography (CT) shows a water density mass (c, **Fig. 30.1C**) with no perceptible wall and sharp demarcation with normal parenchyma.

Diagnosis

Simple renal cyst, Bosniak I

Differential Diagnosis

- Bosniak II cyst
- Bosniak IIF cyst
- Bosniak III cyst
- Bosniak IV cyst

Discussion

Background

Simple renal cysts are common in patients > 30 years of age. Sporadic cysts can be seen in patients < 30 years of age. Multiple bilateral renal cysts in patients < 30 years old should raise suspicion of renal cystic disease [e.g., autosomal dominant polycystic kidney disease (ADPCKD)]. Finding cysts in other parenchymal organs in addition to the kidneys would be confirmatory of ADPCKD.

Clinical Findings

Most simple cysts are asymptomatic, although cysts can become infected or hemorrhage, in which case they may become symptomatic.

Pathology

Simple renal cysts are lined by tubular epithelium and are believed to arise from collected ducts which have become obstructed and no longer function. Contents are an ultrafiltrate of plasma. There is no malignant potential in absence of acquired cystic disease of dialysis (**Fig. 30.2**).

Imaging Findings

RADIOGRAPHY

- IVU detects the majority of renal lesions > 3 cm, but determining enhancement to distinguish between cyst and malignancy is not clear-cut and almost always requires additional studies (e.g., ultrasound or CT) to clarify the finding on IVU.

COMPUTED TOMOGRAPHY

- Bosniak II cysts contain thin septa, have thin "eggshell" calcifications, or are high density (i.e., higher in density than adjacent unenhanced renal parenchyma).
- Bosniak IIF cysts contain minimally thick septa, have calcifications (other than thin), or are high density, totally intrarenal, and measure > 3 cm.

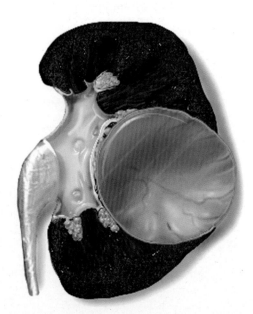

Fig. 30.2   Simple renal cyst.

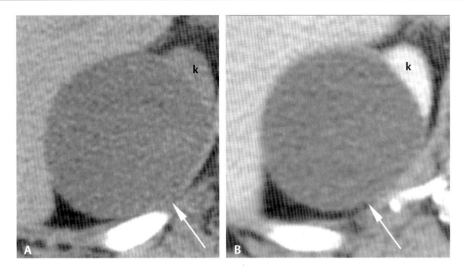

Fig. 30.3 Right upper pole of a simple renal cyst. **(A)** Noncontrast computed tomography (CT) and **(B)** contrast-enhanced CT. The cyst (*arrow*) measured < 20 HU on precontrast CT with no change on postcontrast CT, consistent with a simple cyst (Bosniak I). k, kidney parenchyma.

- Bosniak III cysts contain thick septa and may be multilocular. Enhancement may be detectable in portions of the septa or wall.
- Bosniak IV cysts contain obvious solid tissue and/or enhancement within the solid portions.
- A simple cyst will be a fluid-density [< 20 Hounsfield units (HU)], well-defined lesion arising from the renal cortex with no discernible or measurable enhancement. This is true for routine contrast-enhanced scans (**Fig. 30.1C**) and when noncontrasted and contrast-enhanced scans are obtained for the same exam (**Fig. 30.3**).

ULTRASOUND

- Cysts other than simple cysts will show complicating features, such as internal echoes, septa, calcification, thick walls, or solid tissue and thus do not meet all of the necessary criteria for the diagnosis of simple cyst as listed above (**Fig. 30.1B**). Complex cysts require CT or MRI without and with intravenous contrast for definitive characterization.

MAGNETIC RESONANCE IMAGING

- Simple renal cysts are well-defined round or oval lesions arising from the renal cortex. They follow the signal of simple fluid (e.g., cerebrospinal fluid) on all sequences:
  - High signal on T2-weighted image (**Fig. 30.4A**)
  - Low signal on T1-weighted image (**Fig. 30.4B**)
  - Do not enhance following contrast administration (**Fig. 30.4C**).
- Magnetic resonance imaging performs equally well as CT in characterizing renal cysts and has advantages over CT in patients with iodinated contrast allergy and in very young patients, as well as in females of child-bearing age for whom exposure to ionizing radiation should be minimized.

Treatment

- Simple renal cysts require no specific treatment.

Prognosis

- Excellent

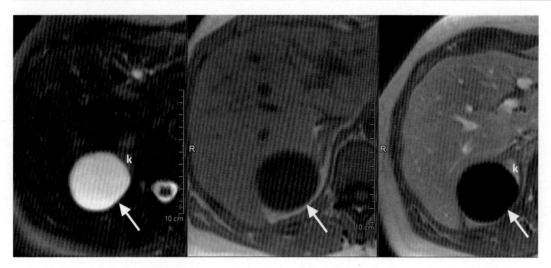

Fig. 30.4 Same patient as in **Fig. 30.3.** Axial magnetic resonance image of the right upper pole shows a simple renal cyst (*arrow*). **(A)** T2-weighted image with fat saturation, **(B)** T1-weighted gradient echo (GRE) without contrast, and **(C)** T1-weighted GRE with contrast. The lesion follows the signal of simple fluid on all sequences and shows no enhancement between **B** and **C**, confirming this is a simple cyst (Bosniak I). k, kidney parenchyma.

PEARLS _____

- When measuring enhancement in a renal lesion that has no visually detectable enhancing elements, the region of interest (ROI) size should be placed within the center of the lesion, including at least 50 to 75% of the lesion's area. Choose your slice halfway between the upper and lower limits of the mass to avoid volume-averaging effects.
- Measure the ROI of the most suspicious portion(s) of the cystic lesion.

Suggested Readings

Bosniak MA. The current radiological approach to renal cysts. Radiology 1986;158(1):1–10.

Bosniak MA. Problems in the radiologic diagnosis of renal parenchymal tumors. Urol Clin North Am 1993;20(2):217–230.

Ho VB, Allen SF, Hood MN, Choyke PL. Renal masses: quantitative assessment of enhancement with dynamic MR imaging. Radiology 2002;224(3):695–700.

Israel GM, Bosniak MA. MR imaging of cystic renal masses. Magn Reson Imaging Clin N Am 2004;12(3):403–412.

Israel GM, Bosniak MA. An update of the Bosniak renal cyst classification system. Urology 2005;66(3):484–488.

Israel GM, Hindman N, Bosniak MA. Evaluation of cystic renal masses: comparison of CT and MR imaging by using the Bosniak classification system. Radiology 2004;231(2):365–371.

CASE 31

Clinical Presentation

Mass on ultrasound

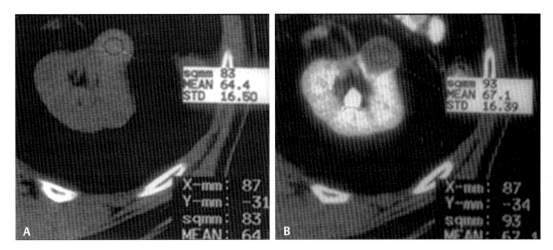

Fig. 31.1 High-density lesion in the left kidney. **(A)** Unenhanced computed tomography (CT) scan shows a high-density lesion (circular region of interest) measuring < 3 cm and 64 Hounsfield units (HU). **(B)** Postcontrast CT shows the lesion with attenuation of 67 HU (circular region of interest).

Radiologic Findings

- High-density renal lesion measuring < 3 cm and predominantly extrarenal with no wall thickening or calcification present (**Fig. 31.1A**)
- No enhancement in the lesion on contrast-enhanced scan (**Fig. 31.1B**)

Diagnosis

High-density renal cyst, Bosniak II

Differential Diagnosis

- Bosniak I
- Bosniak IIF
- Bosniak III
- Bosniak IV

Discussion

Background

Several factors may result in renal cysts having higher density than simple fluid. Infection, hemorrhage, or proteinaceous contents would increase the density of an otherwise simple cyst.

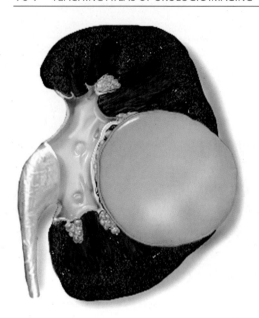

Fig. 31.2 Complex cyst with proteinaceous material.

Clinical Findings

Renal cyst infection may present with flank pain, hematuria, or urinary tract infection. Renal cyst hemorrhage may result in flank pain or a size change in a preexisting renal cyst. Either of these entities may result in a high-density renal cyst even if the patient is asymptomatic.

Pathology

Simple cysts, infected cysts, hemorrhagic cysts, and cysts containing proteinaceous debris are found. No significant risk of malignancy is found in this category (**Fig. 31.2**).

Imaging Findings

RADIOGRAPHY

- Mass effect on intravenous urography (IVU) may be seen if the lesion is large enough. Further work-up is indicated with computed tomography (CT) or ultrasound.

COMPUTED TOMOGRAPHY

- Bosniak I cysts should be < 20 Hounsfield units (HU), less than is seen in this case.
- Bosniak IIF cysts include high-density intrarenal cysts that are > 3 cm. This lesion does not meet size criteria.
- Bosniak III cysts would contain thick septa or a thickened wall, not present in this case.
- Bosniak IV cysts would show solid elements inside the cyst that enhance, also not present in this case.
- Bosniak II cysts also include wholly intrarenal high-density cysts < 3 cm, as in **Fig. 31.3**. No enhancement should be detected on a dedicated renal neoplasm protocol CT performed without and with intravenous (IV) contrast.

Pseudoenhancement

Pseudoenhancement is an important artifact that occurs in renal cysts following IV contrast. It occurs because on nephrogram phase images, high-density contrast in the renal parenchyma surrounding the lesion in question results in a beam-hardening artifact, which the CT reconstruction algorithm

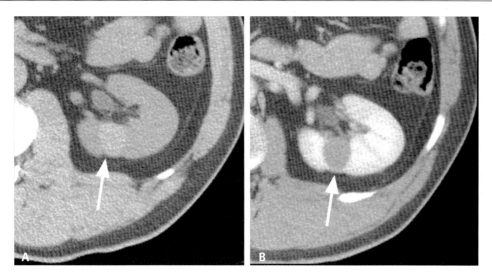

Fig. 31.3 High-density lesion in the left kidney. **(A)** Unenhanced computed tomography (CT) scan shows a high-density wholly intrarenal lesion (*arrow*) measuring < 3 cm and 35 Hounsfield units (HU). **(B)** Postcontrast CT shows the lesion with some overlying cortical thinning (*arrow*) with attenuation of 37 HU, representing no significant enhancement, consistent with a Bosniak II cyst.

cannot correct. This results in a measurable but artifactual increase in cyst attenuation between the unenhanced and enhanced scans. The artifact is encountered with conventional spiral CT scans and is accentuated on multirow detector CT scans. Volume averaging of a cystic lesion with adjacent renal parenchyma can also produce artifact, limiting the accuracy of CT measurements for intrarenal lesions < 1.0 to 1.5 cm. Enhancement > 20 HU is considered true, and borderline enhancement is in the range of 16 to 20 HU.

ULTRASOUND

- High-density lesions may be further evaluated with ultrasound, but ultrasound is often inconclusive because of the internal echoes found within a high-density cyst produced by the proteinaceous or hemorrhagic material.
- Ultrasound may be the initial study, as in this case, with a mildly thickened septum below (**Fig. 31.4**). CT or magnetic resonance imaging (MRI) without and with IV contrast would be required to determine if there is enhancement in the septation, as in **Fig. 31.5**.

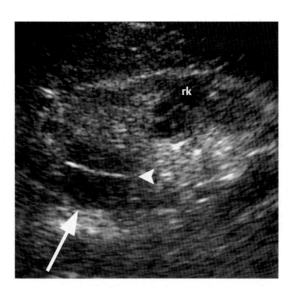

Fig. 31.4 Septated cyst. A single long-axis sonogram of the right kidney (rk) shows a right upper pole cyst (*arrow*) with a prominent septation (*arrowhead*).

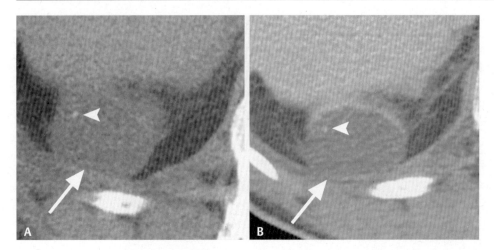

Fig. 31.5 To assess septation found on ultrasound; same patient as in **Fig. 31.4. (A)** Unenhanced and **(B)** contrast-enhanced computed tomography (CT) shows the right upper pole cyst (*arrow*). The septation does not enhance, but there are tiny flecks of calcification within the septation (*arrowhead*). This is consistent with a complex (Bosniak II) renal cyst. It is not unusual for septa to be better seen with ultrasound than with CT.

MAGNETIC RESONANCE IMAGING

- MRI may show more septa than are seen on other imaging modalities, making categorization somewhat problematic. A few nonenhancing hairline-thin septa may be considered Bosniak II (**Fig. 31.6**), but many more than that may elevate the lesion to at least Bosniak IIF (for follow-up).
- Calcifications are not well detected with MRI (**Fig. 31.6**), but calcification is the least predictive factor in determining renal malignancy. So, although MRI may not detect calcification in a renal cyst, it is capable of detecting enhancement without artifact from the calcification as may be encountered with CT.

Treatment

- Bosniak II renal cysts may require treatment depending on the symptoms (e.g., infection), but generally they do not require further evaluation. Bosniak IIF cysts require follow-up imaging to confirm stability or to evaluate for changes.

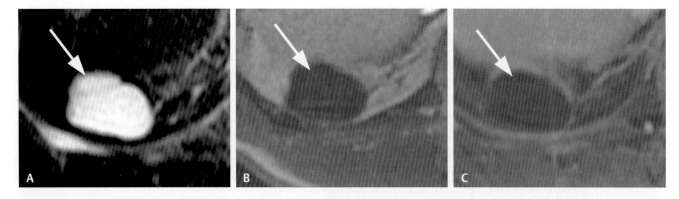

Fig. 31.6 Renal cyst septation; same patient as in **Fig. 31.4** and **Fig. 31.5.** Axial fat saturation magnetic resonance imaging using **(A)** T2-weighted image, **(B)** T1-weighted gradient echo (GRE) image, and **(C)** T1-weighted GRE image postgadolinium showing a renal cyst following signal characteristics of simple fluid on all sequences. Note that the T2-weighted image shows a thin septation (*arrow*) that is not apparent on the T1-weighted image without or with gadolinium. Arrows in **(B)** and **(C)** depict where septation should be but is not seen.

Prognosis

- Excellent

- Dedicated renal imaging with meticulous technique is required when there is a known renal lesion that must be classified as benign versus suspicious. The primary determinant of malignancy in both solid and cystic renal lesions is the detection of enhancement on postcontrast images.
- It may be difficult to obtain reproducible density measurements on CT for intrarenal lesions up to 1.5 cm in size. Such small lesions may be too small to accurately characterize. If definitive diagnosis is clinically important, ultrasound, MRI, or close follow-up may provide additional information.

Suggested Readings

Aronson S, Frazier HA, Baluch JD, Hartman DS, Christenson PJ. Cystic renal masses: usefulness of the Bosniak classification. Urol Radiol 1991;13(2):83–90.

Birnbaum BA, Maki DD, Chakraborty DP, Jacobs JE, Babb JS. Renal cyst pseudoenhancement: evaluation with an anthropomorphic body CT phantom. Radiology 2002;225(1):83–90.

Bosniak MA. Diagnosis and management of patients with complicated cystic lesions of the kidney. AJR Am J Roentgenol 1997;169(3):819–821.

Israel GM, Bosniak MA. Calcification in cystic renal masses: is it important in diagnosis? Radiology 2003;226(1):47–52.

CASE 32

Clinical Presentation

Abdominal pain

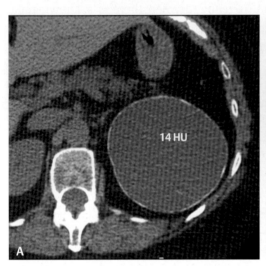 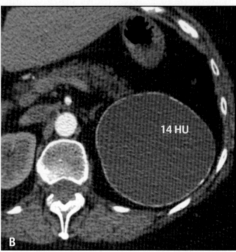

Fig. 32.1 Abdominal pain. Computed tomography **(A)** without and **(B)** with intravenous contrast shows a cystic mass originating from the left upper renal pole. The density of the mass did not change following contrast.

Radiologic Findings

- Renal mass with thick, irregular wall calcification (**Figs. 32.1** and **32.2**)
- No enhancement; 14 Hounsfield units (HU) precontrast and 14 HU postcontrast

Diagnosis

Bosniak IIF calcified cyst, which showed no change over a 4-year follow-up

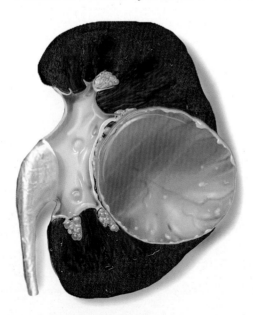

Fig. 32.2 Drawing of a Bosniak IIF calcified cyst.

Differential Diagnosis

- Renal cell carcinoma
- Bosniak I cyst
- Bosniak II cyst
- Bosniak III cyst
- Bosniak IV cyst

Discussion

Background

The Bosniak IIF category for renal cystic lesions was created for lesions that did not easily fit into category II or III. This is the important demarcation between nonsurgical and surgical lesions. The majority of these lesions are benign, but because of their complexity, they require follow-up imaging to ensure stability. This group of lesions has one or more worrisome features (see imaging findings under CT below).

Clinical Findings

Often incidentally discovered lesions

Pathology

Ninety-five percent of Bosniak IIF lesions are benign.

Imaging Findings
COMPUTED TOMOGRAPHY

- Renal cell carcinoma will enhance, and there is no evidence of enhancement in this case. Enhancement is a much more important prognostic feature than the amount of calcification.
- A Bosniak I cyst is a simple cyst with no internal architecture and no calcification.
- A Bosniak II cyst may contain calcification, but it is "eggshell" thin calcification and not as thick as in this case.
- A Bosniak III cyst will show a thick wall or septa, possibly with measurable enhancement.
- A Bosniak IV lesion has enhancement within solid components separable from the walls or septa.
- A Bosniak IIF cystic lesion contains one or more of the following:
  - Increased number of nonenhancing septa
  - Thick calcifications
  - Wall or septa that may be minimally thickened
  - Perceivable but not measurable enhancement in portions of the wall or septa
  - Entirely intrarenal high-density renal cyst > 3 cm (**Fig. 32.3**)

ULTRASOUND

- Ultrasound may detect complex findings, such as thick calcifications, septa, or complex fluid (e.g., fluid debris levels); however, computed tomography (CT) or magnetic resonance imaging (MRI) without and with contrast is required to evaluate for malignant features (**Fig. 32.4**).

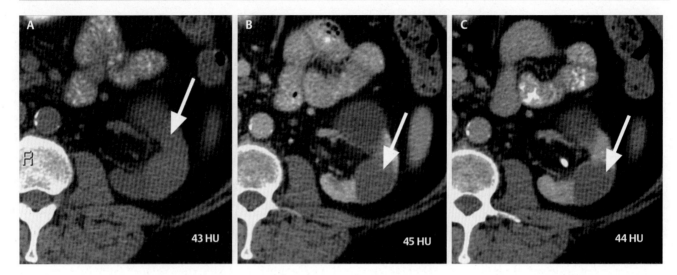

Fig. 32.3   Renal neoplasm protocol computed tomography scans. **(A)** Unenhanced, **(B)** enhanced, and **(C)** delayed images through the left midpole show a completely intrarenal lesion that measures > 3 cm. There is no significant enhancement within the lesion following contrast. This lesion represents a Bosniak IIF renal cyst.

MAGNETIC RESONANCE IMAGING

- Fluid content on both T1- and T2-weighted images will be variable:
  - Simple fluid (i.e., high signal on T2- and low signal on T1-weighted images)
  - Hemorrhagic fluid (i.e., dark signal on T2- and high signal on T1-weighted images)
- Septa are most conspicuous on T2-weighted images (**Fig. 32.5A,B**).
- Wall or septal thickening will be perceivable on both T2- and T1-weighted images.
- "Perceived" enhancement is determined between pre- and postgadolinium T1-weighted images with fat saturation (**Fig. 32.5C,D**). In equivocal cases, subtraction imaging can be helpful to detect enhancement.
- Calcification will not be detected on MRI, or it may result in magnetic susceptibility artifact ("blooming" artifact).

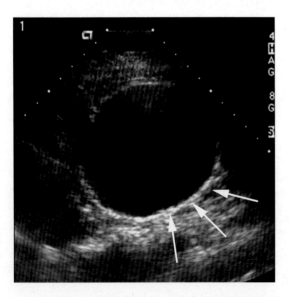

Fig. 32.4   Abdominal pain. Abdominal sonogram of the same patient as in **Fig. 32.1**. The thick echogenic wall structure (*arrows*) corresponds to the thickened, irregular calcified wall seen in **Fig. 32.1**.

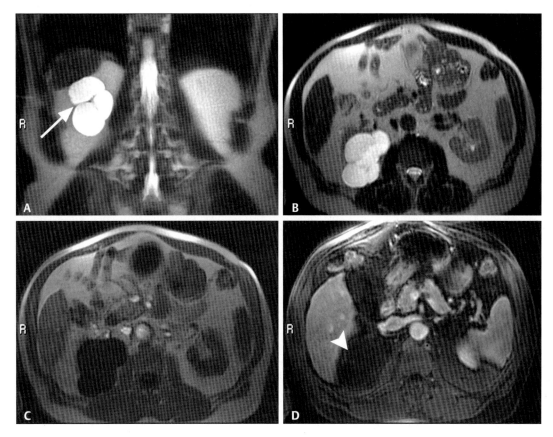

Fig. 32.5   Renal neoplasm protocol magnetic resonance images to evaluate a right upper cystic renal mass. T2-weighted images in **(A)** coronal and **(B)** axial orientations. T1-weighted images in **(C)** axial and **(D)** axial postgadolinium with fat saturation. Images show a multiseptate cystic mass in the right upper pole (*arrow*, **Fig. 32.5A**) with slightly perceivable enhancement in one of the septa (*arrowhead*, **Fig. 32.5D**).

Treatment

- Follow-up imaging is recommended at 6 months after the initial study. If the lesion remains stable, follow-up exams at yearly intervals for at least 5 years are recommended. Optimal follow-up duration has not yet been determined.
- On follow-up studies, if the lesion progresses (e.g., develops more worrisome findings such as measurable enhancement within septa, interval development of solid enhancing elements), the lesion will be upgraded to a Bosniak III or higher category with its associated surgical recommendation. Lesions that become less worrisome (e.g., high-density complex fluid that becomes simple fluid due to resolution of hemorrhage) would be downgraded to Bosniak II or lower with its attendant good prognosis. This type of watchful waiting has been applied successfully to follow lesions that do not fall easily into a benign or malignant category. This strategy can also be followed when a lesion is worrisome (e.g., a Bosniak III cyst), but the patient is initially a poor surgical candidate. On follow-up exams, if the lesion becomes more worrisome and the patient's surgical status has improved, surgery may be entertained. Percutaneous biopsy for diagnosis and initiation of medical oncologic therapy is an alternative. If, however, the lesion remains stable, continued follow-up is appropriate.

Prognosis

- Excellent if follow-up regimen is followed. Bosniak found ~5% of IIF lesions ultimately represent malignant lesions that declare themselves on follow-up imaging.

Suggested Readings

Israel GM, Bosniak MA. Calcification in cystic renal masses: is it important in diagnosis? Radiology 2003;226(1):47–52.

Israel GM, Bosniak MA. Follow-up CT of moderately complex cystic lesions of the kidney (Bosniak category IIF). AJR Am J Roentgenol 2003;181(3):627–633.

Israel GM, Bosniak MA. An update of the Bosniak renal cyst classification system. Urology 2005;66(3):484–488.

Israel GM, Hindman N, Bosniak MA. Evaluation of cystic renal masses: comparison of CT and MR imaging by using the Bosniak classification system. Radiology 2004;231(2):365–371.

CASE 33

Clinical Presentation

Hematuria (**Figs. 33.1, 33.2**)

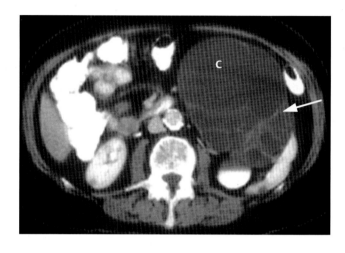

Fig. 33.1 Contrast-enhanced computed tomography scan shows a complex left renal cystic mass (C) with multiple septa (*arrow*).

Radiologic Findings

- Multiseptated left renal cystic mass containing both thin and thick septa with enhancement (**Fig. 33.1**), with no nodular or enhancing soft tissue identified

Diagnosis

Bosniak III indeterminate renal cystic lesion, which proved to be a benign multilocular cyst at surgery

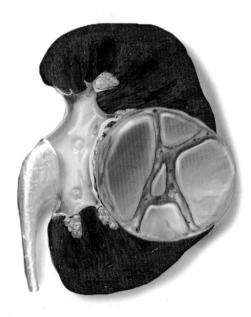

Fig. 33.2 Drawing of the multiseptated cystic mass seen in **Fig. 33.1**.

Differential Diagnosis

- Bosniak I
- Bosniak II
- Bosniak IIF
- Bosniak IV

Discussion

Background

The Bosniak III category represents a variety of cystic renal tumors with a spectrum of pathology from benign to malignant. Entities in adults include multilocular cystic nephroma, multilocular cystic renal cell carcinoma, and localized cystic disease of the kidney. Unfortunately, these lesions cannot be definitively separated based on current imaging or clinical grounds and therefore require surgical resection. Fortunately, most lesions are indolent; thus, nephron-sparing surgery may be undertaken to remove these lesions.

Clinical Findings

Many lesions are discovered incidentally during imaging studies for other reasons. However, hematuria or other urinary tract symptoms may bring the patient to imaging.

Pathology

About 50% of Bosniak III renal lesions represent cystic renal cell carcinoma, and another 50% are benign entities. Benign lesions include infected or hemorrhagic cysts, renal abscesses, and benign multilocular lesions, such as multilocular cystic nephroma.

Imaging Findings

RADIOGRAPHY

- Mass effect on intravenous urography if the lesion is large enough to be visualized but not specific.

COMPUTED TOMOGRAPHY

- Bosniak I lesion should have no complex features (calcification, septation, or enhancement).
- Bosniak II lesion should have no enhancement.
- Bosniak IIF lesion may have septa, but not as thick as in this case and without measurable enhancement.
- Bosniak IV lesion should show solid components with enhancement.
- Bosniak III cystic lesions show enhancement within portions of septa or portions of a thickened wall but no solid nodular enhancing components (**Figs. 33.1** and **33.3**).

ULTRASOUND

- Ultrasound is a common modality for renal imaging; thus, many cystic renal lesions first come to light via ultrasound.
- Simple renal cysts are definitively diagnosed if all sonographic criteria for a simple cyst are met (see Case 30).
- However, characterizing complex renal cystic lesions requires renal neoplasm protocol computed tomography (CT) or magnetic resonance imaging (MRI) without and with contrast to assess for enhancing components (**Fig. 33.4**).

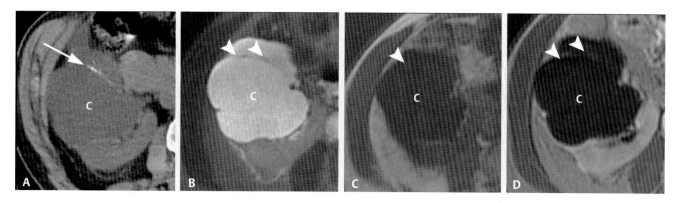

Fig. 33.3 Renal computed tomography (CT) and magnetic resonance imaging (MRI) for the characterization of a complex renal lesion. **(A)** Unenhanced CT scan shows a cyst (c) with a calcified septation (*arrow*). Axial MRI including **(B)** T2-weighted image with fat saturation, **(C)** T1-weighted gradient echo (GRE) image, and **(D)** T1-weighted GRE image postgadolinium show septa (*arrowheads*) with subtle enhancement, consistent with an indeterminate renal cystic lesion (Bosniak III).

MAGNETIC RESONANCE IMAGING

• As on CT, Bosniak III cystic lesions will show enhancement within septa or within portions of a thickened wall but will show no solid nodular components (**Fig. 33.5**).

Treatment

• These lesions should be removed if the patient can tolerate surgery. In patients who cannot tolerate surgery, these lesions can be followed; if there is a significant change in the lesion, treatment options (e.g., chemotherapy, nephron-sparing surgery, or nephrectomy) can be reassessed.

Prognosis

• Most multiseptated malignant lesions (no solid nodular components) have an excellent prognosis.

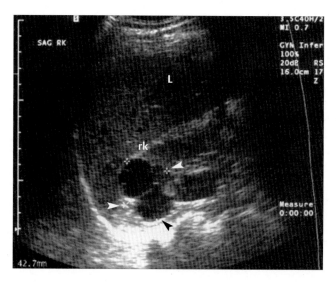

Fig. 33.4 Right upper quadrant (RUQ) pain. RUQ sonogram shows an incidentally detected complex cystic mass projecting from the upper pole of the right kidney (rk). Multiple septa (*arrowheads*) are demonstrated. These complex findings require further evaluation with contrast enhanced computed tomography or magnetic resonance imaging. L, liver (as acoustic window).

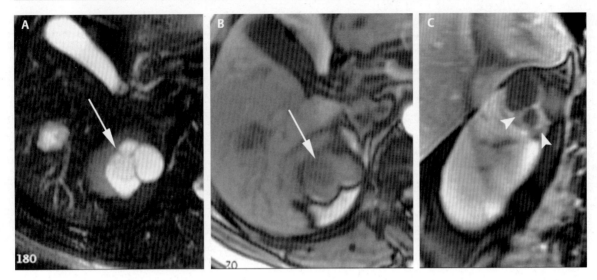

Fig. 33.5   Same patient as in **Fig. 33.4**. Axial magnetic resonance imaging with **(A)** T2-weighted image with fat saturation, **(B)** T1-weighted gradient echo (GRE) image, and **(C)** T1-weighted GRE image postgadolinium show a cystic mass (*arrow*) with septa. Cyst locules of different signal intensities noted on **B** and enhancement within the septa (*arrowheads,* **C**) are consistent with a Bosniak III indeterminate renal cyst, which proved to be cystic renal cell carcinoma at surgery.

PEARLS

- Although the Bosniak classification is a useful one, not all observers agree on how to classify a specific lesion. Differences in classification of cystic lesions can be related to technical performance of the CT scan. The ability to detect enhancement is related to contrast bolus, good nephrographic phase images, thin sections through the lesion, and accurate density measurements.
- It is very difficult to separate benign from malignant multilocular lesions on imaging criteria; therefore, if there is no contraindication to surgery, they should be removed.

Suggested Readings

Bielsa O, Lloreta J, Gelabert-Mas A. Cystic renal cell carcinoma: pathological features, survival and implications for treatment. Br J Urol 1998;82(1):16–20.

Israel GM, Bosniak MA. An update of the Bosniak renal cyst classification system. Urology 2005;66(3):484–488.

Israel GM, Hindman N, Bosniak MA. Evaluation of cystic renal masses: comparison of CT and MR imaging by using the Bosniak classification system. Radiology 2004;231(2):365–371.

CASE 34

Clinical Presentation

Hematuria

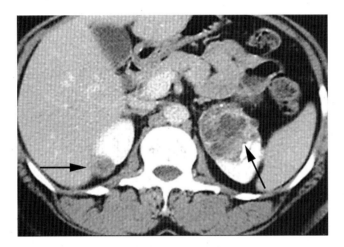

Fig. 34.1 Contrast-enhanced computed tomography scan shows bilateral upper pole complex masses (*arrows*).

Radiologic Findings

- Left cystic mass with thick enhancing septa and solid tissue (Bosniak IV)
- Solid enhancing mass on the right upper kidney representing renal cell carcinoma (RCC)

Diagnosis

Bilateral renal cell carcinoma with Bosniak IV left cystic RCC

Differential Diagnosis

- Left Bosniak III multilocular cyst and right RCC
- Left Bosniak III multilocular cyst and right angiomyolipoma
- Left Bosniak II cyst and right RCC

Discussion

Background

Approximately 15% of RCC cases have some cystic component, often due to hemorrhage or necrosis. Purely cystic renal cell carcinoma (CRCC) (without hemorrhage or necrosis) represents 4 to 10% of RCC. CRCC cannot be reliably distinguished on imaging from RCC with necrosis/hemorrhage, but it does confer a better prognosis. Both types of lesions are malignant and require surgical removal.

Clinical Findings

Hematuria is a common presenting symptom. Incidentally discovered lesions are quite common due to recent increased use of cross-sectional imaging.

Pathology

CRCC is a well-circumscribed lesion containing gelatinous fluid and walls lined by epithelium, where the neoplastic cells are found.

Imaging Findings

COMPUTED TOMOGRAPHY

- Bosniak III lesions can have thick septations, but this lesion goes well beyond what can be accepted for a class III lesion. The thick septa are enhancing, and there is an obvious enhancing solid tissue, consistent with RCC (**Fig. 34.1**).
- Bosniak II lesions have thin septa, which is not a consideration in this case.
- The right upper pole lesion is solid and enhancing and is a typical small RCC. There is no fat present in the lesion to suggest angiomyolipoma (**Fig. 34.1**).
- Bosniak IV lesions will show enhancing solid nodular tissue, sometimes (but not always) with enhancing septa, and enhancing thick walls. On computed tomography (CT) scans performed without and with intravenous contrast, the enhancing elements should show significant change on region of interest (ROI) measurements (**Figs. 34.2, 34.3**).

ULTRASOUND

- Ultrasound may detect complex cystic lesions during routine exam or may be employed when a lesion is detected on another cross-sectional imaging study. However, if the lesion is not a simple cyst, as in **Fig. 34.4**, cross-sectional imaging without and with contrast is required to evaluate for enhancement within any solid components of the mass.

MAGNETIC RESONANCE IMAGING

- Magnetic resonance imaging (MRI) is equal to CT in characterizing renal masses > 1 cm.
- Cystic components of a mass will usually show high signal on T2-weighted images but can be more variable in signal on T1-weighted images.
- Enhancing elements within a cystic or solid renal mass confirm a surgical lesion (**Fig. 34.5**).

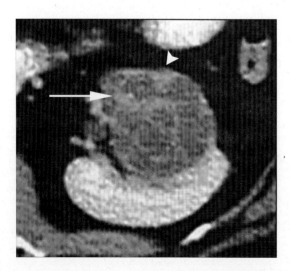

Fig. 34.2   Enhanced computed tomography scan with a multilocular lesion containing enhancing septa (*arrow*) and nodular enhancing soft tissue (*arrowhead*) makes this a Bosniak IV lesion, which was renal cell carcinoma at surgery.

Fig. 34.3 Drawing of the cystic mass seen in **Fig. 34.2.**

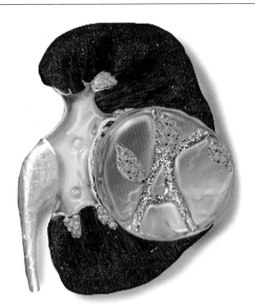

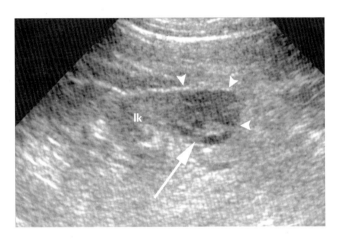

Fig. 34.4 Transverse view of the lower pole of the left kidney (lk) shows a cystic mass (*arrowheads*) with a solid nodule (*arrow*), worrisome for Bosniak IV cyst. Computed tomography (CT) or magnetic resonance imaging would be required to characterize the nodule as enhancing, confirming neoplastic tissue. This lesion did enhance on subsequent renal neoplasm protocol CT and proved to be a cystic renal cell carcinoma at surgery.

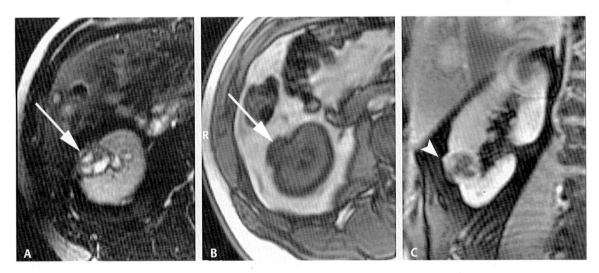

Fig. 34.5 Renal neoplasm protocol magnetic resonance imaging. Axial **(A)** T2-weighted image with fat saturation, **(B)** T1-weighted image, and **(C)** coronal T1-weighted image after gadolinium with fat saturation. On **A** and **B,** the cystic locules follow the signal of simple fluid (*arrow*). On **C,** nodular portions of the cystic mass (*arrowhead*) enhance, consistent with a Bosniak IV renal cyst.

Treatment

- Treatment is primarily surgical resection of the cystic tumor similar to solid renal neoplasms. Unroofing of the neoplasm is not performed, as may be done in some benign cysts, for fear of tumor seeding.

Prognosis

- True cystic RCC has an improved prognosis over solid RCC. The nuclear grade and pathologic stage are lower for cystic RCC. The 5-year survival is as high as 83%.
- Solid RCC with cystic degeneration has a similar prognosis as other solid renal neoplasms.

PEARLS _____

- A poorly enhancing solid renal neoplasm, such as papillary RCC, may simulate a renal cyst due to its low density and well-known poorly enhancing characteristic. Therefore, borderline enhancing lesions should be followed if not removed.

Suggested Readings

Bielsa O, Lloreta J, Gelabert-Mas A. Cystic renal cell carcinoma: pathological features, survival and implications for treatment. Br J Urol 1998;82(1):16–20.

Bosniak MA. Diagnosis and management of patients with complicated cystic lesions of the kidney. AJR Am J Roentgenol 1997;169(3):819–821.

Ho VB, Allen SF, Hood MN, Choyke PL. Renal masses: quantitative assessment of enhancement with dynamic MR imaging. Radiology 2002;224(3):695–700.

Israel GM, Bosniak MA. MR imaging of cystic renal masses. Magn Reson Imaging Clin N Am 2004;12(3):403–412.

Israel GM, Bosniak MA. An update of the Bosniak renal cyst classification system. Urology 2005;66(3):484–488.

Israel GM, Hindman N, Bosniak MA. Evaluation of cystic renal masses: comparison of CT and MR imaging by using the Bosniak classification system. Radiology 2004;231(2):365–371.

CASE 35

Clinical Presentation

A 45-year-old female presents with hypertension.

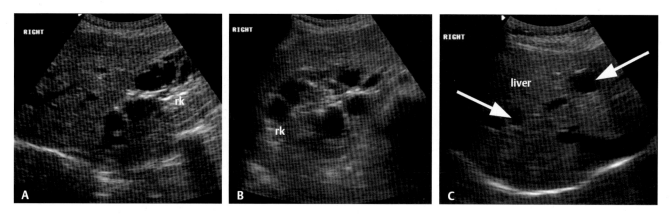

Fig. 35.1 Right upper quadrant ultrasound. Innumerable cysts are seen in the right kidney (rk) on **(A)** longitudinal and **(B)** transverse views, together with **(C)** liver cysts (*arrows*) in the liver.

Radiologic Findings

- Innumerable cysts in the right kidney (rk, **Fig. 35.1A,B**)
- Hepatic cysts (*arrows*, **Fig. 35.1C**)

Diagnosis

Autosomal dominant polycystic kidney disease (ADPKD)

Differential Diagnosis

- Multiple simple cysts
- von Hippel-Lindau disease
- Tuberous sclerosis
- Cystic disease of dialysis

Discussion

Background

ADPKD is one of the most common inherited disorders, with approximately 500,000 people in the United States affected, representing approximately 1 in 800 live births. It is responsible for up to 10% of dialysis-dependent renal failure cases. Men and women are equally affected. Two different genes have been implicated: *ADPK1* and *ADPK2*. Patients with *ADPK2* have less serious complications with improved survival.

Clinical Findings

With this ultrasound appearance (**Fig. 35.1**), a family history of renal disease becomes very important in the diagnosis. This genetic disorder affects primarily the duct-forming structures of the kidney and liver, but the gastrointestinal and cardiovascular systems are also affected. Patients may not be aware they have ADPKD, and the first presentation may be newly diagnosed hypertension or renal failure. In patients with ADPKD, hypertension affects 30% of children, 60% of adults, and 80% of patients with renal failure. Nearly half of all patients will develop renal failure by age 60. Hypertension appears to exacerbate renal failure; thus, control of hypertension is important in these patients.

Chronic pain is probably due to large cysts causing enlarged kidneys. Sixty percent of patients report flank, back, or abdominal pain. Acute exacerbations of pain may be due to acute cyst hemorrhage, cyst infection, pyelonephritis, or renal stones.

Pathology

Cysts form as outpouchings anywhere along the nephron due to a genetic defect in the differentiation of the nephron structures. In addition to renal cysts, cysts are found in the liver, pancreas, ovaries, and spleen. Cardiovascular complications include Berry aneurysms of the intracranial arteries and mitral valve prolapse. There is an increased risk of aneurysms in other arteries as well (e.g., aorta, popliteal).

Imaging Findings

ULTRASOUND

- Multiple simple cysts are a consideration in this case, but the innumerable cysts combined with the hepatic cysts make ADPKD much more likely even though the kidney is not grossly enlarged.
- Von Hippel-Lindau disease has both cysts (which are present) and solid renal tumors, which are not present in this case.
- Tuberous sclerosis has cysts and hyperechoic lesions representing angiomyolipomas; there are no such hyperechoic lesions present in this case.
- A diagnosis of ADPKD should be suggested when multiple bilateral renal cysts are seen in a young patient (< 30 years of age). ADPKD is confirmed if there are cysts in other parenchymal organs or if there is a history of cystic renal disease in a first-degree relative.
- If complex lesions are noted on sonography, computed tomography (CT) or magnetic resonance imaging (MRI) without and with IV contrast would be required to exclude neoplasia, but the patient's renal function must be taken into consideration before using contrast media.

RADIOGRAPHY

- Intravenous pyelography (IVP) will show bilaterally enlarged kidneys with multiple lucencies, representing the cysts, known as "Swiss cheese" kidney. IVU, however, is not the study of choice because of the associated compromised renal function and increased risk of contrast-induced renal failure; more information can be obtained with CT or MRI.

COMPUTED TOMOGRAPHY

- Evaluation of the renal parenchyma requires renal neoplasm protocol CT, as ADPKD demonstrates both simple and complex cysts (**Fig. 35.2B**). Excluding solid enhancing elements is required to rule out an underlying cystic renal cell carcinoma (RCC). Renal function, however, must be considered before using iodinated contrast unless the patient is on dialysis.

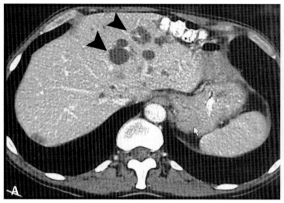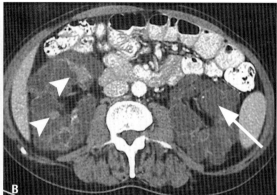

Fig. 35.2 Contrast-enhanced computed tomography scan through the **(A)** liver and **(B)** kidneys. Liver cysts (*black arrowheads*, **A**) and enlarged kidneys are essentially replaced by simple (*arrow*, **B**) and hyperdense (*white arrowheads*, **B**) cysts. The patient had a transplanted kidney, not shown. This indicates renal failure typical of advanced autosomal dominant polycystic kidney disease.

- Simple cysts will present as fluid-containing structures with attenuation < 20 Hounsfield units (HU) without enhancing elements (**Fig. 35.2B**).
- Complex cysts (e.g., hemorrhagic or infected cysts) may present as high-density cysts > 20 HU (**Fig. 35.2B**), but neither type of cyst will show enhancement.
  - Infected cysts can occasionally show an enhancing rim, but the clinical scenario (e.g., fever, dysuria, and/or pyuria) points to the correct diagnosis followed by treatment with antibiotics.
- Multiple renal cysts may represent von Hippel-Lindau disease, tuberous sclerosis, multiple simple renal cysts, acquired cystic disease of dialysis, or ADPKD. Concerning the differential diagnosis:
  - Von Hippel-Lindau disease presents as multiple renal cysts and RCC. It would be difficult to exclude RCC in this example without a noncontrast study, as there are high-density cysts present (arrowheads, **Fig. 35.2B**). The very large kidneys, innumerable cysts, hepatic cysts, and renal failure make ADPKD the likely diagnosis.
  - Tuberous sclerosis consists of renal cysts and angiomyolipomas, not present in this case.
  - There are far too many cysts to consider simple renal cysts as the diagnosis. The large kidneys (**Fig. 35.2B**) and hepatic cysts (**Fig. 35.2A**) also indicate ADPKD and not multiple simple cysts.
  - The large kidneys exclude acquired cystic disease of dialysis, which usually presents with multiple cysts in atrophic native kidneys.

MAGNETIC RESONANCE IMAGING

- MRI has been used previously to assess patients with ADPKD, given that renal function is often impaired (see Case 10 in Part II for Food and Drug Administration (FDA) recommendations regarding gadolinium contraindications in renal insufficiency).
- The kidneys will be enlarged and contain multiple cysts of varying signal intensities (**Fig. 35.3A–C**).
- Simple cysts will follow the signal of simple fluid (e.g., cerebrospinal fluid) on all sequences (i.e., low intensity on T1-weighted and high intensity on T2-weighted images).
- Complex cysts may be high, intermediate, or low signal on both T1- and T2-weighted images (**Fig. 35.3B,C**).
- Simple and complex cysts should not show enhancement following gadolinium.
- Hemorrhage into a renal cyst may have characteristic high signal on T1-weighted and low signal on T2-weighted images.

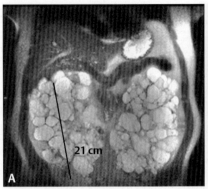 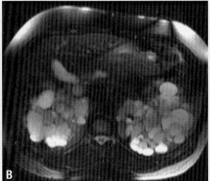 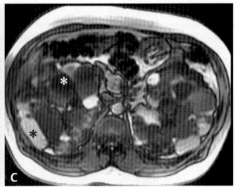

Fig. 35.3 Magnetic resonance imaging in a patient with autosomal dominant polycystic kidney disease. **(A)** Coronal T2-weighted image shows bilaterally enlarged kidneys (both kidneys measure ~21 cm). **(B)** Axial T2-weighted image with fat saturation shows renal parenchyma replaced by fluid-containing cysts. **(C)** Axial T1-weighted image shows the complexity of cysts with intensities ranging from low-signal simple fluid (*white asterisk*) to high-signal complex fluid (*black asterisk*).

Treatment

- Treatment is for symptomatic patients.
  - Pain may be treated with cyst aspiration, although the cysts will frequently recur. Acute pain should instigate a search for cyst infection, cyst hemorrhage, or stone as the cause.
  - Hypertension should be controlled to avoid accelerated renal failure.
  - Renal transplantation is effective in restoring renal function.
  - Berry cerebral aneurysm screening by cerebral vasculature MR angiography for patients with ADPKD and their first-degree relatives is indicated.

Prognosis

- Renal failure and hypertension is common and results in increased morbidity and mortality.

Suggested Readings

Gabow PA. Autosomal dominant polycystic kidney disease. N Engl J Med 1993;329(5):332–342.

Levine E. Autosomal dominant polycystic kidney disease. In: Pollack H, ed. Clinical Urography. Vol 2. Philadelphia: WB Saunders; 1990:1290–1315.

Lonergan GJ, Rice RR, Suarez ES. Autosomal recessive polycystic kidney disease: radiologic-pathologic correlation. Radiographics 2000;20(3):837–855.

Nicolau C, Torra R, Badenas C, et al. Autosomal dominant polycystic kidney disease types 1 and 2: assessment of US sensitivity for diagnosis. Radiology 1999;213(1):273–276.

Wilson PD. Polycystic kidney disease: new understanding in the pathogenesis. Int J Biochem Cell Biol 2004;36(10):1868–1873.

CASE 36

Clinical Presentation

A 30-year-old male presents with gross hematuria.

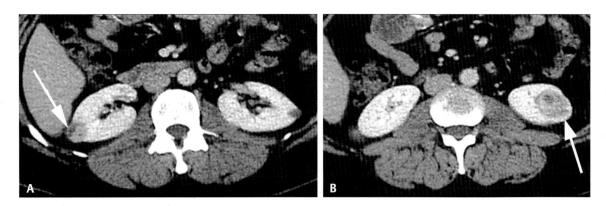

Fig. 36.1 **(A,B)** Enhanced computed tomography scans at two levels show bilateral enhancing renal masses (*arrows*).

Radiologic Findings

- Bilateral enhancing renal masses (**Fig. 36.1**)

Diagnosis

Von Hippel-Lindau disease

Differential Diagnosis

- Autosomal dominant polycystic kidney disease (ADPKD)
- Tuberous sclerosis
- Bilateral sporadic renal cell carcinoma (RCC)

Discussion

Background

Von Hippel-Lindau disease represents autosomal dominant inheritance of mutations in the von Hippel-Lindau tumor suppressor gene. It is associated with central nervous system (CNS) and retinal hemangioblastomas, renal and pancreatic cysts, and RCC and affects 1 in 36,000 people.

Clinical Findings

Autosomal dominant inheritance pattern is seen. Several lesions are characteristic, including RCC, often multiple and recurring. Von Hippel-Lindau disease usually manifests between 18 and 30 years of age. It is the main cause of adult inherited RCC and is the most common cause of death in these patients. Other neoplasms include pheochromocytoma, cerebellar hemangioblastoma, pancreatic cysts and cystic neoplasms, and retinal hemangiomatosis.

Pathology

Simple renal cysts and cystic and solid RCCs are found.

Imaging Findings

COMPUTED TOMOGRAPHY

- ADPKD presents as bilaterally enlarged kidneys with innumerable cysts throughout the renal parenchyma. Cystic neoplasms are a possibility, especially in patients with cystic disease of dialysis, but this patient clearly does not have bilateral renal cysts but rather bilateral solid enhancing renal masses.
- Tuberous sclerosis presents with many renal cysts and, characteristically, renal angiomyolipomas, which are fat-containing renal masses. There is no fat in these renal masses to suggest tuberous sclerosis.
- Bilateral sporadic RCC is a possibility in this case that cannot be differentiated from von Hippel-Lindau disease on renal imaging alone. A family pedigree or imaging of the CNS would help differentiate the two entities.
- Enhancing renal masses are easily detected on computed tomography (CT) as areas of abnormal enhancement (dissimilar from normal renal parenchyma). Equivocal cases may require unenhanced and enhanced imaging (i.e., renal neoplasm protocol CT or MRI) for definitive diagnosis of enhancement.

MAGNETIC RESONANCE IMAGING

- CT and magnetic resonance imaging (MRI) are equally accurate for detection and staging of solid and cystic RCC.
- Solid RCC is isointense to renal parenchyma on T1-weighted images, slightly hyperintense on T2-weighted images, and shows enhancement following intravenous (IV) gadolinium administration (**Fig. 36.2A–C**).
- Hemorrhage and/or necrosis will cause renal masses to have variable signal on T1- and T2-weighted images.
- Cystic RCC (i.e., Bosniak IV renal cyst) may follow the signal of simple fluid on T1- (i.e., low-signal) and T2-weighted (i.e., high-signal) images. Solid portions within the cystic mass will show enhancement following IV gadolinium (**Fig. 36.2A–C**).
- Pancreatic cystic lesions and adrenal lesions (i.e., pheochromocytoma) are also excellently depicted on MRI.

Treatment

- Partial nephrectomy for RCC is required because patients are likely to develop additional RCC throughout their lifetime, making renal sparing surgery essential.
- Yearly screening is indicated to detect RCC in early stages when partial nephrectomy can be easily performed.

Prognosis

- Complications from the numerous features of this syndrome occur throughout life.
  - In the past, 50% of von Hippel-Lindau disease patients died from RCC.

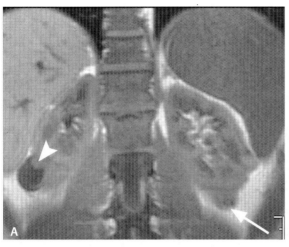 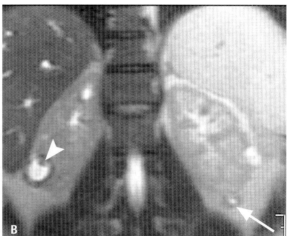

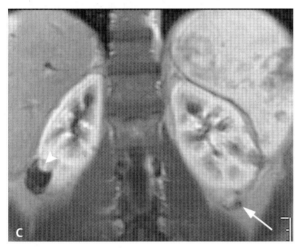

Fig. 36.2 Coronal magnetic resonance images in a patient with von Hippel-Lindau disease. **(A)** T1 gradient echo (GRE), **(B)** T2 turbo spin echo, and **(C)** T1 GRE images following gadolinium show a solid enhancing mass in the lower pole of the left kidney (*arrows*) consistent with renal cell carcinoma. A cystic mass is noted in the lower pole of the right kidney with an enhancing mural nodule (*arrowheads*). Findings are consistent with Bosniak IV cystic renal cell carcinoma on the right.

Suggested Readings

von Choyke P. Hippel-Lindau disease. In: Pollack H, McClennan B, eds. Clinical Urography. Vol 2. 2nd ed. Philadelphia: WB Saunders; 2000:1333–1342.

CASE 37

Clinical Presentation

A 45-year-old male presents with an abnormal ultrasound exam.

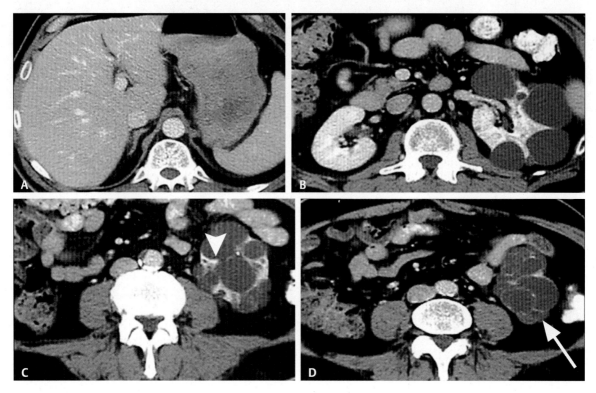

Fig. 37.1 Enhanced computed tomography scans **(A)** through the liver and **(B–D)** three levels through the left kidney.

Radiologic Findings

- No hepatic cysts identified (**Fig. 37.1A**)
- Innumerable cysts in the left kidney (**Fig. 37.1B–D**)
- Normal parenchyma between cysts (*arrowhead*, **Fig. 37.1C**)
- Normal-appearing right kidney (**Fig. 37.1B**)
- Conglomerate cysts in the lower pole without encapsulation (*arrow*, **Fig. 37.1D**)

Diagnosis

Localized cystic disease

Differential Diagnosis

- Autosomal dominant polycystic kidney disease (ADPKD)
- Multilocular cystic nephroma
- Cystic renal cell carcinoma (RCC)

128

Discussion

Background

Localized cystic disease is a rare benign entity, first described in 1989. Classic findings include a collection of cysts involving a portion of one kidney or an entire kidney, with the other kidney normal, with no evidence of ADPKD (e.g., no liver cysts). Men affected more often than women.

Clinical Findings

There is no family history of cystic disease and no association with renal insufficiency. Patients may present with hematuria or a palpable mass, or they may be entirely asymptomatic, and the lesion is discovered incidentally.

Pathology

The thin-walled cysts are not encapsulated into a cystic mass. Cysts are found in the cortex and medulla and are made up of dilated ducts and tubules with flattened cuboidal epithelium. Normal or atrophic renal parenchyma separates the cysts. The cysts closely resemble those of ADPKD.

Imaging Findings

COMPUTED TOMOGRAPHY

- Multiple cysts are seen throughout all or part of only one kidney. The absence of significant cysts in the opposite kidney and the absence of hepatic cysts essentially excludes ADPKD.
- Conglomerate masses of cysts can resemble multilocular cystic nephroma or cystic RCC, but with localized cystic disease there is no true encapsulation, which is seen in multilocular cystic nephroma. Also, there is no enhancement of abnormal tissue, as would be seen in cystic RCC.
- Localized cystic disease involves a portion of the kidney or an entire kidney. Cysts are closely opposed, without encapsulation, with intervening normal or atrophic renal parenchyma.
- Parenchyma between the cysts may enhance in localized cystic disease.

ULTRASOUND

- Multiple cysts are seen throughout all or part of only one kidney. Computed tomography (CT) or magnetic resonance imaging (MRI) may be required for a definitive diagnosis.

MAGNETIC RESONANCE IMAGING

- Findings are similar to CT, but multiplanar capabilities help differentiate localized cystic disease from other possibilities by better showing
  - Localized nature of cysts (**Fig. 37.2A–D**)
  - No encapsulation (**Fig. 37.2C**)
  - Normal or atrophic intervening renal parenchyma (**Fig. 37.2C,D**)
- Cysts may be simple or complex signal intensity.
- Parenchyma between the cysts may enhance.

Treatment

- Observation only

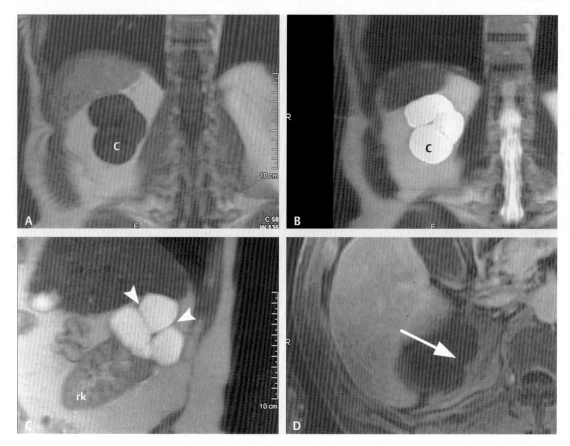

Fig. 37.2 Magnetic resonance imaging utilizing **(A)** coronal T1 gradient echo (GRE), **(B)** coronal T2-weighted half-Fourier acquisition single-shot turbo spin echo (HASTE), **(C)** sagittal T2-weighted HASTE, and **(D)** postgadolinium T1-weighted GRE. A cystic mass (c) is seen in the upper pole of the right kidney (rk). The multilocular, nonencapsulated character of the cysts is clearly depicted on the T2-weighted images **(B,C)** with intervening atrophic parenchyma (*arrowheads*). Only minimal enhancement (*arrow*) is seen in **D** in the intervening atrophic parenchyma.

Prognosis

- Excellent

Suggested Readings

Kim DJ, Kim MJ. Localized cystic disease of the kidney: CT findings. Abdom Imaging 2003;28(4):588–592.

Slywotzky CM, Bosniak MA. Localized cystic disease of the kidney. AJR Am J Roentgenol 2001;176(4):843–849.

CASE 38

Clinical Presentation

A 37-year-old female presents with a history of renal stones. No stones are observed on noncontrast computed tomography (CT).

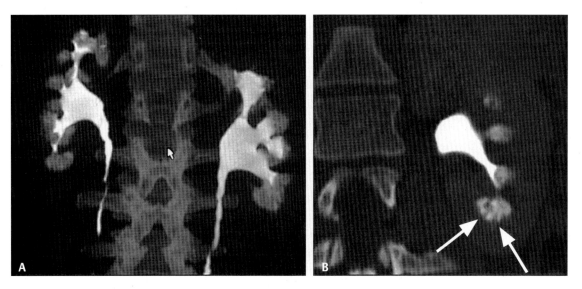

Fig. 38.1 CT-IVP. **(A)** Maximum intensity projection reconstruction in the coronal plane and **(B)** coned multiplanar reconstruction.

Radiologic Findings

- Globular collections of contrast material in essentially all papilla are seen only on the delayed portion of the contrasted CT scan (**Fig. 38.1A**).
- Multiplanar reconstructions of the left kidney provide better detail of globular contrast collections in the left lower pole (*arrows,* **Fig. 38.1B**).

Diagnosis

Medullary sponge kidney

Differential Diagnosis

- Medullary nephrocalcinosis
- Papillary necrosis
- Normal tubular blush

Discussion

Background

Believed to represent a congenital malformation of the collecting tubules that become ectatic, medullary sponge kidney is a radiographic diagnosis. It is an uncommon condition whose prevalence is not exactly known. There are associations with nephrocalcinosis and renal stone formation, urinary tract infection (UTI), and renal failure.

Clinical Findings

Most cases are entirely asymptomatic, and the finding is incidental on intravenous pyelogram (IVP). Some patients with stone disease will have associated hematuria and renal colic when obstruction occurs.

Pathology

Saccular dilatation of the renal collecting tubules is found; generally, it is bilateral, but it can be asymmetric.

Imaging Findings

COMPUTED TOMOGRAPHY

- Medullary nephrocalcinosis can produce multiple calcifications in the pyramids and appear superficially similar to this case. The calcifications would be apparent on the noncontrast images, and the patient's history indicated this was not the case. Medullary nephrocalcinosis can occur with sponge kidney as well as with metabolic disorders such as hyperparathyroidism.
- Calcifications from medullary sponge kidney (or any other cause) are detected with nearly 100% sensitivity by CT.
- Papillary necrosis can produce contrast collections in the pyramids, but not to this extent and not this uniform.
- The contrast in the pyramids is far more than can be considered prominent "blush," even for nonionic contrast. This is the classic sponge kidney appearance.

RADIOGRAPHY/INTRAVENOUS PYELOGRAM

- First described by IVP, classic findings on excretory phase images range from
  - Papillary "blush" with increased but normal contrast noted in the medullary pyramid regions to
  - Papillary striations or "paintbrush" appearance representing linear collections of contrast in the mildly dilated renal tubules (i.e., tubular ectasia) to
  - "Bouquets" of cystically dilated tubules in the medullary regions (sponge kidney, as seen in **Fig. 38.2**)

ULTRASOUND

- Not helpful for diagnosis of medullary sponge kidney

Treatment

- Most cases are asymptomatic. When stones are present, treating acute renal colic symptoms and decreasing the stone burden are therapeutic goals.

Prognosis

- Most are asymptomatic.

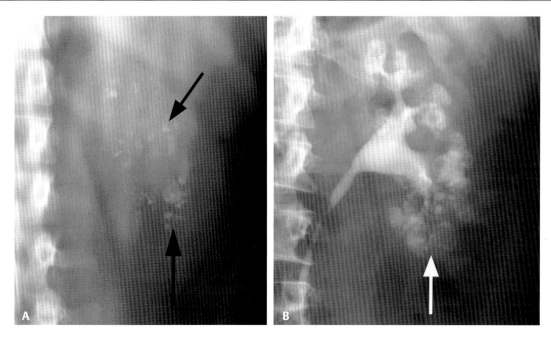

Fig. 38.2   Intravenous pyelogram. **(A)** Precontrast tomogram through the left kidney shows multiple rounded and tubular calcifications in the medullary pyramids representing stones in the dilated renal tubules (*black arrows*). **(B)** Radiograph coned to the left kidney in the excretory phase shows multiple cystically dilated renal tubules filled with contrast (*white arrow*), confirming medullary sponge kidney.

Suggested Readings

Dyer RB, Chen MY, Zagoria RJ. Classic signs in uroradiology. Radiographics 2004;24(Suppl 1):S247–S280.

Gambaro G, Feltrin GP, Lupo A, et al. Medullary sponge kidney (Lenarduzzi-Cacchi-Ricci disease): a Padua Medical School discovery in the 1930s. Kidney Int 2006;69(4):663–670.

Ginalski JM, Schnyder P, Portmann L, Jaeger P. Medullary sponge kidney on axial computed tomography: comparison with excretory urography. Eur J Radiol 1991;12(2):104–107.

Maw AM, Megibow AJ, Grasso M, Goldfarb DS. Diagnosis of medullary sponge kidney by computed tomographic urography. Am J Kidney Dis 2007;50(1):146–150.

CASE 39

Clinical Presentation

Right upper quadrant pain. Ultrasound showed exophytic solid right upper pole renal lesion.

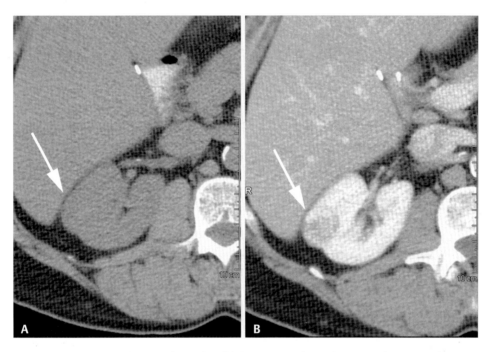

Fig. 39.1 Hematuria. **(A)** Unenhanced and **(B)** contrast-enhanced computed tomography scans through the right upper renal pole show an enhancing intraparenchymal renal lesion (*arrows*). The lesion measured 27 Hounsfield units (HU) precontrast and 108 HU postcontrast.

Radiologic Findings

- Mass enhances following contrast, 27 to 108 Hounsfield units (HU) (**Fig. 39.1A,B**).
- Exophytic mass in the right upper pole measures 1.2 cm (**Fig. 39.1B**).
- No renal vein or inferior vena cava (IVC) involvement
- No demonstrable fat to suggest angiomyolipoma

Diagnosis

Small renal cell carcinoma (RCC) < 7 cm. Nodal disease and distant metastases were not identified on the remainder of the scan.

Differential Diagnosis

- Oncocytoma
- Fat-poor angiomyolipoma
- Hyperdense cyst

135

Discussion

Background

There are nearly 39,000 new cases of renal cell carcinoma (RCC) diagnosed each year in the United States; this represents ~2.6% of all cancers. Kidney cancer accounts for almost 13,000 deaths per year. Risk factors for developing RCC include cigarette smoking, obesity, hypertension, and cystic disease of dialysis. Men are affected twice as often as women. Incidence rates are steadily increasing possibly due to increased obesity in the population.

With improving technology, these lesions are being detected at earlier stages when they are smaller. This offers patients expanded treatment options, including renal sparing surgery with partial nephrectomy and cryotherapy or radiofrequency ablation.

Clinical Findings

RCC presents as hematuria, localized pain, and palpable mass (the so-called classic triad) in only 10% of patients. Many present with symptoms related to advanced disease (e.g., distant metastases or paraneoplastic syndrome). In up to half of all patients, the lesion is discovered incidentally on imaging obtained for reasons other than for the assessment of the kidneys.

Pathology

The most common cell type is conventional clear cell carcinoma (75%), followed by papillary (12%) and chromophobe (4%) RCC and rarer tumor types (**Fig. 39.2**).

Imaging Findings

RADIOGRAPHY

- Can be detected as a mass effect on an intravenous pyelogram if large enough

COMPUTED TOMOGRAPHY

- Oncocytomas present as enhancing masses on computed tomography (CT) and cannot be reliably differentiated from RCC; thus, they are surgically removed.

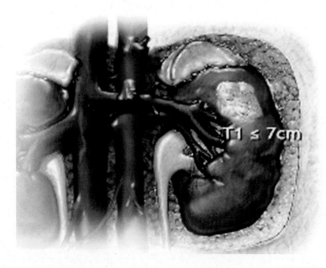

Fig. 39.2 Drawing of a T1 renal cell carcinoma. The T1 RCC is ≤ 7 cm and limited to the kidney.

- Angiomyolipomas require the presence of intratumoral macroscopic fat to make the diagnosis radiologically. A "fat poor" variant will have little discernible fat and cannot be differentiated from other enhancing renal masses; thus, they are surgically removed.

- Hyperdense cysts may show "pseudoenhancement" on the order of < 15 HU, but this case shows enhancement of ~81 HU (27 HU on unenhanced and 108 HU on enhanced scans).

- CT is highly accurate for diagnosing and staging enhancing renal lesions (RCC) when a dedicated renal protocol CT is employed.

- Noncontrast images are most helpful in excluding fat found in angiomyolipoma (**Fig. 39.3A**).

- An unenhanced scan is required to determine if a lesion is truly enhancing. This is done by measuring the lesion's attenuation before and after the administration of intravenous (IV) contrast (**Fig. 39.3A,B**).

- A 5-minute delayed exam is often included to demonstrate the collecting system's relation to the renal mass and to clarify less common lesions, such as calyceal diverticula. Also, "deenhancement" in a renal mass on the delayed scan is further evidence that the lesion is truly enhanced (**Fig. 39.3C**).

ULTRASOUND

- Renal lesions are often detected incidentally on ultrasound, requiring CT or magnetic resonance imaging (MRI) without and with IV contrast to evaluate for enhancing elements.

NUCLEAR MEDICINE

- Although it is not often used, a dimercaptosuccinic acid (DMSA) cortical scan can be helpful in separating a prominent column of Bertin or other atypical area of normal parenchyma from a renal mass. Normal tracer uptake will occur in areas of normal renal parenchyma, but a tumor will show a photopenic defect due to the presence of neoplastic tissue.

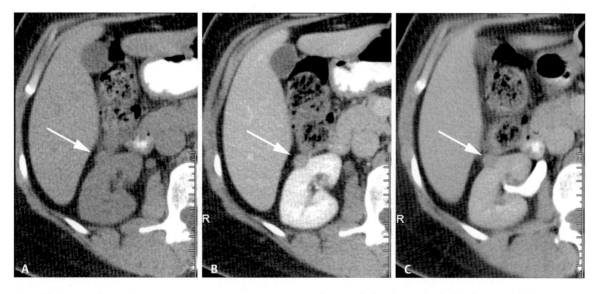

Fig. 39.3 Renal neoplasm protocol computed tomography. **(A)** Unenhanced, **(B)** enhanced, and **(C)** 5-minute delayed scans through the right upper pole show an enhancing lesion (*arrows*). The lesion measured 34, 83, and 59 Hounsfield units, respectively, consistent with a small renal cell carcinoma.

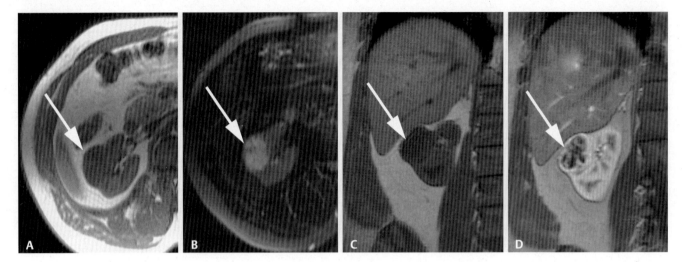

Fig. 39.4 Known renal mass in a patient with contraindication to iodinated contrast materials. **(A)** T1 axial gradient echo (GRE) image shows an exophytic isointense mass (*arrow*). **(B)** T2 axial image with fat saturation shows a slightly hyperintense mass (*arrow*). **(C)** T1 GRE coronal and **(D)** T1 GRE coronal postgadolinium images demonstrate enhancement in the mass consistent with a renal cell carcinoma (*arrows*).

MAGNETIC RESONANCE IMAGING

- MRI is as equally accurate as CT in detecting RCC > 1 cm.
- Detection of adenopathy on MRI is as accurate as with CT.
- Exclusion of a renal vein and IVC thrombus is best performed with MRI. MRI has 100% negative predictive value for vascular invasion.
- RCC presents as an isointense mass on T1-weighted images, is slightly high signal on T2 sequences, and enhances following IV gadolinium (**Fig. 39.4**). Signal may vary on T1- and T2-weighted images depending on the presence of hemorrhage and/or necrosis.

POSITRON EMISSION TOMOGRAPHY

- Positron emission tomography (PET) has an unacceptably high false-negative rate for the detection of primary RCC and RCC metastases.
- PET is less sensitive than CT alone for distant lymph nodes and parenchymal metastases.

Treatment

- Open or laparoscopic nephrectomy is the treatment of choice for T1 RCC. With limited tumor or in patients with compromised renal function, nephron-sparing surgery (e.g., partial nephrectomy, radiofrequency ablation, or cryotherapy) is undertaken with similar survival results.
- Limited nodal sampling may be performed for diagnostic/staging purposes.

Prognosis

- About 64 to 79% 5-year survival overall

Suggested Readings

Bassignani MJ. Understanding and interpreting MRI of the genitourinary tract. Urol Clin North Am 2006;33(3):301–317.

Cohen HT, McGovern FJ. Renal-cell carcinoma. N Engl J Med 2005;353(23):2477–2490.

Guinan P, Sobin LH, Algaba F, et al. TNM staging of renal cell carcinoma: Workgroup No. 3. Union International Contre le Cancer (UICC) and the American Joint Committee on Cancer (AJCC). Cancer 1997;80(5):992–993.

Israel GM, Bosniak MA. Renal imaging for diagnosis and staging of renal cell carcinoma. Urol Clin North Am 2003;30(3):499–514.

Jemal A, Siegel R, Ward E, et al. Cancer statistics, 2006. CA Cancer J Clin 2006;56(2):106–130.

Kang DE, White RL Jr, Zuger JH, Sasser HC, Teigland CM. Clinical use of fluorodeoxyglucose F18 positron emission tomography for detection of renal cell carcinoma. J Urol 2004;171(5):1806–1809.

Lee CT, Katz J, Fearn PA, Russo P. Mode of presentation of renal cell carcinoma provides prognostic information. Urol Oncol 2002;7(4):135–140.

Lipworth L, Tarone RE, McLaughlin JK. The epidemiology of renal cell carcinoma. J Urol 2006;176(6 Pt 1):2353–2358.

Novara G, Martignoni G, Artibani W, Ficarra V. Grading systems in renal cell carcinoma. J Urol 2007;177(2):430–436.

CASE 40

Clinical Presentation

Gross hematuria

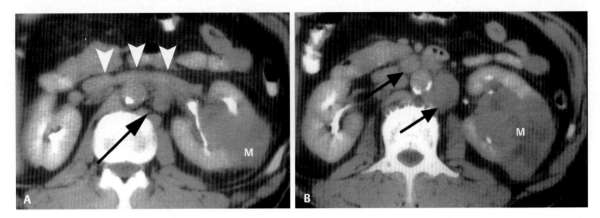

Fig. 40.1 **(A,B)** Enhanced computed tomography scans at two levels show a left renal mass (M). A normal renal vein is seen (*arrowheads*), as well as multiple enlarged lymph nodes (*arrows*). Source: Resnick, Older, Diagnosis of Genitourinary Disease, New York: Thieme, 1997: 367. Reprinted by permission.

Radiologic Findings

- Solid left renal mass (**Fig. 40.1**)
- Multiple pathologic-size periaortic nodes (**Fig. 40.1**)
- Normal left renal vein (**Fig. 40.1A**)

Diagnosis

Renal cell carcinoma (RCC) > 7 cm, with multiple nodal metastases (N2) and no vascular invasion (T2). Distant metastases were not evaluated on the images shown (MX).

Differential Diagnosis

- Stage T2N0
- Stage T2N1
- Stage T3bN2

Discussion

Background

T1 and T2 tumors are those tumors confined to the kidney, meaning confined by the renal capsule. Importantly, maximal tumor dimension should be reported if it is in the anteroposterior, transverse, or longitudinal dimension because the maximal tumor dimension determines the T designation in the TNM system (i.e., T1 tumors are ≤ 7 cm, T2 tumors are > 7 cm).

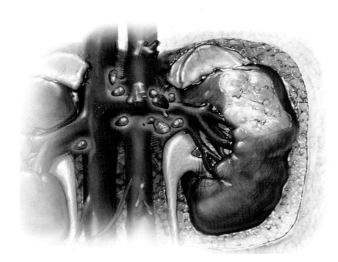

Fig. 40.2 Drawing of T2 renal cell carcinoma (RCC). T2 RCC is > 7 cm and limited to the kidney. Multiple regional lymph node groups are enlarged.

Clinical Findings

Nodal disease is a poor prognostic indication. It is rare that lymphadenectomy will result in cure and thus is usually not undertaken. Lymph node sampling is often performed during nephrectomy to confirm nodal disease and to allow for more accurate pathologic staging of the patient's tumor status.

Pathology

A T2 lesion is > 7 cm. Involvement of more than one regional lymph node groups is consistent with N2 disease (**Fig. 40.2**).

Imaging Findings

COMPUTED TOMOGRAPHY

- T2N0 indicates tumor > 7 cm, which is correct in this case, but also indicates no local adenopathy, which is not correct.
- T2N1 indicates tumor > 7 cm, which is correct in this case, but also indicates that a single local abnormal lymph node and multiple abnormal nodes are present.
- T3bN2 indicates both local adenopathy and venous involvement below the diaphragm and no venous involvement is seen in this case.
- All choices would be labeled MX, indicating that a distant metastasis cannot be assessed.

ULTRASOUND

- Ultrasound is of limited value in staging RCC.

MAGNETIC RESONANCE IMAGING

- Computed tomography (CT) and magnetic resonance imaging (MRI) are equally accurate in staging the primary tumor (**Fig. 40.3**).
- CT and MRI are equally accurate in staging nodal metastases. Nodes may be high signal (**Fig. 40.3A**) and enhance like the primary tumor (**Fig. 40.3D**).
- MRI has 100% negative predictive value for renal vein and inferior vena cava invasion and is an important adjunct to staging in equivocal CT cases.

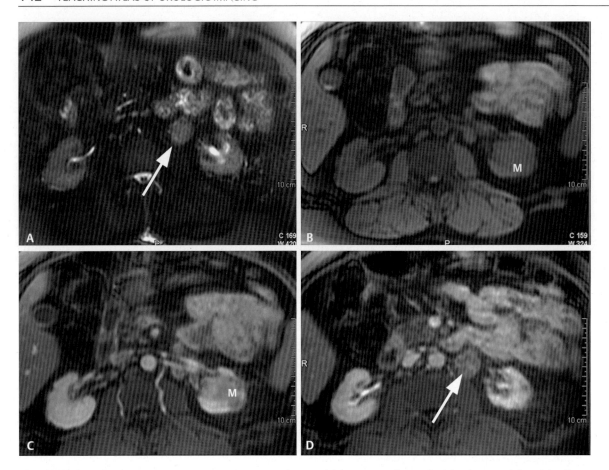

Fig. 40.3   (A–D) Staging magnetic resonance images show nodal metastases (*arrows*) and enhancing left renal cell carcinoma (M). Axial fat saturation **(A)** T2-weighted, **(B)** T1-weighted, and **(C,D)** T1-weighted postgadolinium images at two
levels.

POSITRON EMISSION TOMOGRAPHY

- Positron emission tomography (PET) is of limited value in staging primary or metastatic RCC.

Treatment

- Primary resection is undertaken to decrease primary tumor burden (i.e., nephrectomy).
- Limited nodal sampling may be performed for diagnostic/staging purposes.

Prognosis

- Nodal metastases result in ~5 to 15% 5-year survival rates.

Suggested Readings

Bassignani MJ. Understanding and interpreting MRI of the genitourinary tract. Urol Clin North Am
2006;33(3):301–317.

Cohen HT, McGovern FJ. Renal-cell carcinoma. N Engl J Med 2005;353(23):2477–2490.

Guinan P, Sobin LH, Algaba F, et al. TNM staging of renal cell carcinoma: Workgroup No. 3. Union
International Contre le Cancer (UICC) and the American Joint Committee on Cancer (AJCC). Cancer
1997;80(5):992–993.

Israel GM, Bosniak MA. Renal imaging for diagnosis and staging of renal cell carcinoma. Urol Clin North Am 2003;30(3):499–514.

Jemal A, Siegel R, Ward E, et al. Cancer statistics, 2006. CA Cancer J Clin 2006;56(2):106–130.

Kang DE, White RL Jr, Zuger JH, Sasser HC, Teigland CM. Clinical use of fluorodeoxyglucose F18 positron emission tomography for detection of renal cell carcinoma. J Urol 2004;171(5):1806–1809.

Lee CT, Katz J, Fearn PA, Russo P. Mode of presentation of renal cell carcinoma provides prognostic information. Urol Oncol 2002;7(4):135–140.

Lipworth L, Tarone RE, McLaughlin JK. The epidemiology of renal cell carcinoma. J Urol 2006;176(6 Pt 1):2353–2358.

Novara G, Martignoni G, Artibani W, Ficarra V. Grading systems in renal cell carcinoma. J Urol 2007;177(2):430–436.

CASE 41

Clinical Presentation

Gross hematuria

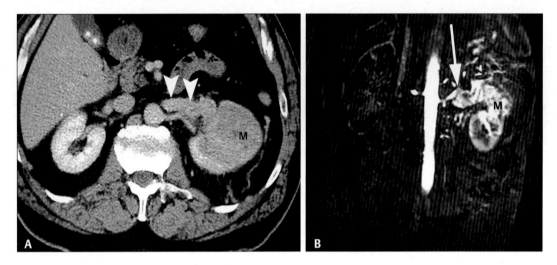

Fig. 41.1 Hematuria. Renal mass (M) and renal vein involvement by tumor on **(A)** enhanced computed tomography (*arrowheads*) and **(B)** enhanced magnetic resonance imaging (*arrow*).

Radiologic Findings

- Prominent left renal vein on computed tomography (CT) (**Fig. 41.1A**)
- Large left renal solid enhancing mass (**Fig. 41.1A,B**)
- Enhancing tumor thrombus in the left renal vein on magnetic resonance imaging (MRI) (**Fig. 41.1B**)

Diagnosis

Renal cell carcinoma (RCC) with gross extension of tumor into renal veins below the diaphragm (T3b). Nodal disease and distant metastases were not evaluated on the images shown.

Differential Diagnosis

- T3c RCC
- T3a RCC
- T2 RCC

Discussion

Background

Newly diagnosed RCC invades the vascular structures in ~4 to 10% of cases.

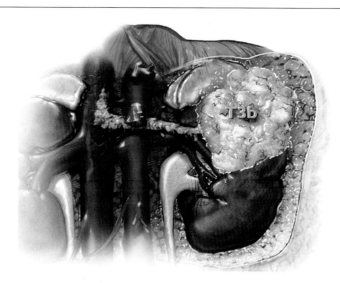

Fig. 41.2 Drawing of T3b renal cell carcinoma. Left renal vein and inferior vena cava invasion below the diaphragm.

Clinical Findings

These tumors can become quite large, at which point symptoms related to mass effect may be noted. Hematuria or pain will bring the patient to imaging. Many tumors are still diagnosed incidentally on imaging for other reasons.

Pathology

A T3 lesion will invade the perinephric fat tissues or the adjacent adrenal gland (T3a), invade a renal vein or the inferior vena cava (IVC) below the diaphragm (T3b) (**Fig. 41.2**), or invade the IVC above the diaphragm (T3c) (**Fig. 41.3**), but will not violate Gerota's fascia.

Imaging Findings

COMPUTED TOMOGRAPHY/MAGNETIC RESONANCE IMAGING

- Stage T3a involves adrenal or perirenal tissues, as in **Fig. 41.4,** but no venous involvement.
- Stage T2 is a lesion > 7 cm, but limited to the renal capsule.
- MRI currently provides the best evaluation of tumor growth into the renal vein and IVC (**Fig. 41.5**).

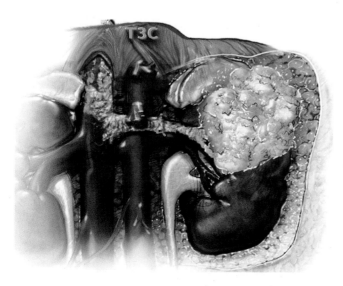

Fig. 41.3 Drawing of T3c renal cell carcinoma. Tumor extension into the renal vein above the diaphragm.

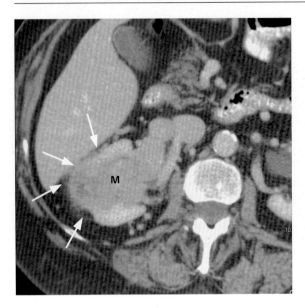

Fig. 41.4 Contrast-enhanced computed tomography scan shows a renal mass (M) with perinephric stranding (*arrows*) beyond the renal capsule consistent with perinephric tumor extension that is not beyond Gerota's fascia. There was no liver invasion at the time of surgery. This is a T3a renal cell carcinoma.

- Stage T3c indicates tumor growth in the IVC extending above the diaphragm, not present in this case. (See an example of T3c in **Figs. 41.5** and **41.6.**)
- Current multidetector CT scanners may provide comparable results to MRI (**Figs. 41.5, 41.6**).

POSITRON EMISSION TOMOGRAPHY

- Positron emission tomography (PET) is insensitive to metastatic disease from RCC.

Treatment

Treatment is primary surgical resection of the tumor and removal of the thrombus from venous structures.

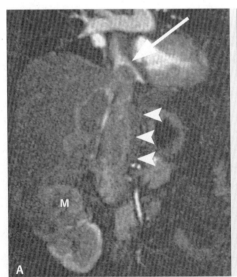
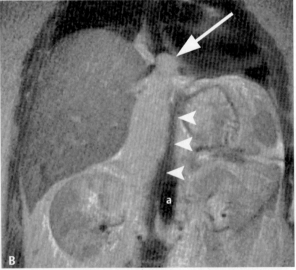

Fig. 41.5 Staging magnetic resonance imaging. **(A)** T1 gradient echo (GRE) coronal arterial phase post-gadolinium fat saturation image and **(B)** T2-weighted coronal image show a right upper pole renal mass (M) with extensive tumor burden in the inferior vena cava (IVC) (*arrowheads*) extending into the right atrium (*arrow*). In **A,** the thrombus is enhancing, suggesting tumor, not bland, thrombus. In **B,** a normal flow void is seen in the aorta (a) but not in the IVC (*arrowheads*) due to the presence of tumor.

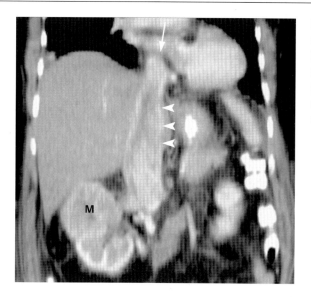

Fig. 41.6 Computed tomography (CT) corollary to **Fig. 41.5** (same patient). Contrast-enhanced CT reconstructed in the coronal plane shows a right upper pole renal mass (M) with extensive tumor burden in the inferior vena cava (*arrowheads*). Extension into the right atrium (*arrow*) was suggested on this CT and confirmed with magnetic resonance imaging (**Fig. 41.5**).

Prognosis

- Approximately 45 to 65% 5-year survival for T3 (a, b, or c) N0M0 disease

PEARLS _____

- Preoperative detection of the cava tumor thrombus is paramount in preoperative planning. If vascular invasion is known in advance, the urologic surgeon may employ a thoracic or vascular surgeon for assistance in removing the thrombus and reconstructing the venous structures.

Suggested Readings

Bassignani MJ. Understanding and interpreting MRI of the genitourinary tract. Urol Clin North Am 2006;33(3):301–317.

Cohen HT, McGovern FJ. Renal-cell carcinoma. N Engl J Med 2005;353(23):2477–2490.

Guinan P, Sobin LH, Algaba F, et al. TNM staging of renal cell carcinoma: Workgroup No. 3. Union International Contre le Cancer (UICC) and the American Joint Committee on Cancer (AJCC). Cancer 1997;80(5):992–993.

Israel GM, Bosniak MA. Renal imaging for diagnosis and staging of renal cell carcinoma. Urol Clin North Am 2003;30(3):499–514.

Jemal A, Siegel R, Ward E, et al. Cancer statistics, 2006. CA Cancer J Clin 2006;56(2):106–130.

Kang DE, White RL Jr, Zuger JH, Sasser HC, Teigland CM. Clinical use of fluorodeoxyglucose F18 positron emission tomography for detection of renal cell carcinoma. J Urol 2004;171(5):1806–1809.

Lee CT, Katz J, Fearn PA, Russo P. Mode of presentation of renal cell carcinoma provides prognostic information. Urol Oncol 2002;7(4):135–140.

Lipworth L, Tarone RE, McLaughlin JK. The epidemiology of renal cell carcinoma. J Urol 2006;176(6 Pt 1):2353–2358.

Novara G, Martignoni G, Artibani W, Ficarra V. Grading systems in renal cell carcinoma. J Urol 2007;177(2):430–436.

CASE 42

Clinical Presentation

Right upper quadrant pain and hematuria. Ultrasound discovered a right renal mass.

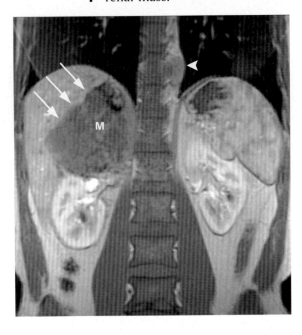

Fig. 42.1 Staging magnetic resonance imaging. T1 gradient echo coronal postgadolinium images show a right upper pole renal mass (M) with an irregular margin between the liver and the mass (*arrows*), consistent with liver invasion. The right adrenal gland was involved by the mass as well.

Radiologic Findings

- An 8 cm right upper pole renal mass (M, **Fig. 42.1**)
- Irregular margin between the liver and the mass consistent with liver invasion (*arrows,* **Fig. 42.1**)
- An enlarged left paraspinal metastatic node (*arrowhead,* **Fig. 42.1**)

Diagnosis

Renal cell carcinoma (RCC) with invasion of the liver and right adrenal gland and nodal metastasis above the diaphragm (T4 N0, M1). No regional lymph nodes were noted; thus, the N0 designation

Differential Diagnosis

T4 RCC (T4 N1, MX)

Discussion

Background

T4 lesions are often larger than lower stage tumors and are more likely to cause symptoms (e.g., palpable mass or pain). Metastatic disease is common at diagnosis, with ~25 to 30% of patients presenting with metastases. Another 50% develop metastases at follow-up.

Clinical Findings

Signs and symptoms related to advanced disease are seen in up to 90% of these patients and depend on the site of metastasis. A palpable mass from mass effect, pain from renal capsule expansion or from invasion into adjacent organs, central nervous system abnormalities due to brain metastasis, and symptoms related to paraneoplastic syndromes are all possible.

Pathology

A T4 lesion will violate Gerota's fascia, which is confirmed in this case with associated invasion into adjacent organs (**Fig. 42.1**). In this case, lymph node enlargement at a distance from regional lymph node groups (i.e., above the diaphragm) indicates metastatic disease (M1). Regional lymph nodes were lacking and thus designated as N0 (**Fig. 42.2**).

Imaging Findings

MAGNETIC RESONANCE IMAGING

- No regional nodal metastases were identified in this case; thus, this is not T4 N1, M0. The nodal metastasis is above the diaphragm, representing distant metastatic disease (M1).
- Magnetic resonance imaging (MRI) is equally accurate as computed tomography (CT) for detecting lymph node enlargement > 1 cm.
- Invasion of renal tumor through Gerota's fascia is seen as tumor tissue infiltration or irregularity beyond the margin of Gerota's fascia.
- Adjacent organ invasion is better depicted on sagittal and coronal images that are a standard part of renal neoplasm protocol MRI.

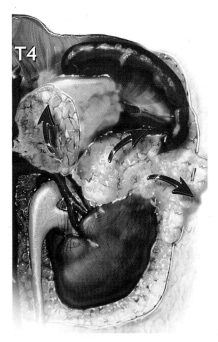

Fig. 42.2 Drawing of T4 renal cell carcinoma. Stage T4 represents extension beyond Gerota's fascia.

COMPUTED TOMOGRAPHY

- Abnormal tumor infiltration beyond Gerota's fascia can be seen on CT, indicative of T4 disease.
- Often adjacent organ involvement is suspected on axial images. Use of multirow detector CT with multiplanar reconstructions in the sagittal and coronal planes is becoming more common and may show tissue planes between the tumor and adjacent organs as well as that seen on MRI.

POSITRON EMISSION TOMOGRAPHY

- Positron emission tomography (PET) is insensitive to metastatic disease from RCC.

Treatment

- The primary tumor will be resected, including removing portions of the patient's liver, because there is some survival benefit to removal of the primary neoplasm and large metastatic deposits (i.e., cytoreduction surgery).

Prognosis

- Approximately 5 to 10% 5-year survival for T4 disease

PEARLS _____

- T4 lesions with adjacent organ invasion may be difficult to determine at imaging. Large tumors will compress adjacent structures, and the desmoplastic response to tumor may blur planes between the tumor and adjacent organs. In equivocal cases, possible invasion beyond Gerota's fascia should be reported to the urologist to assist in surgical planning.

Suggested Readings

Bassignani MJ. Understanding and interpreting MRI of the genitourinary tract. Urol Clin North Am 2006;33(3):301–317.

Cohen HT, McGovern FJ. Renal-cell carcinoma. N Engl J Med 2005;353(23):2477–2490.

Guinan P, Sobin LH, Algaba F, et al. TNM staging of renal cell carcinoma: Workgroup No. 3. Union International Contre le Cancer (UICC) and the American Joint Committee on Cancer (AJCC). Cancer 1997;80(5):992–993.

Israel GM, Bosniak MA. Renal imaging for diagnosis and staging of renal cell carcinoma. Urol Clin North Am 2003;30(3):499–514.

Jemal A, Siegel R, Ward E, et al. Cancer statistics, 2006. CA Cancer J Clin 2006;56(2):106–130.

Kang DE, White RLJr, Zuger JH, Sasser HC, Teigland CM. Clinical use of fluorodeoxyglucose F18 positron emission tomography for detection of renal cell carcinoma. J Urol 2004;171(5):1806–1809.

Lee CT, Katz J, Fearn PA, Russo P. Mode of presentation of renal cell carcinoma provides prognostic information. Urol Oncol 2002;7(4):135–140.

Lipworth L, Tarone RE, McLaughlin JK. The epidemiology of renal cell carcinoma. J Urol 2006;176(6 Pt 1):2353–2358.

Novara G, Martignoni G, Artibani W, Ficarra V. Grading systems in renal cell carcinoma. J Urol 2007;177(2):430–436.

CASE 43

Clinical Presentation

A 68-year-old female presents with hematuria and prior left nephrectomy.

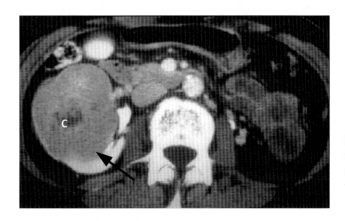

Fig. 43.1 Enhanced computed tomography scan through a right kidney mass (*arrow*). Source: Resnick, Older, Diagnosis of Genitourinary Disease, New York: Thieme, 1997: 383. Reprinted by permission.

Radiologic Findings

- Large, generally homogeneous right renal mass (*arrow,* **Fig. 43.1**)
- Central low density in mass, which measured 27 Hounsfield units (HU) (c, **Fig. 43.1**)

Diagnosis

Oncocytoma

Differential Diagnosis

- Renal cell carcinoma (RCC)
- Bosniak IV cystic mass
- Angiomyolipoma

Discussion

Background

Renal oncocytoma is a benign neoplasm of oncocytic origin (see pathology section below) representing ~3 to 7% of renal neoplasms. Men are affected twice as often as women. It is often discovered incidentally, and patients are usually asymptomatic. Because renal oncocytoma is an enhancing mass, it cannot be reliably differentiated from RCC and therefore is treated surgically.

Clinical Findings

Usually asymptomatic

Pathology

Oncocytomas are well-circumscribed, encapsulated tumors occurring in many parts of the body; they are made up of a homogeneous population of cells that stain brightly eosinophilic with granular cytoplasm. These cells are known as oncocytes and can be found in renal, thyroid, and salivary glands. When the tumor is entirely composed of oncocytes, the lesion is benign. Interestingly, there are case reports of RO with distant metastases, suggesting they can exhibit aggressive behavior.

Imaging Findings

COMPUTED TOMOGRAPHY

- The lesion in this case could represent a solid RCC. The central low density, representing a fibrous scar, suggests the possibility of oncocytoma, but this diagnosis cannot be made with confidence prior to surgery; therefore, these lesions are usually treated as presumed RCC.
- Bosniak IV lesions are cystic with prominent enhancing tissue; this lesion is not cystic.
- Angiomyolipoma would be a consideration if the central low density measured in the range of fat density (–30 to –120 HU), which this lesion does not.
- Renal oncocytoma usually presents as a well-defined solid mass, which can contain a low-attenuation central scar, but these findings are not specific.

MAGNETIC RESONANCE IMAGING

- Low-intensity homogeneous mass on T1-weighted imaging
- Increased intensity on T2-weighted imaging
- The presence of a capsule, central scar, or stellate pattern suggests oncocytoma.
- These findings cannot definitively differentiate between renal oncocytoma and RCC; therefore, the mass should be surgically removed.

ULTRASOUND

- Hypoechoic or heterogeneous mass on ultrasound

ANGIOGRAPHY

- A "spoke wheel" appearance of the feeding arteries can be seen; however, this is not specific for oncocytoma and can be seen in RCC.

Treatment

- Surgical excision or ablative techniques

Prognosis

- Excellent

PEARLS

- Biopsy is not helpful in differentiating this tumor from RCC.

Suggested Readings

Dyer RB, Chen MY, Zagoria RJ. Classic signs in uroradiology. Radiographics 2004;24(Suppl 1):S247–S280.

Harmon WJ, King BF, Lieber MM. Renal oncocytoma: magnetic resonance imaging characteristics. J Urol 1996;155(3):863–867.

Lieber MM. Renal oncocytoma. Urol Clin North Am 1993;20(2):355–359.

Palmer WE, Chew FS. Renal oncocytoma. AJR Am J Roentgenol 1991;156(6):1144.

CASE 44

Clinical Presentation

Incidental finding on abdominal ultrasound

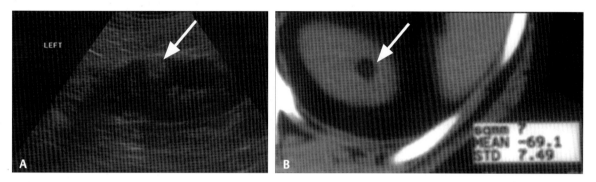

Fig. 44.1 **(A)** Longitudinal ultrasound of the left kidney. **(B)** Follow-up noncontrast computed tomography scan.

Radiologic Findings

- Hyperechoic lesion on ultrasound (*arrow*, **Fig. 44.1A**) with mild acoustic shadowing posterior to the lesion
- Fat density lesion on computed tomography (CT) measuring –69 Hounsfield units (HU) (*arrow*, **Fig. 44.1B**)

Diagnosis

Renal angiomyolipoma (AML)

Differential Diagnosis

- Renal cell carcinoma (RCC)
- Oncocytoma
- Stone debris in a calyceal diverticulum

Discussion

Background

Angiomyolipoma is rare and found in two scenarios: 80% are sporadic and usually unilateral and single, and 20% are multiple and bilateral in patients with tuberous sclerosis. Prevalence is from 0.3 to 3.0%. Women are affected 4 times more often than men. The mean age of diagnosis is the mid-40s.

Clinical Findings

- Renal AML is usually asymptomatic (60%) and discovered incidentally on imaging studies.
- Larger lesions tend to bleed. Bleeding can be severe and life threatening.

Pathology

AML in the kidney is a benign tumor composed of mature fat tissue, smooth muscle, and blood vessels. It is considered a choristoma because it is composed of tissues not normally found in the kidney. There is no malignant potential, although the larger the lesion, the more likely it is to hemorrhage. Some AML will contain no discernible fat; these are known as "fat-poor" AMLs. Because macroscopic fat is not detectable, these fat-poor AMLs cannot be differentiated from other enhancing renal masses, such as RCC. Multiple and bilateral AMLs are seen associated with multiple renal cysts in patients with tuberous sclerosis.

Imaging Findings

COMPUTED TOMOGRAPHY

- Although an echogenic lesion is typically considered to be AML, a small RCC can have an identical echogenic appearance. Documentation of fat on CT or magnetic resonance imaging (MRI) is therefore necessary to prove AML and exclude RCC.
- Oncocytoma can, on occasion, be hyperechoic, but it would not demonstrate fat on CT, as in this case.
- Stone debris will be echogenic, but typically more echogenic than in this case and with greater acoustic shadowing. Stone debris would be high density on the CT, with density most likely 300 HU or greater.
- AML often presents as a heterogeneous mass containing both low-density fat elements and soft tissue (**Fig. 44.2**). The key to imaging diagnosis is demonstrating mature fat in a renal cortical mass. Fat density on CT is in the range of –30 to –120 HU. There are case reports of RCCs with

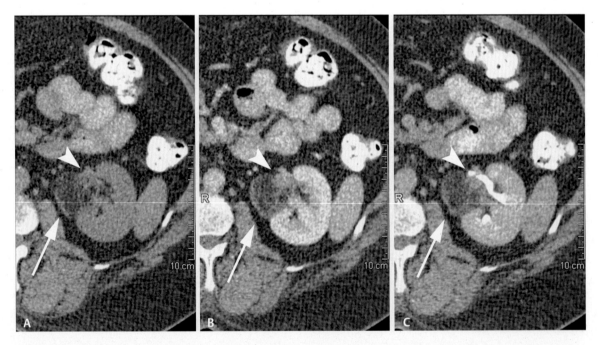

Fig. 44.2   Fatty renal mass. Renal mass protocol computed tomography (CT) utilizing **(A)** unenhanced, **(B)** contrast-enhanced, and **(C)** 5-minute delayed axial images showing a fatty mass (*arrow*) with soft tissue elements (*arrowhead*) arising from the left midrenal cortex. The mass was predominantly fatty with a small enhancing soft tissue element (*arrowhead*) that did not represent a soft tissue mass engulfing renal sinus fat.

bony metaplasia containing marrow fat and also reports of large RCCs engulfing renal sinus fat. To exclude RCC, the fatty mass should not contain bone, nor should a renal mass invading the renal sinus fat be mistaken for AML.

- The amount of soft tissue within the AML will determine how much the AML enhances following contrast (**Fig. 44.2**).

RADIOGRAPHY

- AML would present, if detected, as a space-occupying lesion on intravenous pyelogram, which would require further work-up with CT or MRI.
- Occasionally, fat may be detected in larger AMLs.

ULTRASOUND

- AML will be a well-defined, sharply marginated cortical mass that is as hyperechoic as the renal sinus fat. Shadowing may be seen (**Fig. 44.1A**).
- Ultrasound findings, however, are not specific and thus require CT or MRI to confirm the presence of macroscopic fat. Keep in mind that ~30% of small RCCs will present as hyperechoic masses.

MAGNETIC RESONANCE IMAGING

- AML will be high signal on a T1-weighted image without fat saturation, which becomes low signal on fat-saturated T1-weighted imaging (**Fig. 44.3**).
- Soft tissue portions of the AML may enhance.
- A small AML may be difficult to detect with MRI compared with CT due to slightly poorer spatial resolution.

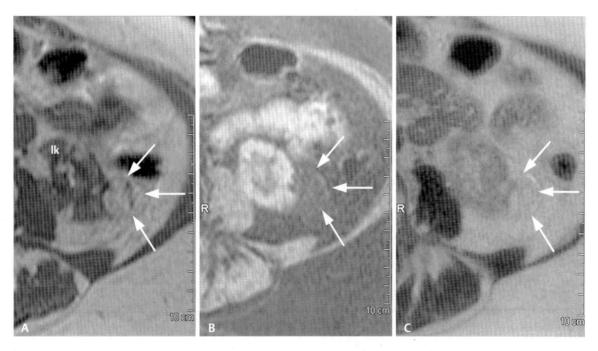

Fig. 44.3 Axial magnetic resonance imaging. **(A)** T1-weighted images without fat saturation and **(B)** postgadolinium with fat saturation show a fatty mass (*arrows*) arising from the lower pole of the left kidney (lk). The mass is high signal, like the retroperitoneal and subcutaneous fat on T1-weighted imaging, and it gets darker on fat saturation sequences, consistent with angiomyolipoma. **(C)** On a T2-weighted image, the lesion's signal intensity is similar to the surrounding retroperitoneal fat.

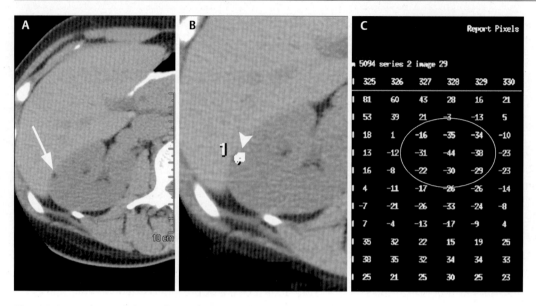

Fig. 44.4   Pixel map. **(A)** Unenhanced computed tomography (CT) scan shows a tiny low-density lesion in the right lateral renal midpole (*arrow*). **(B)** Image capture from the CT console with the region of interest (ROI) drawn over the lesion (*arrowhead*). **(C)** Pixel map from the ROI. Note the low-attenuation numbers (*circle*) measuring fat (i.e., < −30 HU) corresponding to this small low-density renal lesion and confirming a fat-containing angiomyoplipoma.

Treatment

- Small AMLs require no specific treatment. Lesions > 4 cm are prophylactically removed or embolized due to the risk of hemorrhage.
- Multiple bilateral AMLs should raise the possibility of tuberous sclerosis.

Prognosis

- Excellent, if no complications of hemorrhage

PEARLS _____

- Pixel mapping on CT (**Fig. 44.4**) is an ideal way to confirm small amounts of fat in an indeterminate lesion that is felt to represent an AML. On the CT console, the CT technologist draws a region of interest to completely surround the suspected fatty lesion. The pixel map function then displays all the attenuation values for that region of interest. If the numbers are in the range of macroscopic fat (−30 to −120 HU), the presence of fat is confirmed.

Suggested Readings

Forman HP, Middleton WD, Melson GL, McClennan BL. Hyperechoic renal cell carcinomas: increase in detection at US. Radiology 1993;188(2):431–434.

Helenon O, Merran S, Paraf F, et al. Unusual fat-containing tumors of the kidney: a diagnostic dilemma. Radiographics 1997;17(1):129–144.

Israel GM, Bosniak MA, Slywotzky CM, Rosen RJ. CT differentiation of large exophytic renal angiomyolipomas and perirenal liposarcomas. AJR Am J Roentgenol 2002;179(3):769–773.

Siegel CL, Middleton WD, Teefey SA, McClennan BL. Angiomyolipoma and renal cell carcinoma: US differentiation. Radiology 1996;198(3):789–793.

Silverman SG, Pearson GD, Seltzer SE, et al. Small (≤ 3 cm) hyperechoic renal masses: comparison of helical and convention CT for diagnosing angiomyolipoma. AJR Am J Roentgenol 1996;167(4):877–881.

Smirniotopoulos J, Hartman D. Renal cystic disease associated with tuberous sclerosis. In: Pollack H, McClennan B, eds. Campbell's Urology. St. Louis: Elsevier; 2002:1359–1367.

Wagner BJ, Wong-You-Cheong JJ, Davis CJ Jr. Adult renal hamartomas. Radiographics 1997;17(1):155–169.

CASE 45

Clinical Presentation

A 12-year-old female

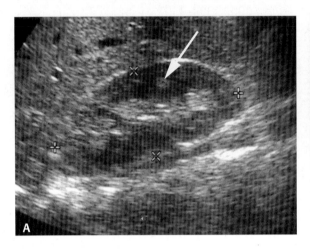
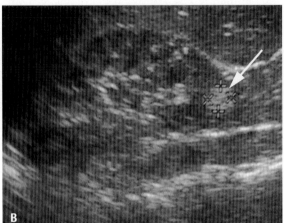

Fig. 45.1 **(A,B)** Renal ultrasound.

Radiologic Findings

- Multiple hyperechoic masses on ultrasound (*white arrows*, **Fig. 45.1**)
- Bilateral fat-containing lesions on computed tomography (CT) (*black arrows*, **Fig. 45.2**)

Diagnosis

Tuberous sclerosis

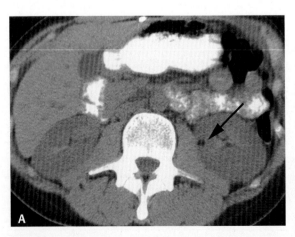
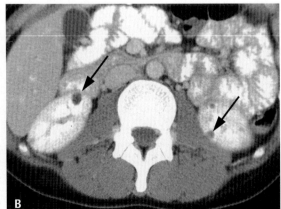

Fig. 45.2 **(A,B)** Pre- and postcontrast computed tomography.

Differential Diagnosis

- Polycystic kidneys
- Von Hippel-Lindau disease
- Simple cysts

Discussion

Background

Tuberous sclerosis is an autosomal dominant inherited multisystem disorder that requires a combination of major (e.g., renal angiomyolipomas) and minor clinical features to confirm the diagnosis.

Clinical Findings

Renal angiomyolipomas (AMLs) are multiple and bilateral and can be found in up to 75% of patients with tuberous sclerosis. AMLs are often seen in association with multiple bilateral renal cysts. Small

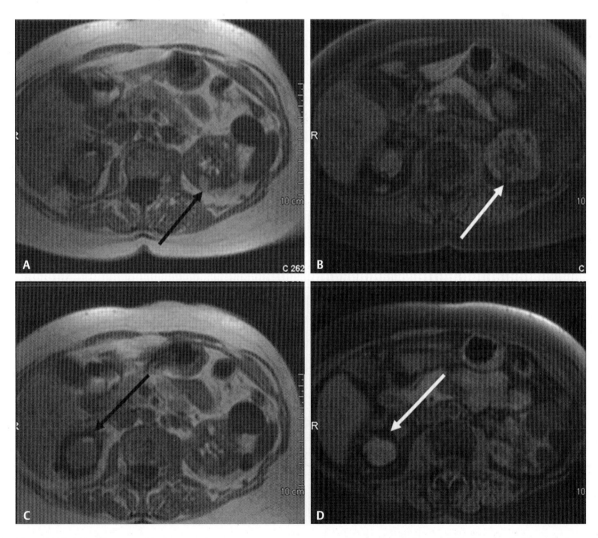

Fig. 45.3 Renal magnetic resonance imaging. T1-weighted images **(A,C)** without and **(B,D)** with fat saturation. Note the bilateral high-signal renal cortical lesions on non-fat-saturated images (*black arrows*). These lesions become dark on fat-saturated images (*white arrows*).

AMLs are usually asymptomatic but may hemorrhage as they grow larger. Thus, lesions > 4 cm are treated with prophylactic angiographic embolization to prevent the complication of life-threatening spontaneous hemorrhage. Central nervous system lesions (i.e., cortical tubers and subependymal nodules) can result in neurologic disorders, including epilepsy and cognitive impairment. Skin lesions (i.e., facial angiofibromas) and cardiac rhabdomyomas are also very common.

Pathology

AML in the kidney is a benign tumor composed of mature fat tissue, smooth muscle, and blood vessels. It is considered a choristoma because it is composed of tissues not normally found in the kidney. There is no malignant potential, although the larger a lesion, the more likely it is to hemorrhage. Some AMLs will contain no discernible fat; these are known as "fat-poor" AMLs. If macroscopic fat is not detectable, these fat-poor AMLs cannot be differentiated from other enhancing renal masses, such as renal cell carcinomas (RCCs).

Imaging Findings

COMPUTED TOMOGRAPHY

- Fat-containing renal lesions are pathognomonic of AMLs; therefore, tuberous sclerosis is the diagnosis and not von Hippel-Lindau disease.
- AML often presents as a heterogeneous mass containing both low-density fat elements and soft tissue. The key to imaging diagnosis is demonstrating mature fat in a renal cortical mass. Fat density on CT is in the range of –30 to –120 Hounsfield units. There are case reports of RCCs with bony metaplasia containing marrow fat and also reports of large RCCs engulfing renal sinus fat. To exclude RCC, the fatty mass should not contain bone, nor should a mass invading the renal sinus fat be mistaken for AML.

ULTRASOUND

- The absence of cysts excludes polycystic kidneys.
- AML is a well-defined, sharply marginated cortical mass that is as hyperechoic as the renal sinus fat. Shadowing may be seen.
- Hyperechoic lesions may represent AML or RCC. Documentation of fat on CT or magnetic resonance imaging (MRI) is therefore necessary to prove AML and to exclude RCC.

MAGNETIC RESONANCE IMAGING

- Alternate method to show fat in lesions.
- The fat within the AML will be high signal on T1-weighted imaging without fat saturation (*arrows,* **Fig. 45.3A,C**), which becomes dark on fat-saturated T1-weighted imaging (*arrows,* **Fig. 45.3B,D**).
- Soft tissue portions of the AML may enhance.
- Small AMLs may be difficult to detect with MRI compared with CT due to slightly poorer spatial resolution (**Fig. 45.3**).

Treatment

- Small AMLs require no specific treatment. Lesions > 4 cm are treated with prophylactic embolization because of the risk of hemorrhage.
- AMLs are followed with imaging to confirm stability.

Prognosis

- There is no increased malignant potential in the AML. The patient's other tuberous sclerosis sequelae may dominate the clinical picture.

PEARLS _____

- When incidentally discovered multiple bilateral AMLs are noted on an imaging study, the possibility of tuberous sclerosis should be raised with the ordering clinician.

Suggested Readings

Crino PB, Nathanson KL, Henske EP. The tuberous sclerosis complex. N Engl J Med 2006;355(13):1345–1356.

Helenon O, Merran S, Paraf F, et al. Unusual fat-containing tumors of the kidney: a diagnostic dilemma. Radiographics 1997;17(1):129–144.

Smirniotopoulos J, Hartman D. Renal cystic disease associated with tuberous sclerosis. In: Pollack H, McClennan B, eds. Campbell's Urology. St. Louis: Elsevier; 2002:1359–1367.

Wagner BJ, Wong-You-Cheong JJ, Davis CJ Jr. Adult renal hamartomas. Radiographics 1997;17(1):155–169.

CASE 46

Clinical Presentation

A 45-year-old male presents with an abnormal intravenous pyelogram (IVP) and hematuria. The presence or absence of pyuria or positive cytology is important to consider in the diagnosis.

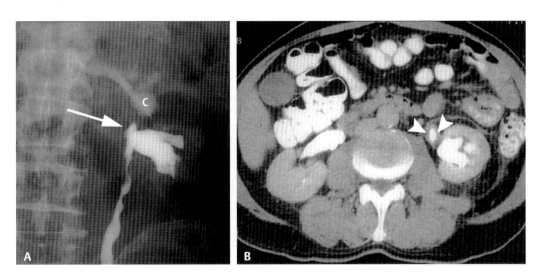

Fig. 46.1   **(A)** Retrograde pyelogram. **(B)** Delayed enhanced computed tomography scan.

Radiologic Findings

- Amputated upper pole infundibulum seen on a retrograde pyelogram (*arrow,* **Fig. 46.1A**)
- Partial filling of the upper pole calyx (c, **Fig. 46.1A**)
- Circumferential ureteral thickening seen on a computed tomography (CT) scan (*arrowheads,* **Fig. 46.1B**)

Diagnosis

Transitional cell carcinoma (TCC)

Differential Diagnosis

- Tuberculosis
- Nonspecific infundibular stricture
- Infundibular stone

Discussion

Background

Transitional cell carcinoma of the renal pelvis and ureter is uncommon compared with bladder cancer. TCCs of the renal pelvis and ureter accounts for 4 to 15% and 1% of all TCCs of the urinary tract, respectively. Risk factors are similar to those for bladder cancer and include smoking, chemical exposure in certain industries (e.g., dye, leather, rubber), chronic irritation from stones or infection, cyclophosphamide treatment, and analgesic abuse. Males are affected more often than females. Most tumors are seen in the 6th to 7th decade. Multifocal tumor is found pathologically in up to 30% of patients originally thought to have a solitary tumor. From 25 to 75% of patients with upper tract TCC may subsequently develop bladder cancer.

Clinical Findings

Patients present with gross hematuria (75%), flank pain (30%), or a palpable mass (10%), but some present with no specific sign or symptom.

Pathology

Ninety percent of upper tract lesions are TCCs. Both papillary and flat growth patterns are encountered. Tumors are staged based on the TNM (tumor size, node involvement, and metastasis status) system (see Section K in Appendix). Squamous cell and adenocarcinomas make up 7 and 1% of upper tract neoplasms, respectively.

Imaging Findings

RADIOGRAPHY/RETROGRADE PYELOGRAM/INTRAVENOUS PYELOGRAM

- A radiopaque stone should be noted on the scout film.
- Partial occlusion with a sharp cutoff of an infundibulum is termed an amputation, suggesting tuberculosis or TCC (**Fig. 46.1A**). Urine culture and cytologic analysis plus retrograde pyelogram represents appropriate work up.
- Upper tract tumors are seen as radiolucent irregular filling defects attached to the urothelium on the pyelogram phase of retrograde or intravenous urography (IVU).
- Tumor may produce incomplete or nonfilling infundibulum or calyx, as in **Fig. 46.1A.** Amputation can be caused by external compression of the collecting system by crossing a vessel, blood clot, radiolucent stone, sloughed renal papilla, stricture, or fungus ball.
- Multifocality is common in TCC (**Fig. 46.1A,B**).
  - Up to 30% of cases will have a synchronous TCC.
  - IVU may not detect up to 40% of urothelial abnormalities.

COMPUTED TOMOGRAPHY

- A stricture from a stone would not have circumferential wall thickening.
- Both tuberculosis and TCC can have circumferential wall thickening (**Fig. 46.1B**), making cytology and culture important determinants in the diagnosis.
- Multirow detector CT scan using a CT/IVP technique can detect up to 89% of urothelial tumors.
  - The detection of lesions on three-dimensional (3D) reconstructed images is reported to be limited, so axial data should still be reviewed for a primary diagnosis.
  - Reasons for failing to detect ureteral TCC include a ureteral segment in which the tumor is located is not distended, is not opacified, or both.
  - TCC may be inconspicuous on unenhanced CT scans (although secondary findings, such as ureteral dilatation, may be present).
  - TCC enhances poorly following contrast, so delayed images with complete ureteral filling are required to optimally evaluate for filling defects.
- Adenopathy and distant metastases are best evaluated with CT (**Fig. 46.2**).

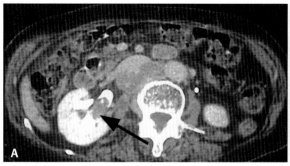
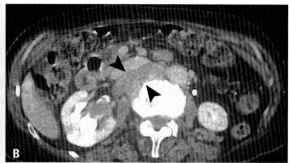

Fig. 46.2 (A,B) An 81-year-old female with hematuria. Computed tomography (CT) scans at two levels during the pyelogram phase from a CT-IVP show a right renal pelvis filling defect (*black arrow*) and retrocaval adenopathy (*arrowheads*).

ULTRASOUND

- Ultrasound is not used in the primary diagnosis of TCC, but it may detect secondary signs, such as dilated calyx, hydronephrosis, and hydroureter (**Fig. 46.3**).

MAGNETIC RESONANCE IMAGING

- Magnetic resonance urography (MRU) uses heavily T2-weighted sequences with fat saturation, which show dilated collecting systems quite well, although normal, nondistended systems are less well evaluated (**Fig. 46.4A,B**).
- TCC may enhance, indicating a neoplasm, but TCC enhances poorly following contrast (**Fig. 46.4C**).
- For nondilated systems, postgadolinium T1-weighted imaging, using fat-saturated gradient echo (GRE) volumetric acquisition and 3D reconstruction following furosemide, can provide exquisite images of the collecting systems.

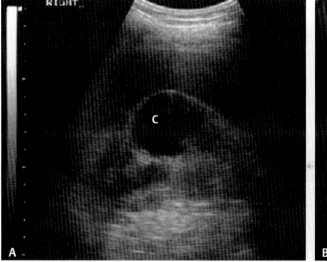
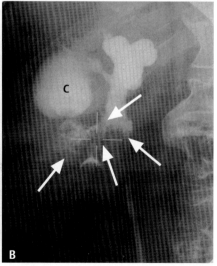

Fig. 46.3 (A) Sonogram of the right kidney shows a cystic mass (c) that proved to be a hydronephrotic calyx secondary to extensive transitional cell carcinoma, seen as **(B)** multiple irregular filling defects (*arrows*) shown on a retrograde pyelogram.

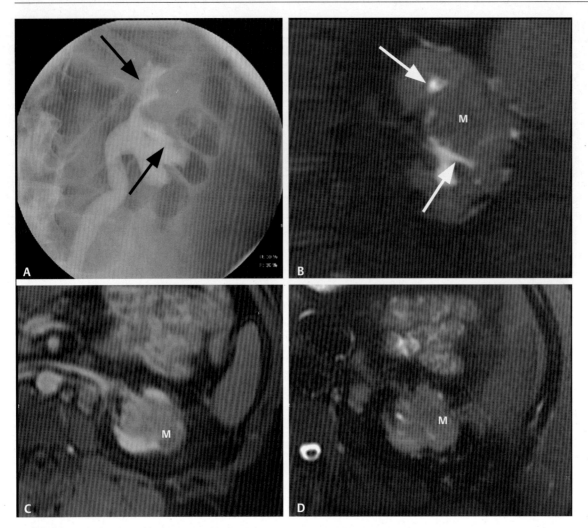

Fig. 46.4 History of advanced bladder carcinoma status post cystectomy now with abnormal screening cytology. **(A)** Retrograde ureterogram shows a left midpole mass splaying the collecting system of the upper and midpole (*arrows*). **(B–D)** Magnetic resonance urography. **(B)** Coronal T2-weighted image with fat saturation from MRU shows a mass (M) splaying the collecting system of the upper and midpole (*arrows*). Fat saturation axial **(C)** T1-weighted image following gadolinium and **(D)** T2-weighted fat saturation image show a collecting system mass (M).

- TCC of the renal pelvis or ureter will appear as a filling defect in the collecting system on either sequence (**Fig. 46.4B,D**). The differential diagnosis for a collecting system filling defect includes TCC, blood clot, stone, or fungus ball (rare).

- The detection of small urothelial lesions is limited, however, due to limited spatial resolution of MRU. Thus, MRU is proven useful as a second-tier imaging strategy in patients who cannot undergo CT-IVP. Indications for MRU over CT-IVP usually represent some contraindication to iodinated contrast materials (i.e., allergy) or in an effort to limit ionizing radiation (children, women of child-bearing age).

POSITRON EMISSION TOMOGRAPHY

- Limited data suggest positron emission tomography (PET) may be useful in detecting distant metastatic disease but may be imperfect in detecting a primary tumor due to tracer excretion into the collecting system, which may obscure the tumor.

Treatment

- Treatment for TCC of the renal pelvis and ureter is nephroureterectomy, which includes excision of the involved ureter and its kidney, as well as a cuff of bladder around the ipsilateral trigone.
- Cystoscopy and imaging follow-up (e.g., IVP or CT-IVP) are performed to screen the remaining urothelium (renal pelvis and ureter of the contralateral system, and the bladder) for recurrent or new TCC for up to 5 years after the initial tumor resection.

Prognosis

- Prognosis is based on the tumor stage (T designation) and pathologic cell-type grading.
- Patients with low-grade noninvasive tumors have an increased risk of recurrent and new TCC, but long-term survival is excellent.
- T1 disease has an ~74 to 95% 5-year survival rate, and T3/T4 disease has an ~15% 5-year survival rate.

PEARLS _____

- Filling defects that move within the collecting system represent a blood clot or nonopaque stones. Other filling defects require ureteroscopy with biopsy for definitive diagnosis.
- Short-term follow-up can also be used to determine if a filling defect resolves.

Suggested Readings

Baron RL, McClennan BL, Lee JK, Lawson TL. Computed tomography of transitional-cell carcinoma of the renal pelvis and ureter. Radiology 1982;144(1):125–130.

Caoili EM, Cohan RH, Inampudi P, et al. MDCT urography of upper tract urothelial neoplasms. AJR Am J Roentgenol 2005;184(6):1873–1881.

Genega EM, Porter CR. Urothelial neoplasms of the kidney and ureter: an epidemiologic, pathologic, and clinical review. Am J Clin Pathol 2002;117(Suppl):S36–S48.

Obuchi M, Ishigami K, Takahashi K, et al. Gadolinium-enhanced fat-suppressed T1-weighted imaging for staging ureteral carcinoma: correlation with histopathology. AJR Am J Roentgenol 2007;188(3):W256–W261.

Urban BA, Buckley J, Soyer P, Scherrer A, Fishman EK. CT appearance of transitional cell carcinoma of the renal pelvis, I: Early-stage disease. AJR Am J Roentgenol 1997;169(1):157–161.

Urban BA, Buckley J, Soyer P, Scherrer A, Fishman EK. CT appearance of transitional cell carcinoma of the renal pelvis, II: Advanced-stage disease. AJR Am J Roentgenol 1997;169(1):163–168.

Zhang J, Lefkowitz RA, Bach A. Imaging of kidney cancer. Radiol Clin North Am 2007;45(1):119–147.

CASE 47

Clinical Presentation

A 50-year-old female presents with persistent hematuria.

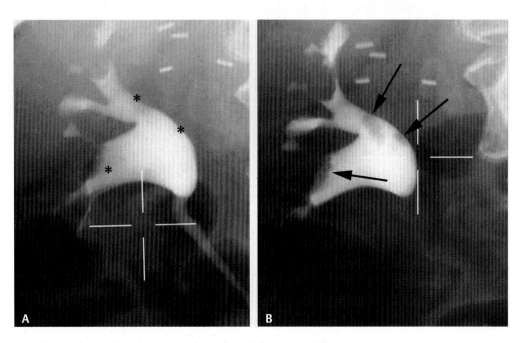

Fig. 47.1 Retrograde pyelogram. **(A)** Initial and **(B)** 9-month follow-up.

Radiologic Findings

- Multiple filling defects are seen in the renal pelvis on the initial study (*asterisks,* **Fig. 47.1A**).
- Defects have increased in size and conspicuity on follow-up (*arrows,* **Fig. 47.1B**).

Diagnosis

Progressive transitional cell carcinoma (TCC) of the renal pelvis

Differential Diagnosis

- Pyelitis cystica
- Nonopaque stones
- Blood clot

Discussion

Background

Transitional cell carcinomas of the renal pelvis and ureter are uncommon compared with bladder cancer. TCCs of the renal pelvis and ureters account for 4 to 15% and 1% of all TCCs of the urinary tract, respectively. Risk factors are similar to those for bladder cancer and include smoking, chemical exposure in certain industries (e.g., dye, leather, rubber), chronic irritation from stones or infection, cyclophosphamide treatment, and analgesic abuse. Males are affected more often than females. Most tumors are seen in the 6th to 7th decade. Multifocal tumor is found pathologically in up to 30% of patients originally thought to have a solitary tumor. From 25 to 75% of patients with upper tract TCC may subsequently develop bladder cancer.

Clinical Findings

Patients present with gross hematuria (75%), flank pain (30%), or a palpable mass (10%), but some present with no specific sign or symptom.

Pathology

Ninety percent of upper tract lesions are TCC. Both papillary and flat growth patterns are encountered. Tumors are staged based on the TNM (tumor size, node involvement, and metastasis status) system (see the appendix). Squamous cell and adenocarcinomas make up 7 and 1% of upper tract neoplasms, respectively.

Imaging Findings

RADIOGRAPHY/RETROGRADE PYELOGRAM/INTRAVENOUS PYELOGRAM

- Pyelitis cystica is an inflammatory process that produces smooth, well-marginated urothelial filling defects, which would not show this type of growth.
- Stones could produce enlarging filling defects with stone growth; nonopaque stones cannot be completely excluded on the intravenous pyelogram (IVP). Opaque stones would be detected on initial scout KUB.
- Blood clots are unlikely to grow and remain in the same positions in the renal pelvis.
- Persistent hematuria in the presence of progressive filling defects would make TCC the most likely diagnosis.
- Filling defects on contrasted studies like IVP are most often calculi, cancer, or clots, known as "the three C's." Progressive enlargement strongly favors TCC.

COMPUTED TOMOGRAPHY

- A stone would be very high density, not seen in this case.
- A clot or a polyp can appear as soft tissue density, similar to TCC, but it will not produce the "goblet sign" (see Case 48) with distal dilatation of the ureter.

ULTRASOUND

- Ultrasound would be a simple test to exclude nonopaque stones, as they would be hyperechoic and produce shadowing.

MAGNETIC RESONANCE IMAGING

- TCC of the renal pelvis or ureter will appear as a filling defect in the collecting system. The differential diagnosis for a collecting system filling defect includes blood clot, stone, or fungus ball (rare).
- The detection of small urothelial lesions is limited, however, due to limited spatial resolution of magnetic resonance urography (MRU). Thus, MRU is proven useful as a second-tier imaging strategy in patients who cannot undergo CT-IVP. Indications for MRU over CT-IVP usually represent some contraindication to iodinated contrast material (i.e., contrast sensitivity) or an effort to limit ionizing radiation (e.g., in children or women of child-bearing age).

Treatment

- Treatment for TCC of the renal pelvis and/or ureter is nephroureterectomy, which includes excision of the involved ureter and its kidney, as well as a cuff of bladder around the ipsilateral trigone.

Prognosis

- Prognosis is based on the tumor stage (T designation) and cell-type grading.
- Patients with low-grade noninvasive tumors have an increased risk of recurrent and new TCC, but long-term survival is excellent.
- T1 disease has an ~74 to 95% 5-year survival rate, and T3/T4 disease has an ~15% 5-year survival rate.

PEARLS _____

- Filling defects that move within the collecting system represent blood clots or nonopaque stones. Other filling defects require ureteroscopy with biopsy for a definitive diagnosis.

Suggested Readings

Baron RL, McClennan BL, Lee JK, Lawson TL. Computed tomography of transitional-cell carcinoma of the renal pelvis and ureter. Radiology 1982;144(1):125–130.

Caoili EM, Cohan RH, Inampudi P, et al. MDCT urography of upper tract urothelial neoplasms. AJR Am J Roentgenol 2005;184(6):1873–1881.

Genega EM, Porter CR. Urothelial neoplasms of the kidney and ureter: an epidemiologic, pathologic, and clinical review. Am J Clin Pathol 2002;117(Suppl):S36–S48.

Obuchi M, Ishigami K, Takahashi K, et al. Gadolinium-enhanced fat-suppressed T1-weighted imaging for staging ureteral carcinoma: correlation with histopathology. AJR Am J Roentgenol 2007;188(3):W256–W261.

Urban BA, Buckley J, Soyer P, Scherrer A, Fishman EK. CT appearance of transitional cell carcinoma of the renal pelvis, I: Early-stage disease. AJR Am J Roentgenol 1997;169(1):157–161.

Urban BA, Buckley J, Soyer P, Scherrer A, Fishman EK. CT appearance of transitional cell carcinoma of the renal pelvis, II: Advanced-stage disease. AJR Am J Roentgenol 1997;169(1):163–168.

Zhang J, Lefkowitz RA, Bach A. Imaging of kidney cancer. Radiol Clin North Am 2007;45(1):119–147.

CASE 48

Clinical Presentation

A 65-year-old male presents with hematuria. The scout radiograph is negative.

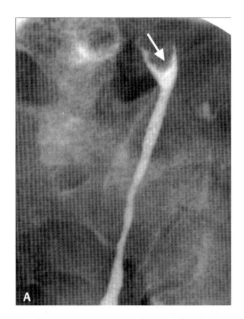

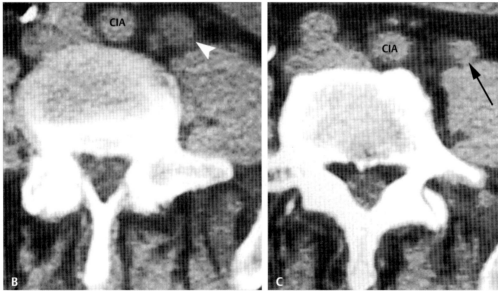

Fig. 48.1 **(A)** Retrograde pyelogram. Enhanced computed tomography scans **(B)** just above the retrograde filling defect and **(C)** at the level of the retrograde filling defect. CIA, common iliac artery.

Radiologic Findings

- On a retrograde pyelogram, a ureteral filling defect creating the goblet sign is present (*arrow*, **Fig. 48.1A**).
- On computed tomography (CT), a dilated ureter is seen immediately above the filling defect (*arrowhead*, in **Fig. 48.1B**).

- A solid enhancing ureteral tumor (*arrow*, **Fig. 48.1C**) is seen on CT and at the level of the filling defect on the retrograde pyelogram (**Fig. 48.1A**).

Diagnosis

Transitional cell carcinoma (TCC) of the ureter

Differential Diagnosis

- Ureteral stone
- Ureteral clot
- Ureteral polyp

Discussion

Background

Transitional cell carcinoma of the ureter is uncommon compared with bladder cancer. Ureteral TCC accounts for ~1% of all TCCs of the urinary tract. Risk factors are similar to those for bladder cancer and include smoking, chemical exposure in certain industries (e.g., dye, leather, rubber), chronic irritation from stones or infection, cyclophosphamide treatment, and analgesic abuse. Males are affected more often than females. Most tumors are seen in the 6th to 7th decade. Multifocal tumor is found pathologically in up to 30% of patients originally thought to have a solitary tumor. From 25 to 75% of patients with upper tract TCC may subsequently develop bladder cancer.

Clinical Findings

Patients present with gross hematuria (75%), flank pain (30%), or a palpable mass (10%), but some present with no specific sign or symptom.

Pathology

Ninety percent of upper tract lesions are TCCs. Both papillary and flat growth patterns are encountered. Tumors are staged based on the TNM (tumor size, node involvement, and metastasis status) system (see Section M, Renal Pelvis and Ureter Tumor Staging, in Appendix). Squamous cell and adenocarcinomas make up 7 and 1% of upper tract neoplasms, respectively.

Imaging Findings

RADIOGRAPHY/RETROGRADE PYELOGRAM

- A ureteral stone will dilate the ureter proximal to the stone but not distal to the stone because of ureteral spasm produced by the stone. On retrograde studies, this would appear as a narrowed region of the ureter.
- A stone would be seen on the scout film, not seen in this case.
- A clot or polyp can appear as soft tissue density, similar to TCC, as seen in **Fig. 48.1C,** but it will not produce the goblet sign with distal dilatation of the ureter on retrograde pyelogram.
- A filling defect with dilatation of the ureter below the defect produces the goblet sign, which is essentially diagnostic of TCC.

COMPUTED TOMOGRAPHY

- A stone would be very high density, not seen in this case.
- A clot or polyp can appear as soft tissue density but will not produce the goblet sign.

Treatment

- Treatment for TCC of the ureter is nephroureterectomy, which includes excision of the involved ureter and its kidney, as well as a cuff of bladder around the ipsilateral trigone.
- Cystoscopy and imaging follow-up [e.g., intravenous pyelogram (IVP) or CT-IVP] is performed to screen the remaining urothelium (renal pelvis and ureter of the contralateral system, and the bladder) for recurrent or new TCC for up to 5 years after the initial tumor resection.

Prognosis

- Prognosis is based on the tumor stage (T designation) and pathologic cell-type grading.
- Patients with low-grade noninvasive tumors have an increased risk of recurrent and new TCC, but long-term survival is excellent.
- T1 disease has an ~74 to 95% 5-year survival rate, and T3/T4 disease has an ~15% 5-year survival rate.

Suggested Readings

Daniels RE. The goblet sign. Radiology 1999;210(3):737–738.

CASE 49

Clinical Presentation

A 45-year-old male presents with an abnormal bladder ultrasound.

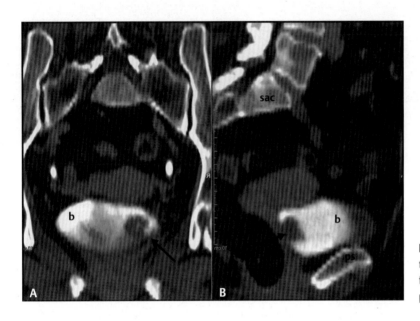

Fig. 49.1 Coronal **(A)** and sagittal **(B)** reconstruction of the bladder from CT-IVP. sac, sacrum; b, bladder; ps, pubic symphysis

Radiologic Findings

- Polypoid left bladder filling defect (*arrows,* **Fig. 49.1A,B**)

Diagnosis

Transitional cell carcinoma (TCC) of the bladder

Differential Diagnosis

- Bladder stone
- Bladder clot
- Ureterocele

Discussion

Background

Bladder cancer is the most common type of urothelial cancer. Men are affected 3 to 4 times more often than women, and Caucasian patients ~2 times more often than African-American patients. The median age of diagnosis is 70 years. Risk factors include smoking and industrial exposure (dye, leather, rubber industries) to chemicals, which are excreted into the urine. Pelvic irradiation or previous cyclophosphamide treatments both increase bladder cancer risks. Twenty-five to 75% of patients with upper tract urothelial carcinoma will develop bladder cancer. Patients with bladder cancer, however, may develop subsequent upper tract urothelial neoplasms in only ~5% of cases.

Clinical Findings

The most common presenting sign (85% of patients) is gross but painless hematuria. Urinary frequency and/or urgency or dysuria will be seen due to tumor irritation and/or reduced bladder capacity.

Pathology

Most (> 90%) bladder cancers are urothelial neoplasms (arising from the epithelial lining of the genitourinary tract). Squamous cell carcinoma (3–7%) often occurs in patients with chronic irritation to the bladder, such as that seen with chronic cystitis, due to long-standing indwelling catheters or bladder stones. Adenocarcinomas (2%) include urachal adenocarcinoma arising from a urachal remnant at the anterior bladder dome.

Imaging Findings

COMPUTED TOMOGRAPHY

- Bladder-filling defects on computed tomography (CT) (**Fig. 49.1**) are often nonspecific, with cystoscopy needed to confirm the diagnosis.
- Stones, however, would be apparent on the noncontrast images as very high density structures.
- Noncontrast bladder images may show a high-density blood clot or soft tissue density if the lesion is large, but these entities may not be distinguishable on late-phase images with the bladder filled with contrast (i.e., they will both appear as filling defects).
- Immediate post-enhancement images may show an enhancing tumor (**Fig. 49.2**).
- A ureterocele typically is more sharply marginated than a neoplasm, as in this case.
- See Section C, "Genitourinary Specific Imaging" in the Appendix for the CT-IVP protocol.

RADIOGRAPHY

- Most bladder-filling defects on IVP are not specific and can represent tumor, stones, or clot; they require cystoscopy for a definitive diagnosis.
- Stones most often will have a smooth surface and be apparent on the scout radiograph.
- A clot can have an irregular appearance and cannot always be distinguished from tumor on IVP.
- A stippled appearance of the lesion due to contrast within the interstices of the frondlike surface of the tumor is consistent with TCC (**Fig. 49.3**). A blood clot may have a similar appearance.

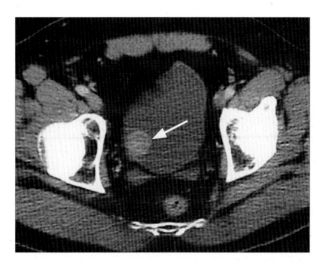

Fig. 49.2 An immediate enhanced pelvic computed tomography scan shows an enhancing right bladder mass (*arrow*), indicative of transitional cell carcinoma.

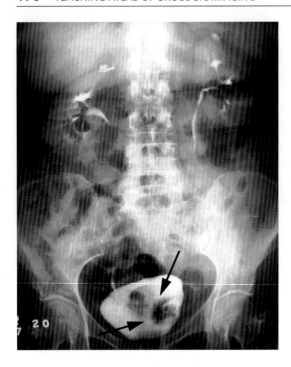

Fig. 49.3 A 20-minute intravenous pyelogram radiograph demonstrates a left bladder mass with a stippled appearance (*arrows*).

ULTRASOUND

- Ultrasound can be used to detect an echogenic but nonopaque stone.
- Other lesions on the differential diagnosis may be difficult to differentiate with ultrasound.

POSITRON EMISSION TOMOGRAPHY

- Excretion of tracer into the bladder limits positron emission tomography (PET) as a useful staging modality for primary bladder cancer.
- PET's role is limited to the evaluation of metastatic disease.

Treatment

- Treatment for noninvasive bladder cancer involves local tumor excision via cystoscopy [transurethral resection of bladder tumor (TURBT)] with fulguration of the surrounding area by Bovie electrocautery.
- Intravesical bacille Calmette-Guérin (BCG) instillation may also be given.
- Follow-up screening imaging studies of the urothelium (CT-IVP) are performed for up to 5 years due to the high incidence of recurrent and/or metachronous lesions.

Prognosis

- A major determinant is the depth of tumor invasion into the bladder wall (i.e., tumor T stage), along with bladder tumor cytologic grading, but this grading system is not yet universally utilized.
- One grading system includes grade 1 (low grade, well differentiated) to grade 3 (high grade, poorly differentiated).
- Tumors that do not violate the muscular layer are considered noninvasive, with up to 80% 5-year survival rate.
- Muscle invasive cancer survival rate is much reduced (~40% at 5 years).

PEARLS

- BCG is an attenuated mycobacterium that has demonstrated antitumor activity and is used as intravesical chemotherapy in nonmuscle invasive bladder cancer.

Suggested Readings

Dietbert H. Neoplasms of the urinary bladder. In: Pollack H, ed. Clinical Urography. Vol 2. Philadelphia: WB Saunders; 1990:1353–1380.

Dyer RB, Chen MY, Zagoria RJ. Intravenous urography: technique and interpretation. Radiographics 2001;21(4):799–821, discussion 822–794.

Jemal A, Siegel R, Ward E, Murray T, Xu J, Thun MJ. Cancer statistics, 2007. CA Cancer J Clin 2007;57(1):43–66.

Messing E. Urothelial tumors of the bladder. In: Wein, ed. Campbell-Walsh Urology. St. Louis: Elsevier; 2007:2407–2446.

Zhang J, Gerst S, Lefkowitz RA, Bach A. Imaging of bladder cancer. Radiol Clin North Am 2007;45(1):183–205.

CASE 50

Clinical Presentation

A 45-year-old female presents with gross hematuria.

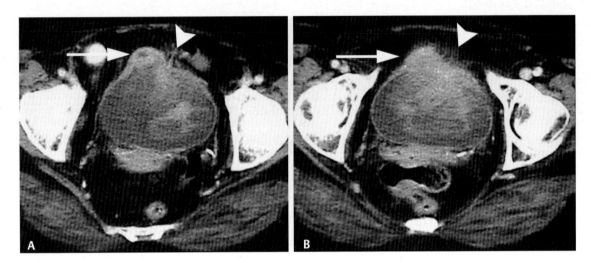

Fig. 50.1 Enhanced computed tomography scans at two levels through the bladder.

Radiologic Findings

- Enhancing bladder mass (*arrows,* **Fig. 50.1**)
- Mass is anterior, superior, and midline.
- Stranding of fat around the anterior bladder (*arrowheads,* **Fig. 50.1**)

Diagnosis

Urachal adenocarcinoma (UAC)

Differential Diagnosis

- Transitional cell carcinoma (TCC) of the bladder
- Extrinsic tumor invading the bladder
- Blood clot
- Infected urachal remnant

Discussion

Background

The urachus is an embryologic structure that connects the allantois (primitive gut) to the cloaca (precursor to the fetal bladder). The urachus obliterates and becomes the median umbilical ligament as the bladder moves into the fetal pelvis. When the urachus persists, varying structures may be seen to arise from the anterosuperior aspect of the bladder, including a patent urachus (50%), urachal cyst (30%), vesicourachal sinus (15%), and urachal diverticulum (5%) (**Fig. 50.2**). Most of these lesions (except for patent urachus) are asymptomatic, although they may become infected. Malignancy aris-

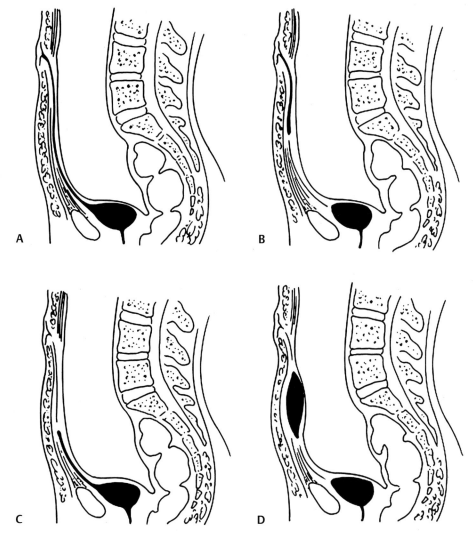

Fig. 50.2   Drawings of various urachal abnormalities. **(A)** Patent urachus. **(B)** Vesicourachal sinus. **(C)** Urachal diverticulum. **(D)** Urachal cyst.

ing in the urachus is derived from glandular tissue, and 90% of cases are adenocarcinomas. UAC represents < 1% of bladder cancer.

Clinical Findings

UAC is a rare neoplasm. Hematuria is the most common clinical finding in > 80% of cases.

Pathology

UAC is an aggressive adenocarcinoma in most cases.

Imaging Findings

COMPUTED TOMOGRAPHY

- Tumor in this case has only minimal extension outside the bladder (*arrowheads*, **Fig. 50.1**), and nonurachal bladder adenocarcinoma and TCC of the bladder could have a similar appearance.

- Extrinsic tumor invading the bladder is unlikely with the bulk of the tumor within the bladder lumen, as in this case.
- A blood clot would not enhance.
- A differentiation between infected urachal remnant and UAC cannot be made based on imaging findings alone.
- UAC typically presents as a midline mass, seen at the bladder dome, extending outside the bladder. It often contains calcifications.
- The anterior midline position in this case is suggestive of, but not conclusive for, urachal tumor.

RADIOGRAPHY

- A filling defect at the bladder dome on intravenous urography suggests the possibility of UAC.

ULTRASOUND

- Ultrasound will show a heterogeneous mass in the appropriate position for the urachus.
- Calcifications will demonstrate typical echogenic interface with posterior acoustic shadowing.
- Mucin within the cystic components will be heterogeneous or echogenic (i.e., the cystic components are not anechoic as one might expect because the fluid is not simple but rather is mucinous).

Treatment

- Resection of the urachal mass and adjacent bladder is the treatment of choice.

Prognosis

- Survival is poor (< 20%) at 5 years.

Suggested Readings

Ashley RA, Inman BA, Sebo TJ, et al. Urachal carcinoma: clinicopathologic features and long-term outcomes of an aggressive malignancy. Cancer 2006;107(4):712–720.

Mengiardi B, Wiesner W, Stoffel F, Terracciano L, Freitag P. Case 44: adenocarcinoma of the urachus. Radiology 2002;222(3):744–747.

Yu JS, Kim KW, Lee HJ, et al. Urachal remnant diseases: spectrum of CT and US findings. Radiographics 2001;21(2):451–461.

CASE 51

Clinical Presentation

A 60-year-old male presents with hematuria and a history of bladder cancer.

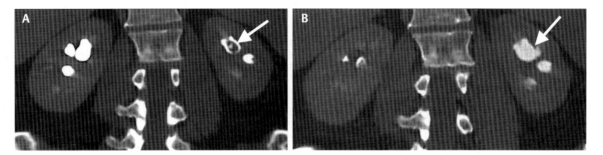

Fig. 51.1 Computed tomography urography with delayed phase imaging. **(A)** Initial study and **(B)** 1-month follow-up without interval therapy.

Radiologic Findings

- Filling defect in the left upper pole calyx (*arrow,* **Fig. 51.1A**)
- Significant decrease in the defect on 1-month follow-up (*arrow,* **Fig. 51.1B**)

Diagnosis

Blood clot

Differential Diagnosis

- Transitional cell carcinoma (TCC)
- Stone
- Fungus ball
- Papillary necrosis

Discussion

Background

Hematuria is the presence of blood in the urine. It is a common indication for a genitourinary (GU) work-up, especially in adult patients where GU malignancy must be excluded. Gross hematuria is more likely to yield a positive finding on a GU work-up than is microscopic hematuria.

Clinical Findings

Microscopic hematuria is detected on urinalysis and may be asymptomatic. Gross hematuria usually brings the patient to medical attention. Both entities should result in a urologic work-up to exclude GU malignancy. Blood clots present in the urine may be amorphous (and may originate from the bladder, prostate, or urethra), or they may be wormlike, suggesting they are from the ureter. If flank pain is found in association with hematuria, the leading diagnosis is that of calculus disease with obstruction.

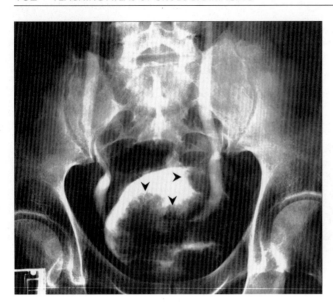

Fig. 51.2 Gross hematuria. Conventional intravenous pyelogram coned to the bladder shows polypoid filling defects in the bladder (*arrowheads*). A differential diagnosis includes bladder tumor, blood clot, and fungus balls. Hydroureter was noted bilaterally. Following copious bladder irrigation, a bladder ultrasound showed a normal bladder consistent with blood clots, which resolved.

Pathology

Microscopic hematuria is defined as significant if there are three or more red blood cells per high-power field on microscopy. Gross hematuria is visibly red urine with or without blood clots.

Imaging Findings

COMPUTED TOMOGRAPHY

- TCC is a possibility on the initial computed tomography (CT) study (**Fig. 51.1A**), but not after there is significant improvement, as shown on the 1-month follow-up (**Fig. 51.1B**).
- Low-density stones could produce the filling defects seen, but the rapid improvement is much more indicative of resolving blood clots. Stones would also be apparent on the noncontrast phase of the CT-IVP (not shown).
- Fungus balls are an uncommon cause of a filling defect, and rapid resolution would not be expected, especially as no specific therapy was instituted against fungus.
- Papillary necrosis is usually found in diabetic patients often in association with urinary tract infection and/or obstruction, which is not the clinical presentation in this case.

RADIOGRAPHY

- Bladder filling defects as well as renal collecting system filling defects on IVP can represent a clot, cancer, calculi (the three Cs), or fungus ball. Other than opaque stones, these entities often cannot be distinguished on the initial study. Retrograde pyelogram versus ureteroscopy may be required for a definitive diagnosis (**Fig. 51.2**).

Treatment

- If blood clots in the bladder cause obstruction, bladder lavage may be performed with instillation of high volumes of sterile saline and bladder catheter drainage.
- Treat the underlying cause of the bleeding.

Prognosis

- Depends on the underlying cause

PEARLS _____

- The etiology of noncalcified renal collecting system filling defects is not always apparent, and short-term follow-up is a simple method to determine the etiology of these filling defects, separating blood clots from neoplasm.

Suggested Readings

Gerber G, Brendler C. Evaluation of the urologic patient: history, physical examination, and urinalysis. In: Wein A, ed. Campbell-Walsh Urology. 9th ed. Philadelphia: Saunders Elsevier; 2007:81–105.

Joffe SA, Servaes S, Okon S, Horowitz M. Multi-detector row CT urography in the evaluation of hematuria. Radiographics 2003;23(6):1441–1455, discussion 1455–1456.

CASE 52

Clinical Presentation

A 45-year-old male presents with hematuria.

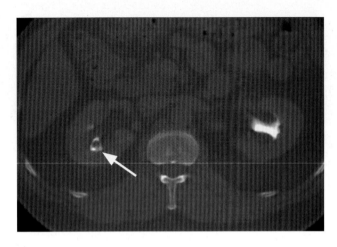

Fig. 52.1 Delayed image from CT-IVP.

Radiologic Findings

- A smooth, sharply marginated filling defect in the right posterior calyx (*arrow,* **Fig. 52.1**)

Diagnosis

Prominent papilla

Differential Diagnosis

- Transitional cell carcinoma (TCC)
- Blood clot
- Stone

Discussion

Background

Filling defects in the contrast of a CT-IVP, IVP, or retrograde and antegrade pyelogram include stones, tumor, clot, and fungus ball. In the calyceal system, a prominent renal papilla may mimic any of these entities.

Clinical Findings

The findings should be correlated with the reason the patient is having the genitourinary (GU) exam, but findings are nonspecific for a prominent papilla.

Pathology

Compound calyces and their papilla seen most commonly at the polar regions may present as disconcerting filling defects. An occasional aberrant papilla in an unexpected location may also present as a mass. Oblique imaging on IVP often will uncover the true nature of the finding, as it melds imperceptibly with the medullary pyramid. In equivocal cases, additional studies may be required.

Imaging Findings

COMPUTED TOMOGRAPHY

- The filling defect in this case has the position of a papilla, but it was larger than all other papillae. This finding is not specific, and neither blood clot nor tumor can be reliably excluded.
- Most calcium stones are similar in density to contrast and do not produce a lucent filling defect, as seen in this case. Even a uric acid stone would be more opaque than the defect in this case. Stones would also be excluded on the noncontrast phase of the CT-IVP.
- The diagnosis in this case was made with ureteroscopy.

Treatment

- Once a benign diagnosis is made, no specific treatment is necessary.

Prognosis

- Excellent

Suggested Readings

Dyer RB, Chen MY, Zagoria RJ. Intravenous urography: technique and interpretation. Radiographics 2001;21(4):799–821, discussion 822–824.

CASE 53

Clinical Presentation

A 50-year-old male on allopurinol presents with hematuria.

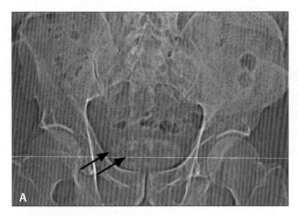

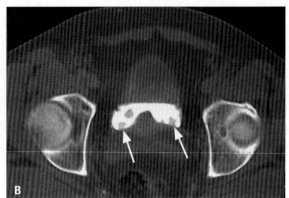

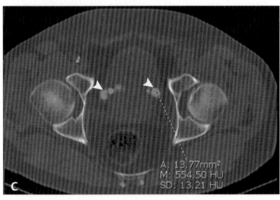

Fig. 53.1 CT-IVP **(A)** Scout view, **(B)** delayed enhanced images, and **(C)** initial unenhanced images through the bladder.

Radiologic Findings

- Mildly opaque stones on the scout view (*black arrows,* **Fig. 53.1A**)
- Bladder filling defects on delayed CT-IVP (*white arrows,* **Fig. 53.1B**)
- Bladder stones on unenhanced images (*arrowheads,* **Fig. 53.1C**). Density of the stones is ~554 Hounsfield units (HU) (region of interest measurement), most likely representing uric acid stones, which are generally in the 400 to 500 HU range.

Diagnosis

Bladder stones

Differential Diagnosis

- Bladder tumors
- Clots
- Cystitis glandularis

Discussion

Background

Bladder calculi may be migrant, primary, or secondary. Migrant calculi represent stones from the upper genitourinary (GU) tract that have migrated to the bladder. Secondary stones are by far the most common; they are found in the bladder in up to 5% of adults with urolithiasis caused by urinary stasis, foreign bodies, or infection due to bladder outlet obstruction (75% of cases). Neurogenic bladder is a source of secondary stones. Primary stones are idiopathic and rare, and are found in children in underdeveloped countries.

Clinical Findings

Most bladder stones are asymptomatic and found incidentally. Most patients are male, with the most common cause being bladder outlet obstruction from benign prostatic hypertrophy.

Pathology

The pathology depends on the cause of the stone formation. The most common stone type is calcium oxalate. Uric acid stones may be found in acidic urine. Infection stones are typically ammonium magnesium phosphate.

Imaging Findings

COMPUTED TOMOGRAPHY

- Filling defects are not specific once contrast fills the bladder. They could represent any of the differential diagnoses listed.
- The scout view shows mildly opaque stones, and noncontrast CT clearly demonstrates stones.
- Neither tumor, clot, nor cystitis glandularis would appear as high density on noncontrast CT, as in this case. Also, none would appear opaque on a scout view. A fresh blood clot could appear as highly dense but < 100 HU and not in the 500 HU range, as in this case. Therefore, tumor, clot, and cystitis glandularis are excluded.
- Bladder stones are best identified on unenhanced CT scan (**Fig. 53.1C**), where all stones, except for rare Indinavir and protein matrix stones, will be visibly dense.

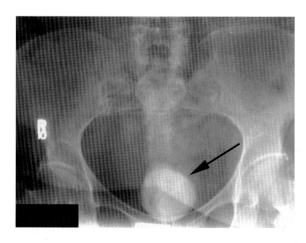

Fig. 53.2 Intravenous pyelogram scout film coned to the bladder. A large, dense stone is seen within the bladder (*arrow*). On contrast-enhanced images, the stone was inconspicuous.

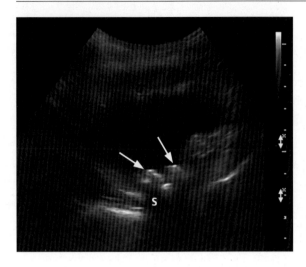

Fig. 53.3   Sonogram of the bladder. In the dependent portion of the bladder, multiple echogenic foci (*arrows*) with strong posterior acoustic shadowing (S) represent bladder calculi.

- Not all bladder stones will be visible on CT after contrast fills the bladder. Stone conspicuity in the contrast-filled bladder depends on the density of the stone relative to the density of contrast.

RADIOGRAPHY

- Opaque stones are often visible on abdominal radiographs (**Fig. 53.2**).
- Bladder stones may or may not be visible on IVP with the bladder filled with contrast. Stone conspicuity in the contrast-filled bladder depends on the density of the stone relative to the density of the contrast.

ULTRASOUND

- Essentially, all bladder stones will present as echogenic foci with acoustic shadowing (**Fig. 53.3**).

Treatment

- Symptomatic stone removal via cystoscopy, lithotripsy, or dissolution is appropriate. The underlying cause should be sought and treated as well.

Prognosis

- Generally good

Suggested Readings

Caoili EM, Cohan RH, Korobkin M, et al. Urinary tract abnormalities: initial experience with multidetector row CT urography. Radiology 2002;222(2):353–360.

Ho K, Segura J. Lower urinary tract calculi. In: Wein A, ed. Campbell-Walsh Urology. 9th ed. Philadelphia: Saunders Elsevier; 2007:2663–2673.

CASE 54

Clinical Presentation

A patient in a motor vehicle collision presents with microscopic hematuria.

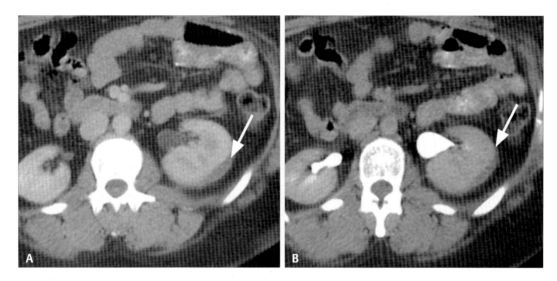

Fig. 54.1   Grade 1 renal injury. **(A)** A contrast-enhanced computed tomography (CT) scan and **(B)** a 10-minute delayed CT.

Radiologic Findings

- Small subcapsular fluid collection indenting the left lateral renal cortex (*arrow*, **Fig. 54.1**), consistent with a small subcapsular hematoma

Diagnosis

Grade 1 renal injury, subcapsular hematoma

Differential Diagnosis

- Grade 1 renal contusion
- Grade 2 renal laceration
- Grade 3 renal laceration

Discussion

Background

The majority of renal injuries result from blunt abdominal trauma, with motor vehicle collisions being the most common cause. The second most common cause of renal injury is penetrating trauma (e.g., a gunshot wound). Eighty percent of renal injuries are minor, but in the setting of penetrating trauma, the severity of injury (e.g., vascular injury) increases.

To quantify the renal injury, assist in treatment decision making, and estimate prognosis, a grading scale is helpful. The American Association for the Surgery of Trauma (AAST) has validated a renal injury scale (www.aast.org) that corresponds to the abbreviated injury scale used to determine a patient's injury severity score (see Section I, "Adrenal Organ Injury Scale" in the Appendix).

Clinical Findings

Hematuria is present in up to 95% of cases where there is a renal injury. However, there is no direct relationship between the presence or absence of hematuria and the severity of the renal injury.

Pathology

If the renal capsule is not torn, blood collects underneath it, which results in mass effect on the adjacent renal parenchyma (**Fig. 54.2**).

Imaging Findings

The technique of choice for imaging the hemodynamically stable patient is contrast-enhanced computed tomography (CT) of the abdomen and pelvis performed in the portal venous phase and again with 10-minute delayed imaging through the kidneys, ureters, and bladder if there is suspicion of a genitourinary (GU) injury. CT accurately identifies vascular and parenchymal injuries, perinephric hematomas, and urine extravasation. The main objectives of imaging are to (1) grade the injury, (2) identify any preexisting renal lesion separable from the acute traumatic injury, (3) document a normal contralateral kidney, and (4) document associated injuries.

COMPUTED TOMOGRAPHY

- A renal contusion will present as an ill-defined or discrete area of patchy or poor renal enhancement in the setting of trauma, not seen in this case.
- No laceration is present in this case excluding grade 2 or grade 3 injury.

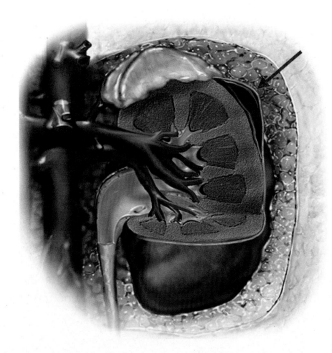

Fig. 54.2 Drawing of a grade 1 renal injury with a subcapsular hematoma (*arrow*).

- An acute subcapsular hematoma, grade 1 injury, will appear as a crescent or lens-shaped area of fluid between the renal parenchyma and the renal capsule (**Fig. 54.1**). The hematoma will be high density precontrast but will appear visually low density postcontrast compared with the enhancing renal parenchyma. If the renal capsule is not torn, blood collects underneath it, which results in mass effect on the adjacent renal parenchyma, resulting in the characteristic lens-shaped or crescentric collection.

ULTRASOUND

- Ultrasound has little role in the evaluation of an acute renal injury, although it can be used to follow known fluid collections or to follow up on hydronephrosis.

MAGNETIC RESONANCE IMAGING

- There is little use for magnetic resonance imaging in the evaluation of GU injury in the acute trauma setting.

Treatment

- Observation

Prognosis

- Excellent prognosis for the preservation of renal function

PEARLS

- Acute subcapsular hematoma will appear relatively low density compared with enhancing renal parenchyma even though it is high-density fresh blood.

Suggested Readings

Al-Qudah HS, Santucci RA. Complications of renal trauma. Urol Clin North Am 2006;33(1):41–53.

Kawashima A, Sandler CM, Corl FM, et al. Imaging of renal trauma: a comprehensive review. Radiographics 2001;21(3):557–574.

McAninch J, Santucci R. Renal and ureteral trauma. In: Wein A, ed. Campbell-Walsh Urology. 9th ed. Philadelphia: Saunders Elsevier; 2007:1274–1278.

Park SJ, Kim JK, Kim KW, Cho KS. MDCT Findings of renal trauma. AJR Am J Roentgenol 2006;187(2):541–547.

Santucci RA, McAninch JW, Safir M, et al. Validation of the American Association for the Surgery of Trauma organ injury severity scale for the kidney. J Trauma 2001;50(2):195–200.

Santucci RA, Wessells H, Bartsch G, et al. Evaluation and management of renal injuries: consensus statement of the renal trauma subcommittee. BJU Int 2004;93(7):937–954.

CASE 55

Clinical Presentation

Blunt abdominal trauma with hematuria

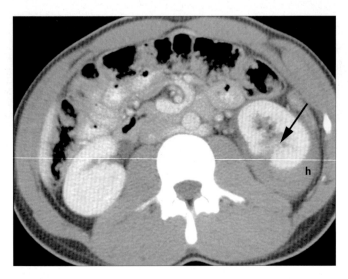

Fig. 55.1 Contrast-enhanced computed tomography scan.

Radiologic Findings

- Moderately sized high-density perinephric hematoma (h, **Fig. 55.1**) confined to Gerota fascia with an associated small (< 1 cm) renal cortical laceration (*arrow,* **Fig. 55.1**)
- Left kidney displaced anteriorly by the perinephric hematoma

Diagnosis

Grade 2 renal injury, laceration < 1 cm, and perinephric hematoma

Differential Diagnosis

- Subcapsular hematoma
- Urinoma
- Ruptured abdominal aorta
- Grade 3 renal injury

Discussion

Background

Grades 2 and 3 renal injuries represent ~10 to 15% of all renal injuries.

Clinical Findings

Similar to grade 1 renal injury

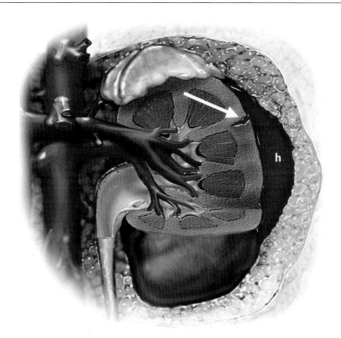

Fig. 55.2 Drawing of a type 2 renal injury with a perinephric hematoma (h) and laceration < 1 cm (*arrow*).

Pathology

- Nonexpanding perirenal hematoma confined to the renal retroperitoneum (**Fig. 55.2**)
- Cortical laceration < 1 cm without urinary extravasation

Imaging Findings

COMPUTED TOMOGRAPHY

- A subcapsular hematoma compresses the kidney rather than displacing the kidney, as in this case.
- Urinoma is excluded, as it would be water density on the early enhanced images.
- Type 3 renal injury includes laceration > 1 cm, not present in this case.
- A ruptured abdominal aortic aneurysm may present with a high-density collection in the left retroperitoneum, as seen in this case, but the scenarios are quite different. In the absence of an aneurysm, a ruptured aorta is less likely.
- Type 2 renal injury includes a perinephric hematoma confined to Gerota fascia (h, **Fig. 55.1**), as seen in this case. This may or may not be seen in association with a renal parenchymal laceration that is no more than 1 cm deep (*arrow,* **Fig. 55.1**) and does not involve the renal vessels or collecting system (i.e., no urinary extravasation).

Treatment

- In hemodynamically stable patients, observation of a perinephric hematoma to ensure that it is not expanding is acceptable.
- Follow-up imaging (i.e., 6 to 24 hours) is required to ensure there are no delayed complications (e.g., expanding hematoma, urinomas).

Prognosis

- Good for preservation of renal function

PEARLS _____

- Perinephric hematoma displaces the kidney, and subcapsular hematoma compresses the kidney.

Suggested Readings

Al-Qudah HS, Santucci RA. Complications of renal trauma. Urol Clin North Am 2006;33(1):41–53.

Kawashima A, Sandler CM, Corl FM, et al. Imaging of renal trauma: a comprehensive review. Radiographics 2001;21(3):557–574.

McAninch J, Santucci R. Renal and ureteral trauma. In: Wein A, ed. Campbell-Walsh Urology. 9th ed. Philadelphia: Saunders Elsevier; 2007:1274–1278.

Park SJ, Kim JK, Kim KW, Cho KS. MDCT Findings of renal trauma. AJR Am J Roentgenol 2006;187(2):541–547.

Santucci RA, McAninch JW, Safir M, et al. Validation of the American Association for the Surgery of Trauma organ injury severity scale for the kidney. J Trauma 2001;50(2):195–200.

Santucci RA, Wessells H, Bartsch G, et al. Evaluation and management of renal injuries: consensus statement of the renal trauma subcommittee. BJU Int 2004;93(7):937–954.

CASE 56

Clinical Presentation

A 30-year-old male in a motor vehicle collision

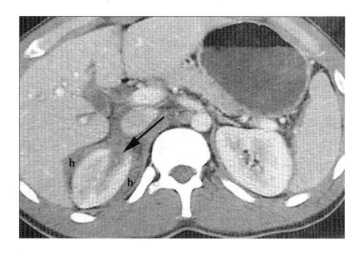

Fig. 56.1 Enhanced computed tomography scan through the kidneys.

Radiologic Findings

- Anterior linear defect in the right renal cortex consistent with a cortical laceration > 1 cm (*arrow,* **Fig. 56.1**)
- Perinephric fluid collections (h, **Fig. 56.1**)

Diagnosis

Grade 3 renal injury with a laceration > 1 cm and a perinephric hematoma

Differential Diagnosis

- Renal injury grade 2
- Subcapsular hematoma
- Shattered kidney

Discussion

Background

With greater traumatic mechanism, injury severity and associated injuries increase. Renal lacerations result from direct contact with the kidney or a secondary collision with the ribs or vertebrae or their fracture fragments.

Clinical Findings

Hematuria

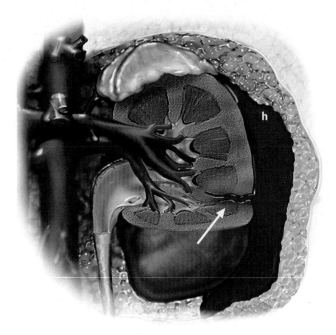

Fig. 56.2 Drawing of a type 3 renal injury with a laceration > 1 cm (*arrow*) and a perirenal hematoma (h).

Pathology

- Cortical laceration > 1 cm without urinary extravasation (**Fig. 56.2**)

Imaging Findings

COMPUTED TOMOGRAPHY

- Laceration seen anteriorly is > 1 cm, excluding a grade 2 injury.
- A subcapsular hematoma compresses the kidney, not evident in this case.
- Multiple deep lacerations are not present, excluding a shattered kidney (grade 5 injury).
- Grade 3 renal injury includes a renal parenchyma laceration > 1 cm.
- Delayed images are necessary to exclude extravasation of contrast (**Fig. 56.3**).

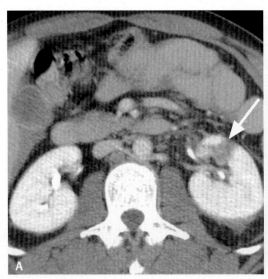
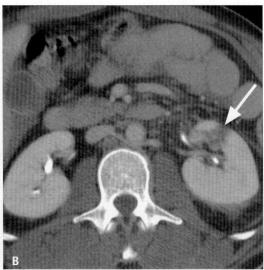

Fig. 56.3 Grade 3 renal injury. A 10-minute delayed contrast-enhanced computed tomography scan in **(A)** soft tissue windows and **(B)** wider windows shows a 2 cm laceration of the left midpole renal cortex (*arrows*) without associated urinary extravasation.

Treatment

- Observation in hemodynamically stable patients
- Follow-up dedicated genitourinary (GU) imaging should be performed when there is clinical concern for a delayed complication (e.g., renal abscess or renal arteriovenous fistula).

Prognosis

- Good prognosis for renal function

PEARLS _____

- When imaging GU trauma, delayed images should always be obtained to determine if perinephric fluid collections represent urinary extravasation or hematoma.

Suggested Readings

Al-Qudah HS, Santucci RA. Complications of renal trauma. Urol Clin North Am 2006;33(1):41–53.

Kawashima A, Sandler CM, Corl FM, et al. Imaging of renal trauma: a comprehensive review. Radiographics 2001;21(3):557–574.

McAninch J, Santucci R. Renal and ureteral trauma. In: Wein A, ed. Campbell-Walsh Urology. 9th ed. Philadelphia: Saunders Elsevier; 2007:1274–1278.

Park SJ, Kim JK, Kim KW, Cho KS. MDCT Findings of renal trauma. AJR Am J Roentgenol 2006;187(2):541–547.

Santucci RA, McAninch JW, Safir M, et al. Validation of the American Association for the Surgery of Trauma organ injury severity scale for the kidney. J Trauma 2001;50(2):195–200.

Santucci RA, Wessells H, Bartsch G, et al. Evaluation and management of renal injuries: consensus statement of the renal trauma subcommittee. BJU Int 2004;93(7):937–954.

CASE 57

Clinical Presentation

Automobile accident

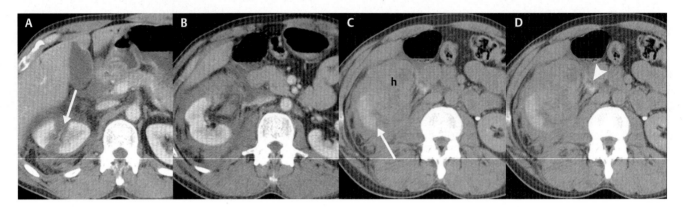

Fig. 57.1 **(A,B)** Contrast-enhanced computed tomography scans and **(C,D)** 10-minute delayed images through the right kidney.

Radiologic Findings

- Laceration of the right kidney > 1 cm extending to the collecting system (*arrow,* **Fig. 57.1A**)
- Large, high-density perinephric hematoma (h, **Fig. 57.1C**)
- Urinary contrast extravasation at the ureteropelvic junction (UPJ) (*arrowhead,* **Fig. 57.1D**)

Diagnosis

Grade 4 renal injury with a deep laceration and urinary contrast extravasation

Differential Diagnosis

- Grade 2 renal injury
- Grade 3 renal injury
- Grade 5 renal injury

Discussion

Background

Grades 4 and 5 injuries more often require surgical exploration, but conservative management for genitourinary (GU) trauma is generally indicated in stable patients.

Clinical Findings

The presence of hematuria does not correlate well with the stage of renal injury. In up to one third of patients with renal vascular injuries, hematuria may be absent.

198

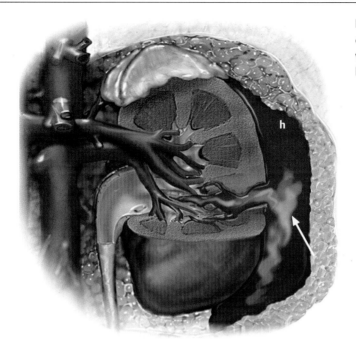

Fig. 57.2   Drawing of grade 4 renal trauma with a deep laceration extending to the collecting system with urinary extravasation (*arrow*) and perinephric hematoma (h).

Pathology

- Parenchymal laceration involving the cortex, medulla, and collecting system
- Limited vascular injury with contained hemorrhage (**Fig. 57.2**)

Imaging Findings

COMPUTED TOMOGRAPHY

- Grades 2 and 3 lacerations are excluded with the presence of urine extravasation.
- Shattered kidney diagnosis (grade 5) is reserved for severe renal parenchymal destruction where the kidney is fragmented, fragments are dispersed by intervening hematoma, vascular and collecting system structures are irreparably damaged, and little functional tissue remains, not seen in this case.
- Grade 4 renal injury includes laceration involving the cortex (**Fig. 57.1A**), medulla, and collecting system with associated urinary extravasation seen on delayed imaging (**Fig. 57.1C,D**). Grade 4 renal injury can also include segmental vascular injury, as in **Fig. 57.3**.

RADIOGRAPHY

- Urinary extravasation may be apparent on intravenous pyelogram, as in **Fig. 57.4**.
- A "single-shot IVP" may be performed in the operating room (OR) when a critically injured patient's other injuries are being treated. IVP on the OR table gives the trauma surgeon useful information about the integrity of the GU system.

Treatment

- If hemodynamic instability is the result of hemorrhage from the renal injury, surgery must be directed at the repair or removal of the kidney. Nephrectomy rates in these patients approach 100%.
- Urine extravasation is not an absolute indication for surgery, as most collecting system leaks will heal spontaneously in up to 90% of patients.

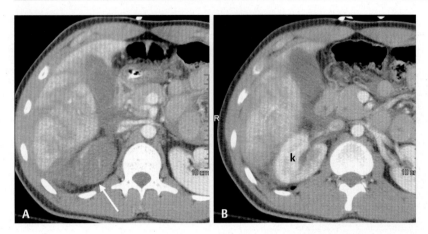

Fig. 57.3 Contrast-enhanced computed tomography scan through **(A)** the upper pole and **(B)** the midpole of the right kidney. Segmental renal infarction of the right upper pole is shown as no contrast enhancement (*arrow,* **A**). This is likely due to a segmental renal artery injury. Image of the right midpole shows a normally enhancing remainder of the kidney (k, **B**).

- Persistent urine leak, expanding urinoma, or sepsis will require intervention, usually with percutaneous nephrostomy, ureteral stenting, or both.
- Significant trauma may result in large parenchymal avascular fragments that become devitalized and are a setup for infection. These may require surgical removal.
- Rebleeding or other vascular complications are seen in grades 3 and 4 renal injuries in up to one quarter of patients. Continued or rebleeding, arteriovenous fistula, and pseudoaneurysm formation are treated with angiographic embolization.

Prognosis

- Variable

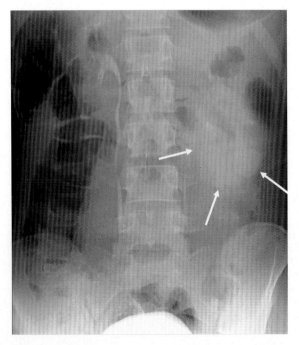

Fig. 57.4 Single-shot intravenous pyelogram performed in the operation room 10 minutes following rapid intravenous bolus infusion of iodinated contrast shows a left collecting system injury with extravasation of contrast (*arrows*) into the left retroperitoneum. Normal excretion is seen on the right.

- There is some overlap between grades 4 and 5 renal injuries, as both will have deep lacerations and large hematomas. Grade 5 is reserved for a totally devitalized or shattered kidney.

Suggested Reading

Al-Qudah HS, Santucci RA. Complications of renal trauma. Urol Clin North Am 2006;33(1):41–53.

Kawashima A, Sandler CM, Corl FM, et al. Imaging of renal trauma: a comprehensive review. Radiographics 2001;21(3):557–574.

McAninch J, Santucci R. Renal and ureteral trauma. In: Wein A, ed. Campbell-Walsh Urology. 9th ed. Philadelphia: Saunders Elsevier; 2007:1274–1278.

Park SJ, Kim JK, Kim KW, Cho KS. MDCT Findings of renal trauma. AJR Am J Roentgenol 2006;187(2):541–547.

Santucci RA, McAninch JW, Safir M, et al. Validation of the American Association for the Surgery of Trauma organ injury severity scale for the kidney. J Trauma 2001;50(2):195–200.

Santucci RA, Wessells H, Bartsch G, et al. Evaluation and management of renal injuries: consensus statement of the renal trauma subcommittee. BJU Int 2004;93(7):937–954.

CASE 58

Clinical Presentation

Motor vehicle collision with multiple injuries

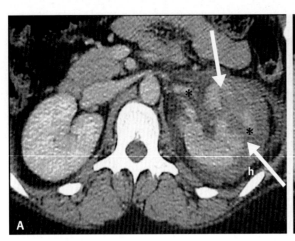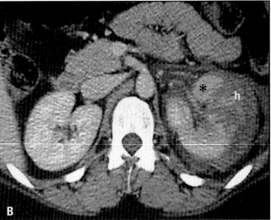

Fig. 58.1 **(A,B)** Enhanced computed tomography scans at two levels.

Radiologic Findings

- Multiple left renal deep lacerations (*arrows,* **Fig. 58.1A**)
- Perinephric hematoma (h, **Fig. 58.1A,B**)
- Multiple left renal fragments that enhance (*asterisks,* **Fig. 58.1A,B**)

Diagnosis

Shattered kidney, grade 5 renal injury

Differential Diagnosis

- Grade 4 renal injury
- Grade 3 renal injury

Discussion

Background

Grade 5 renal injuries account for < 5% of renal trauma and generally require surgical exploration, often with nephrectomy. Thrombosis from renal arterial dissection or avulsion of the renal pedicle occurs as a result of rapid deceleration forces (e.g., in motor vehicle collisions).

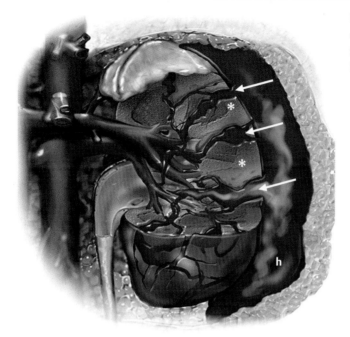

Fig. 58.2 Drawing of a shattered kidney showing deep lacerations (*arrows*), devitalized fragments of the renal parenchyma (*asterisks*), and a perinephric hematoma (h).

Clinical Findings

Multiple associated parenchymal and bony injuries. Hematuria may be absent.

Pathology

- Shattered kidney with multiple large lacerations and many parenchymal fragments (**Fig. 58.2**).
- Avulsion of the renal pedicle that devitalizes the kidney.

Imaging Findings

COMPUTED TOMOGRAPHY

- Both grades 3 and 4 renal injuries include lacerations, but not of the number and severity seen in the shattered kidney in this case.
- Grade 5 shattered kidney is characterized by fragmentation of the renal parenchyma (*asterisks,* **Fig. 58.1**). Multiple enhancing or nonenhancing fragments of the renal cortex will be present, perhaps widely separated by an intervening high-density hematoma (h, **Fig. 58.1**).
- Renal vascular pedicle injury is also a feature of grade 5 injury and will be indicated by a lack of enhancement in the renal artery or kidney or visualization of an arterial dissection or laceration of the renal artery or vein, with active bleeding or perivascular hematoma (**Fig. 58.3**).
- Avulsion of the ureteropelvic junction (UPJ) is also a grade 5 injury (**Fig. 58.4**).

ANGIOGRAPHY

- May be required to embolize a pedicle injury
- Revascularization of renal arterial dissection may be attempted if the organ is ischemic < 4 to 8 hours (**Fig. 58.5**).

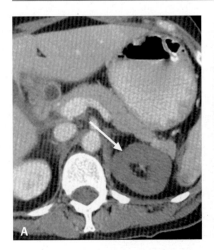
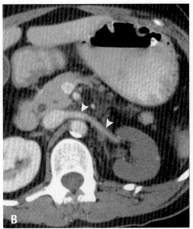

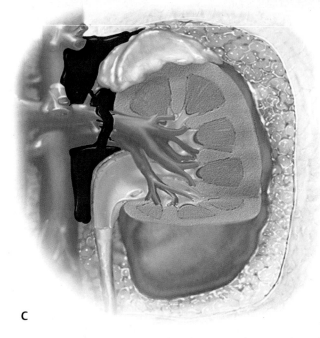

C

Fig. 58.3 **(A)** Contrast-enhanced computed tomography scan through the left kidney shows no enhancement of the renal parenchyma (*arrow*), consistent with a renal vascular injury. The renal artery (not shown) also did not enhance. **(B)** At the level of the left renal vein (*arrowheads*), reflux of contrast from the inferior vena cava is noted into the left renal vein. **(C)** Drawing of a major vessel injury with essentially no renal blood flow with blood extravasating into the retroperitoneum.

Treatment

- Actively bleeding vascular injury requires surgery or angiographic embolization.
- Repair of a UPJ avulsion is mandatory.

Prognosis

- There is high morbidity (e.g., renal function loss and/or kidney loss) and mortality associated with this injury and its concomitant injuries in other organs.

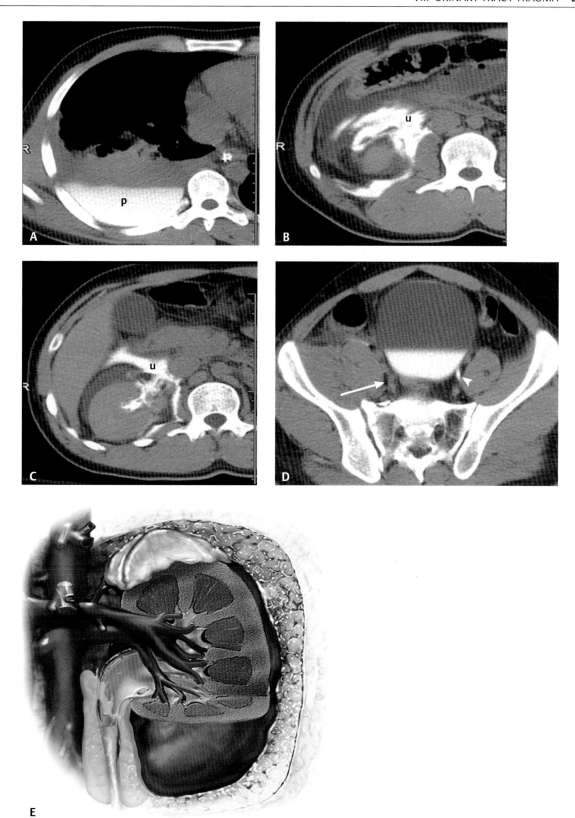

Fig. 58.4 Contrast-enhanced computed tomography (CT) scans. **(A)** A 10-minute delayed CT scan through the lung base shows extravasated contrast-enhanced urine in the pleural space (p) in this patient with a diaphragmatic rupture. **(B,C)** Disruption of the right renal hilum with extensive extravasated contrast enhanced urine in the perirenal space (u). **(D)** No filling of the right ureter (*arrow*) compared with normally filling left ureter (*arrowhead*), consistent with right ureteropelvic junction (UPJ) avulsion. **(E)** Drawing of UPJ avulsion and urine extravasation into the retroperitoneum.

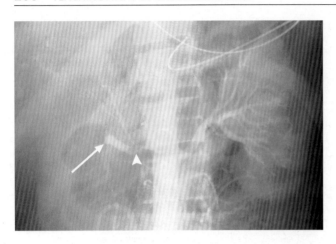

Fig. 58.5 Aortogram at the level of the renal arteries shows proximal right renal artery dissection (*arrowhead*) and abrupt termination of the artery in the renal hilum (*arrow*), consistent with a renal pedicle injury.

Suggested Readings

Al-Qudah HS, Santucci RA. Complications of renal trauma. Urol Clin North Am 2006;33(1):41–53.

Kawashima A, Sandler CM, Corl FM, et al. Imaging of renal trauma: a comprehensive review. Radiographics 2001;21(3):557–574.

McAninch J, Santucci R. Renal and ureteral trauma. In: Wein A, ed. Campbell-Walsh Urology. 9th ed. Philadelphia: Saunders Elsevier; 2007:1274–1278.

Park SJ, Kim JK, Kim KW, Cho KS. MDCT Findings of renal trauma. AJR Am J Roentgenol 2006;187(2):541–547.

Santucci RA, McAninch JW, Safir M, et al. Validation of the American Association for the Surgery of Trauma organ injury severity scale for the kidney. J Trauma 2001;50(2):195–200.

Santucci RA, Wessells H, Bartsch G, et al. Evaluation and management of renal injuries: consensus statement of the renal trauma subcommittee. BJU Int 2004;93(7):937–954.

CASE 59

Clinical Presentation

Male in a motor vehicle collision

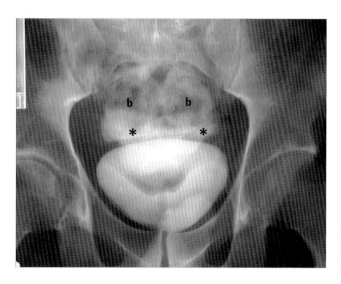

Fig. 59.1 Cystogram. Extravasation of contrast is seen into the peritoneum (*asterisks*) outlining bowel loops (b).

Radiologic Findings

- Contrast extending above the bladder (*asterisks*, **Fig. 59.1**)
- Contrast outlining bowel loops (b, **Fig. 59.1**)

Diagnosis

Intraperitoneal bladder rupture (IPBR)

Differential Diagnosis

- Extraperitoneal bladder rupture (EPBR)
- Vesicoenteric fistula

Discussion

Background

IPBR is the most common type of bladder rupture, seen in > 80% of such cases. EPBR is seen in < 20% of cases, and a combination can be seen in ~10%.

Clinical Findings

Pelvic injury without or with fracture

Pathology

Pelvic injury with a full bladder typically is associated with IPBR through the peritoneal lining adjacent to the dome of the bladder (**Fig. 59.2**).

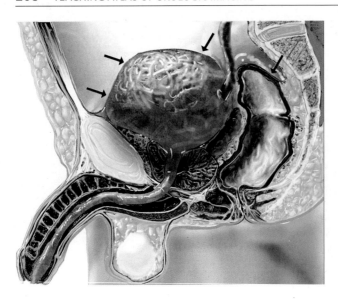

Fig. 59.2 Drawing of the bladder shows how the peritoneum drapes over the superior bladder surface (*arrows*), leading to intraperitoneal bladder rupture following blunt pelvic trauma.

Imaging Findings

RADIOGRAPHY/CYSTOGRAM

- An extraperitoneal rupture shows contrast extravasation typically lateral to or below the bladder, but it can extend superiorly. Computed tomography (CT) clarifies these cases.
- A vesicoenteric fistula during a cystogram would result in contrast within the bowel, not around it.
- Cystogram is the gold standard test. It is performed with a bladder catheter in place. Contrast is drip instilled under gravity assistance.
- Classic signs of IPBR are
  - Contrast outlining bowel loops (b, **Fig. 59.1**)
  - Contrast in the paracolic gutters (**Fig. 59.3**)
  - Contrast typically superior to the bladder (*asterisks,* **Fig. 59.1**)

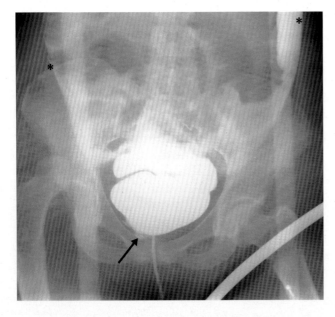

Fig. 59.3 Trauma. The cystogram shows signs of both intraperitoneal and extraperitoneal bladder rupture. Extraperitoneal bladder rupture findings include a contained leak at the bladder base (*arrow*). Intraperitoneal bladder rupture findings include urine in the bilateral paracolic gutters (*asterisks*).

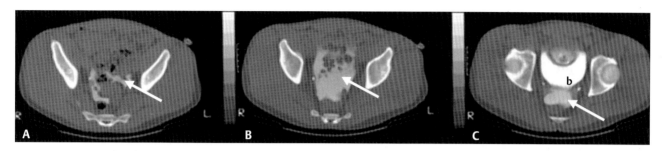

Fig. 59.4 Contrast-enhanced computed tomography (CT) in the delayed phase, shown in bone windows at three levels. **(A–C)** CT clearly demonstrates contrast in the peritoneal cavity outlining bowel loops (*arrows*). b, bladder.

COMPUTED TOMOGRAPHY

- CT offers a better demonstration of contrast in the peritoneal cavity surrounding loops of the small bowel (**Fig. 59.4**).
- A CT cystogram using retrograde instillation of bladder contrast is more reliable than routine contrast-enhanced CT with delayed images and is the CT study of choice.
- A CT cystogram can be performed together with three-dimensional reconstructions and detects bladder rupture as well as or better than a conventional cystogram. Drip infusion of contrast into the bladder via a bladder catheter is performed as with a conventional cystogram. The bladder should be under pressure to unmask a bladder rupture.

Treatment

- IPBR and combined injuries are treated with surgical repair.

Prognosis

- Good

Suggested Readings

Chan DP, Abujudeh HH, Cushing GL Jr, Novelline RA. CT cystography with multiplanar reformation for suspected bladder rupture: experience in 234 cases. AJR Am J Roentgenol 2006;187(5):1296–1302.

Morey A, Rozanski T. Genital and lower urinary tract trauma. In: Wein A, ed. Campbell-Walsh Urology. 9th ed. Saunders Elsevier; 2007:2649–2658.

Peng MY, Parisky YR, Cornwell EE III, Radin R, Bragin S. CT cystography versus conventional cystography in evaluation of bladder injury. AJR Am J Roentgenol 1999;173(5):1269–1272.

CASE 60

Clinical Presentation

Motor vehicle collision with pelvic fractures

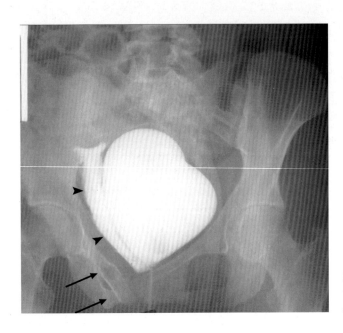

Fig. 60.1 Cystogram. Contrast extravasation along the right lateral aspect and inferior to bladder (*arrowheads*) together with pelvic fractures (*arrows*).

Radiologic Findings

- Contrast extravasation lateral and inferior to bladder (*arrowheads,* **Fig. 60.1**)
- Pelvic fractures (*arrows,* **Fig. 60.1**)

Diagnosis

Extraperitoneal bladder rupture (EPBR)

Differential Diagnosis

- Intraperitoneal bladder rupture (IPBR)
- Type 2 urethral injury
- Type 3 urethral injury

Discussion

Background

Most bladder injuries are the result of rapid deceleration forces, such as those seen in motor vehicle collisions. They are associated with significant nonurologic injuries. EPBR is seen in < 20% of bladder ruptures.

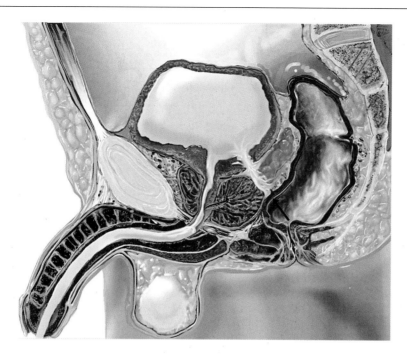

Fig. 60.2 Drawing showing an extraperitoneal bladder rupture with posteroinferior extravasation (*arrow*).

Clinical Findings

A history of trauma with pelvic fractures is usually present. Hematuria is present in nearly 100% of cases.

Pathology

Due to deceleration forces, the bladder tears at its fascial attachment, allowing for posterior and inferior extravasation of urine into the extraperitoneal space (**Fig. 60.2**).

Imaging Findings

RADIOGRAPHY/CYSTOGRAM

- Classic signs of intraperitoneal rupture (i.e., contrast outlining bowel loops and contrast in the paracolic gutters) are not present in this case.
- A type 2 urethral injury produces extravasation above the urogenital diaphragm, but typically on a retrograde urethrogram, not on a cystogram.
- A type 3 urethral injury produces extravasation above and below the urogenital diaphragm, but also on a retrograde urethrogram with the urethra filled. There is no contrast in the urethra in this case.
- Extraperitoneal ruptures typically occur lateral to or below the bladder (*arrowheads,* **Fig. 60.1**), as in this case.
- With EPBR, contrast is confined to the pelvic retroperitoneum and does not outline bowel loops or layer in the paracolic gutters.

COMPUTED TOMOGRAPHY

- Computed tomography offers a better demonstration of contrast in the extraperitoneal spaces and is particularly helpful when contrast extends superiorly.

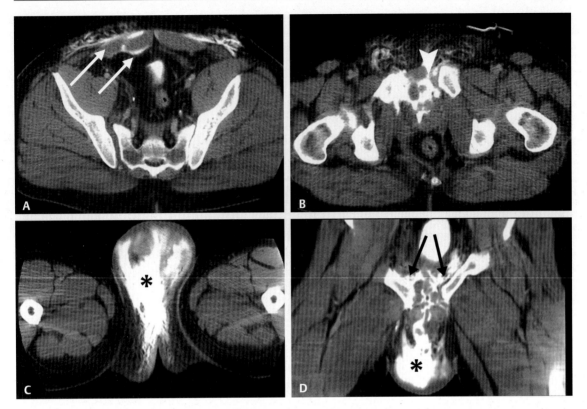

Fig. 60.3   Trauma. Contrast-enhanced CT in the delayed phase at **(A–C)** three levels and **(D)** three-dimensional (3D) coronal reconstruction. **(A)** Cephalad to the bladder, contrast from the ruptured bladder tracks into the extraperitoneal space/rectus sheath (*white arrows*). **(B)** Disruption of the bladder base with extraperitoneal extravasation (*arrowhead*). **(C)** Image below the bladder shows contrast tracking into the scrotum (*asterisk*). **(D)** 3D coronal reconstruction shows pubic symphysis diastasis (*arrows*) and extraperitoneal extravasation into the scrotum (*asterisk*).

- An examination is performed with a bladder catheter in place, with contrast drip infused into the bladder.
- Three-dimensional reconstructions may improve the ability to differentiate the types of bladder rupture (**Fig. 60.3**).
- Contrast extravasation is confined to the extraperitoneal spaces (**Fig. 60.3**).

Treatment

- Bladder catheter drainage until healed

Prognosis

- Good

Suggested Readings

Chan DP, Abujudeh HH, Cushing GL Jr, Novelline RA. CT cystography with multiplanar reformation for suspected bladder rupture: experience in 234 cases. AJR Am J Roentgenol 2006;187(5):1296–1302.

Morey A, Rozanski T. Genital and lower urinary tract trauma. In: Wein A, ed. Campbell-Walsh Urology. 9th ed. Philadelphia: Saunders Elsevier; 2007:2649–2658.

Peng MY, Parisky YR, Cornwell EE III, Radin R, Bragin S. CT cystography versus conventional cystography in evaluation of bladder injury. AJR Am J Roentgenol 1999;173(5):1269–1272.

CASE 61

Clinical Presentation

Young male in automobile accident

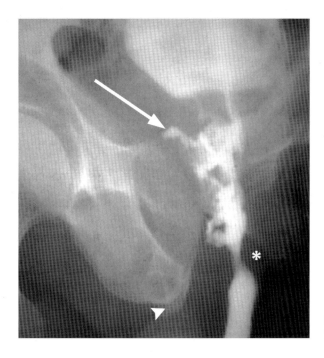

Fig. 61.1 Retrograde urethrogram. Membranous urethra (*asterisk*).

Radiologic Findings

- Contrast extravasation above the urogenital diaphragm (*arrow*, **Fig. 61.1**)
- Pelvic fracture (*arrowhead*, **Fig. 61.1**)

Diagnosis

Type 2 urethral injury

Differential Diagnosis

- Type 3 urethral injury
- Type 1 urethral injury
- Straddle injury

Discussion

Background

Most urethral injuries occur in association with pelvic fractures (especially ischiopubic fractures). Blunt trauma from a motor vehicle collision is the most common cause. Posterior urethral injuries result from a shearing force, pelvic fracture, and disruption of the membranous urethra. Because of the force required for this type of injury, there are often associated critical injuries.

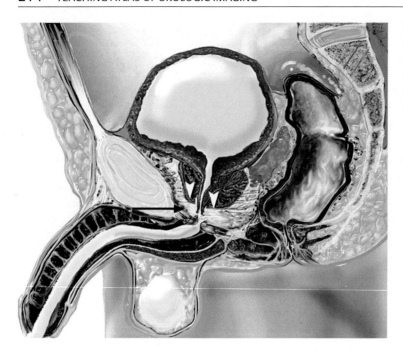

Fig. 61.2 Drawing of a type 2 urethral injury with disruption of the urethra above the urogenital diaphragm (*arrow*) and extravasation only above the urogenital diaphragm (*arrowheads*).

Clinical Findings

Any of these findings may suggest urethral injury:

- Blood at the meatus
- Pelvic fracture
- Palpably distended bladder and/or inability to void

Pathology

With a type 2 urethral injury, there is disruption of the urethra above the urogenital diaphragm (*arrow,* **Fig. 61.2**) with extravasation of urine only above the urogenital diaphragm.

Imaging Findings

RADIOGRAPHY

- A type 3 injury disrupts the urogenital diaphragm and produces extravasation above and below the urogenital diaphragm.
- A type 1 injury is stretching of the urethra without tear. There are no definitive radiographic findings in type 1 injuries.
- A straddle injury is produced by a direct blow to the bulbar urethra with extravasation localized to that region.
- Extravasation only above the urogenital diaphragm (**Fig. 61.1**), as seen in this case, indicates a urethral tear above the urogenital diaphragm, which is a type 2 injury.

Retrograde Urethrogram

- With the pelvis 30 to 45% oblique, contrast is instilled into the urethra through a balloon catheter held in the fossa navicularis by minimal balloon distension with a few cubic centimeters of saline.
- Contrast fills the anterior urethra, including the bulbous urethra, but often does not fill the posterior urethra, including the membranous urethra and the prostatic urethra.
- Tapering of the bulbous urethra to a conical appearance is normal (**Fig. 61.3**).

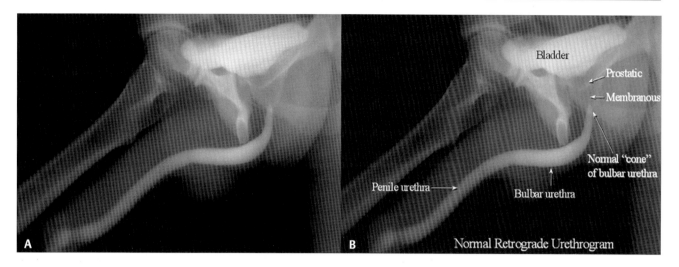

Fig. 61.3   Normal retrograde urethrogram (study of choice). Source: Resnick, Older, Diagnosis of Genitourinary Disease, New York: Thieme, 1997: 72. Reprinted by permission.

Voiding Cystourethrogram

- The bladder is filled with contrast (**Fig. 61.4**).
- The patient is asked to void during the exam.
- The posterior urethra, including the prostatic and membranous urethra, fills as well as the anterior urethra (**Fig. 61.4**).

Treatment

- Surgical repair of urethral injury.

Prognosis

- Depends on associated injuries

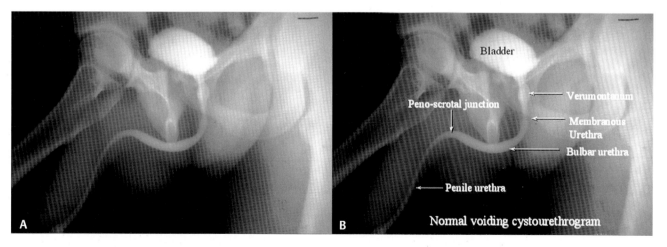

Fig. 61.4   Normal antegrade urethrogram (voiding cystourethrogram). Source: Resnick, Older, Diagnosis of Genitourinary Disease, New York: Thieme, 1997: 70. Reprinted by permission.

PEARLS

In the setting of a strong clinical suspicion (e.g., pelvic fracture or blood at the meatus), bladder catheterization should not be performed until a retrograde urethrogram excludes a urethral injury.

Suggested Readings

Goldman SM, Sandler CM, Corriere JN Jr, McGuire EJ. Blunt urethral trauma: a unified, anatomical mechanical classification. J Urol 1997;157(1):85–89.

Morey A, Rozanski T. Genital and lower urinary tract trauma. In: Wein A, ed. Campbell-Walsh Urology. 9th ed. Philadelphia: Saunders Elsevier; 2007:2649–2658.

Kawashima A, Sandler CM, Wasserman NF, et al. Imaging of urethral disease: a pictorial review. Radiographics 2004;24(Suppl 1):S195–S216.

Rosenstein DI, Alsikafi NF. Diagnosis and classification of urethral injuries. Urol Clin North Am 2006;33(1):73–85.

CASE 62

Clinical Presentation

Pelvic trauma

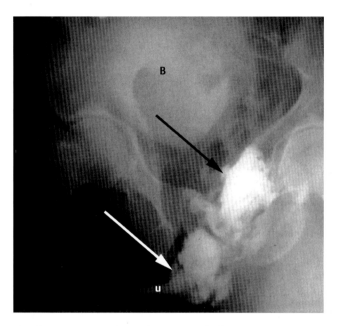

Fig. 62.1 Retrograde urethrogram. u, bulbous urethra.

Radiologic Findings

- Contrast extravasation above (*black arrow*, **Fig. 62.1**) and below (*white arrow*, **Fig. 62.1**) the urogenital diaphragm
- High-riding bladder ("pie in the sky" bladder) (B, **Fig. 62.1**)

Diagnosis

Type 3 urethral injury

Differential Diagnosis

- Type 2 urethral injury
- Type 1 urethral injury (stretch injury)
- Straddle injury

Discussion

Background

Most urethral injuries occur in association with pelvic fractures (especially ischiopubic fractures). Blunt trauma from a motor vehicle collision is the most common cause. Posterior urethral injuries result from a shearing force, pelvic fracture, and disruption of the membranous urethra. Due to the force required for this type of injury, there are often associated critical injuries.

217

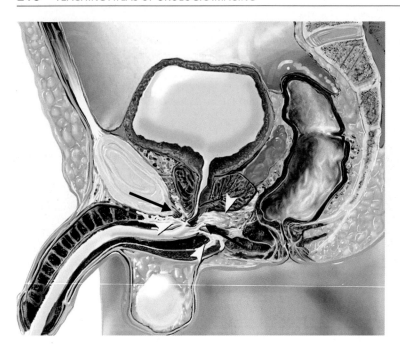

Fig. 62.2 Drawing of a type 3 urethral injury with disruption of the pelvic floor (*arrows*) and extravasation above and below the urogenital diaphragm (*arrowheads*).

Clinical Findings

Any of these findings may suggest urethral injury:

- Blood at the meatus
- Pelvic fractures
- Palpably distended bladder and/or inability to void

Pathology

With a type 3 urethra injury, there is disruption of the urethra and the urogenital diaphragm (*arrows,* **Fig. 62.2**), with extravasation of urine above and below the urogenital diaphragm.

Imaging Findings

See Case 61 for normal retrograde urethrogram and antegrade urethrogram studies.

RADIOGRAPHY/RETROGRADE URETHROGRAM

- Extravasation both above and below the urogenital diaphragm excludes a type 2 urethral injury, which produces extravasation only above the urogenital diaphragm.
- A type 1 injury is stretching of the urethra without tearing. There are no definitive radiographic findings in type 1 injuries.
- A straddle injury is produced by a direct blow to the bulbar urethra with extravasation localized to that region.
- A type 3 injury disrupts the urogenital diaphragm and produces extravasation above and below the urogenital diaphragm (*arrows,* **Fig. 62.1**). A high-riding bladder (B, **Fig. 62.1**), also known as "pie in the sky" bladder, is related to ligamentous and urethral disruption.

Treatment

- Surgical repair

Prognosis

- Depends on associated injuries

- In the setting of a strong clinical suspicion (e.g., pelvic fracture or blood at the meatus), bladder catheterization should not be performed until a retrograde urethrogram excludes a urethral injury.

Suggested Readings

Goldman SM, Sandler CM, Corriere JN Jr, McGuire EJ. Blunt urethral trauma: a unified, anatomical mechanical classification. J Urol 1997;157(1):85–89.

Kawashima A, Sandler CM, Wasserman NF, et al. Imaging of urethral disease: a pictorial review. Radiographics 2004;24(Suppl 1):S195–S216.

Morey A, Rozanski T. Genital and lower urinary tract trauma. In: Wein A, ed. Campbell-Walsh Urology. 9th ed. Philadelphia: Saunders Elsevier; 2007:2649–2658.

Rosenstein DI, Alsikafi NF. Diagnosis and classification of urethral injuries. Urol Clin North Am 2006;33(1):73–85.

CASE 63

Clinical Presentation

Direct trauma to the base of the penis

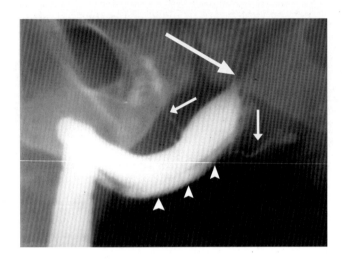

Fig. 63.1 Retrograde urethrogram. Local contrast extravasation of contrast (*arrowheads*) confined by Buck's fascia. Normal filling of Cowper ducts (*arrows*). Normal tapered cone of the bulbous urethra at the urogenital diaphragm (*long white arrow*).

Radiologic Findings

- Local contrast extravasation of contrast (*arrowheads,* **Fig. 63.1**) confined by Buck's fascia
- Normal filling of Cowper ducts (*arrows,* **Fig. 63.1**)
- Normal tapered cone of the bulbous urethra at the urogenital diaphragm (*long white arrow,* **Fig. 63.1**)

Diagnosis

Straddle injury of the urethra

Differential Diagnosis

- Type 1, type 2, or type 3 urethral injury

Discussion

Background

Most straddle injuries are due to blunt trauma to the perineum. A motor vehicle collision, bicycle accident, landing atop a fence railing, or kick to the groin represent the usual etiologies. Bulbous urethra is the most common site, as blunt trauma to the perineum crushes the urethra against the fixed pubic bone. Trauma may be minor enough for the patient to not seek medical attention. Delayed symptoms (up to 10 years) will eventually bring the patient to the urologist.

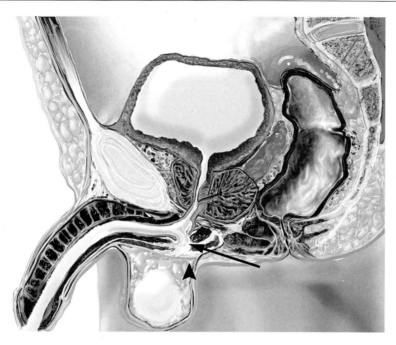

Fig. 63.2 Drawing of a straddle injury with extravasation (*arrow*) from the bulbous urethra confined by Buck's fascia (*arrowhead*).

Clinical Findings

Perineal trauma with (1) blood at the meatus, or (2) an inability to void, or (3) dysuria or hematuria can be presenting signs and symptoms. Delayed stricturing from a urethral injury usually presents as anterior urethral stricturing and voiding symptoms (see below).

Pathology

A straddle injury usually results from blunt trauma to the anterior urethra, commonly the bulbous urethra (*arrow*, **Fig. 63.2**). Disruption of the anterior urethra results in local extravasation of urine/contrast contained by Buck's or Colles fascia (**Fig. 63.2**).

Imaging Findings

RADIOGRAPHY/RETROGRADE URETHROGRAM

- No extravasation above the urogenital diaphragm excludes both type 2 and type 3 urethral injuries, which both demonstrate extravasation above the urogenital diaphragm.
- The presence of extravasation excludes a type 1 urethral injury, which is stretching of the urethra without extravasation.
- Straddle injury features:
  - Involves anterior urethra, commonly the bulbous urethra
  - Local extravasation contained by Buck's or Colles fascia
  - Pelvic fracture not required

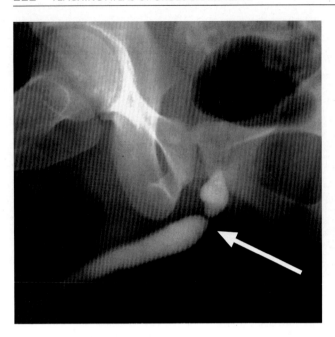

Fig. 63.3 History of remote trauma. Retrograde urethrogram shows a short stricture of the bulbous urethra (*arrow*) in a patient with urinary symptoms remote from his urethral trauma.

VOIDING CYSTOURETHROGRAM

- Normal prostatic and membranous urethra seen on a voiding cystourethrogram
- Anterior urethra with extravasation locally contained by fascial planes

Treatment

- Initial treatment includes suprapubic tube drainage to bypass the urethra and allow healing. Acute phase strictures are repaired by resection and reanastomosis of the stricture-free segments.
- Delayed urethral stricture (**Fig. 63.3**) may occur, requiring surgical repair.

Prognosis

- Good with initial therapy. Early and delayed repair of a urethral stricture has a 95% success rate.

PEARLS _____

- If there is a strong clinical suspicion of urethral trauma, no attempt should be made at bladder catheterization before a retrograde urethrogram excludes a urethral injury.

Suggested Readings

Goldman SM, Sandler CM, Corriere JN Jr, McGuire EJ. Blunt urethral trauma: a unified, anatomical mechanical classification. J Urol 1997;157(1):85–89.

Kawashima A, Sandler CM, Wasserman NF, et al. Imaging of urethral disease: a pictorial review. Radiographics 2004;24(Suppl 1):S195–S216.

Morey A, Rozanski T. Genital and lower urinary tract trauma. In: Wein A, ed. Campbell-Walsh Urology. 9th ed. Philadelphia: Saunders Elsevier; 2007:2649–2658.

Rosenstein DI, Alsikafi NF. Diagnosis and classification of urethral injuries. Urol Clin North Am 2006;33(1):73–85.

CASE 64

Clinical Presentation

Patient presents with a lung mass and an adrenal mass.

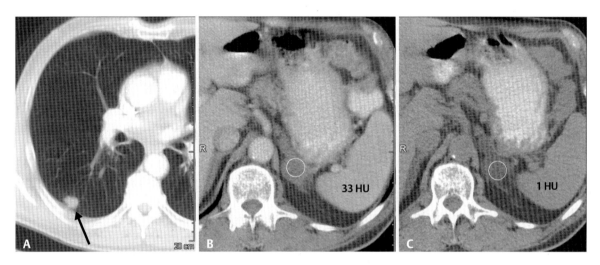

Fig. 64.1 Lung cancer staging work-up. **(A)** Lung windows from a contrast-enhanced chest computed tomography (CT) scan. **(B)** Soft tissue windows through the adrenal glands in the portal venous phase. **(C)** Follow-up adrenal protocol CT scan without intravenous contrast.

Radiologic Findings

Routine chest computed tomography (CT) scans with intravenous (IV) contrast found the following:

- Classic stellate mass at the right lung base consistent with a T1 bronchogenic carcinoma (*arrow,* **Fig. 64.1A**)
- Incidentally discovered left adrenal mass (*circle*) that measured 33 Hounsfield units (HU) on the portal venous phase CT scan (**Fig. 64.1B**)
- Follow-up adrenal protocol CT scan without IV contrast (**Fig. 64.1C**) shows the mass (*circle*) measuring 1 HU, consistent with a lipid-rich adrenal adenoma. The remainder of the adrenal protocol did not need to be performed because the unenhanced scan was diagnostic and conclusive of adrenal adenoma.

Diagnosis

Lipid-rich adrenal adenoma

Differential Diagnosis

- Adrenal metastasis
- Pheochromocytoma
- Adrenal cortical carcinoma

Discussion

Background

Incidentally discovered adrenal masses are found in ~5% of abdominal CT scans done for reasons other than for the assessment of the adrenal glands and are therefore referred to as adrenal "incidentalomas." Most are nonfunctioning adrenal adenomas. Adrenal size is an important differentiating factor between benign and malignant disease. Most adrenal adenomas are small (< 3 cm). Lesions > 6 cm are almost universally malignant and are treated primarily with surgical resection. Two thirds of small adrenal incidentalomas are usually benign in the absence of a primary malignancy. However, 70% of adrenal masses in patients with primary malignancy are metastases.

The lipid contained within adenomas is cholesterol, which is the precursor to the production of steroid hormones. Cholesterol imparts low density to adrenal adenomas on an unenhanced CT scan, which is the preferred imaging method of diagnosis. Importantly, 20 to 30% of adrenal adenomas are lipid poor and must be characterized based on the rapid washout of iodinated contrast materials that is observed with adrenal adenomas.

Clinical Findings

Functioning adrenal adenomas are rare but usually present early due to their hormone or metabolic imbalance. If the patient is asymptomatic, recommendations are for an endocrinology work-up in patients who have adenomas at imaging to identify potential subclinical Cushing syndrome and pheochromocytoma. If there is hypertension and hypokalemia, an aldosterone-secreting adrenal tumor is likely.

Pathology

* Adrenal adenomas are lipid rich (70–80%) or lipid poor (20–30%).

Imaging Findings

COMPUTED TOMOGRAPHY

* Adrenal metastasis would not have such a low precontrast attenuation, as in **Fig. 64.1C.** This low attenuation is diagnostic of a lipid-rich adrenal adenoma.
* Pheochromocytomas may contain sufficient lipid to present with low attenuation on an unenhanced CT scan, but a functional pheochromocytoma should present with at least one symptom from the classic clinical triad of palpitations, diaphoresis, and headache plus hypertension.
* Adrenal cortical carcinomas are often quite large at diagnosis, usually > 6 cm.
* Most (70–80%) adrenal adenomas can be diagnosed on unenhanced CT scans due to their high lipid content (**Fig. 64.1C**).
* Diagnosis of adrenal adenoma is confirmed when the adrenal mass density measures < 10 HU with a specificity of 100% (**Fig. 64.2**).

Adrenal Incidentaloma Work-Up

When an adrenal lesion is incidentally discovered on a routine contrast-enhanced CT, washout is determined with a 15-minute delayed scan through the adrenal mass, at which point relative percentage washout (RPW) is calculated based on the formula [(Enhanced – Delayed)/(Enhanced)] × 100%, with a threshold of > 40% RPW, yielding a sensitivity and specificity of 82 and 92%, respectively, for adenoma. *Note:* Some authors use a 10-minute delayed scan for calculation of RPW and absolute percentage washout (APW) (**Fig. 64.3**).

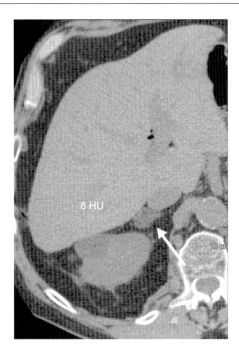

Fig. 64.2 Unenhanced computed tomography scan through the right adrenal gland shows a low-density mass (*arrow*), which measures 8 HU, consistent with a lipid-rich adrenal adenoma.

For known adrenal lesions, a formal adrenal protocol CT scan is performed with an unenhanced scan, followed by an enhanced portal venous phase CT followed by a 15-minute delayed scan (**Fig. 64.4**). APW is calculated based on the formula [(Enhanced – Delayed)/(Enhanced – Unenhanced)] × 100%, with a threshold of > 60% APW, yielding a sensitivity and specificity of 86 and 92%, respectively, for adenoma (**Fig. 64.4**).

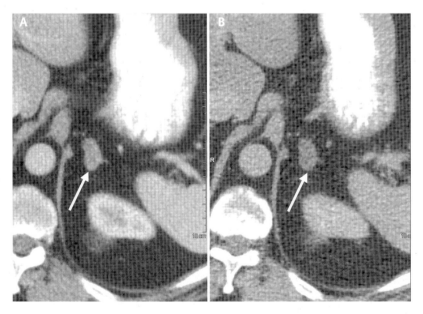

Fig. 64.3 History of a pelvic mass, contrast-enhanced computed tomography (CT) scans. **(A)** Portal venous phase staging CT in a patient with a pelvic mass revealed an incidentally discovered left adrenal mass (*arrow*). **(B)** A 15-minute delayed image through the adrenal gland was obtained. Enhanced attenuation = 57 HU, delayed attenuation = 19 HU, relative percentage washout = 67%, consistent with an adrenal adenoma.

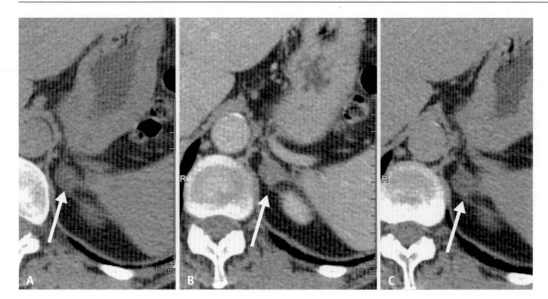

Fig. 64.4 Standard adrenal protocol computed tomography (CT) scans. The patient originally presented with abdominal pain. A left adrenal mass (*arrows*) was not immediately recognized while the patient was still on the CT table. The patient returned for a dedicated adrenal protocol CT. **(A)** Unenhanced attenuation = 14 HU, **(B)** enhanced attenuation = 53 HU, and **(C)** delayed attenuation = 24 HU. Absolute percentage washout = 74%, consistent with adrenal adenoma.

ULTRASOUND

- Ultrasound has little role in the diagnosis of adrenal adenoma.

MAGNETIC RESONANCE IMAGING

- Chemical shift artifact causes the signals from lipid and soft tissue to cancel one another on the opposed phase (OP) gradient echo T1 sequences when compared with the in phase (IP) sequence (i.e., the signal in the adrenal adenoma seen in IP decreases on the OP sequence).

  On magnetic resonance imaging (MRI), we take advantage of an artifact that occurs when there are equal amounts of intracytoplasmic lipid and soft tissue in the same picture element (i.e., pixel) as we find in adrenal adenomas. With window/level settings identical, we visually compare the two sequences; if the adrenal mass gets darker on OP images, the mass is an adrenal adenoma, using this qualitative measurement (**Fig. 64.5**).

  Most cases are able to be diagnosed visually as long as the windowing and leveling of the images are the same (**Fig. 64.5**). In equivocal cases, a signal intensity index (SII) may be calculated using the spleen as an internal control. To diagnose an adrenal adenoma, ~25% drop is required for a sensitivity and specificity of 100 and 82%, respectively, for adenoma. The formula for the adrenal-spleen SII is

$$[(OPSI\ adr)/(OPSI\ spl)\ /\ (IPSI\ adr)/(IPSI\ spl)] - 1 \times 100\%,$$

where OPSI is opposed phase signal intensity and IPSI is in phase signal intensity (adr, adrenal; spl, spleen).

Treatment

- Benign nonfunctioning adrenal adenomas require no specific treatment.
- The National Institutes of Health consensus panel on adrenal incidentalomas suggests 1-year imaging follow-up to confirm stability in the adrenal mass and endocrine work-up to exclude subclinical Cushing syndrome.

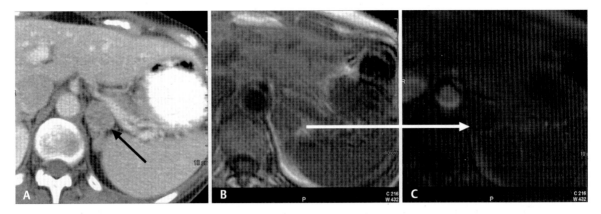

Fig. 64.5 **(A)** A patient with a known neurogenic tumor with an incidentally discovered left adrenal mass (*black arrow*) on a staging computed tomography scan. **(B)** Magnetic resonance imaging shows a left adrenal mass on the **(B)** in phase (IP) image that drops in signal on **(C)** the opposed phase (OP) image consistent with an adrenal adenoma. (Window center and width level settings are the same between the IP and OP images.)

Prognosis

- Nonfunctioning adrenal adenomas are benign.

PEARLS _____

- Lipid-poor adrenal adenomas need follow-up, as washout criteria are not 100% sensitive and specific.

Suggested Readings

Blake MA, Kalra MK, Sweeney AT, et al. Distinguishing benign from malignant adrenal masses: multi-detector row CT protocol with 10-minute delay. Radiology 2006;238(2):578–585.

Caoili EM, Korobkin M, Francis IR, et al. Adrenal masses: characterization with combined unenhanced and delayed enhanced CT. Radiology 2002;222(3):629–633.

Dunnick NR, Korobkin M. Imaging of adrenal incidentalomas: current status. AJR Am J Roentgenol 2002;179(3):559–568.

Grumbach MM, Biller BM, Braunstein GD, et al. Management of the clinically inapparent adrenal mass ("incidentaloma"). Ann Intern Med 2003;138(5):424–429.

Hussain HK, Korobkin M. MR imaging of the adrenal glands. Magn Reson Imaging Clin N Am 2004;12(3):515–544.

Korobkin M, Brodeur FJ, Francis IR, et al. CT time-attenuation washout curves of adrenal adenomas and nonadenomas. AJR Am J Roentgenol 1998;170(3):747–752.

Mayo-Smith WW, Lee MJ, McNicholas MM, et al. Characterization of adrenal masses (< 5 cm) by use of chemical shift MR imaging: observer performance versus quantitative measures. AJR Am J Roentgenol 1995;165(1):91–95.

Nawar R, Aron D. Adrenal incidentalomas—a continuing management dilemma. Endocr Relat Cancer 2005;12(3):585–598.

Shen WT, Sturgeon C, Duh QY. From incidentaloma to adrenocortical carcinoma: the surgical management of adrenal tumors. J Surg Oncol 2005;89(3):186–192.

Yamada T, Ishibashi T, Saito H, et al. Adrenal adenomas: relationship between histologic lipid-rich cells and CT attenuation number. Eur J Radiol 2003;48(2):198–202.

CASE 65

Clinical Presentation

Endometrial carcinoma

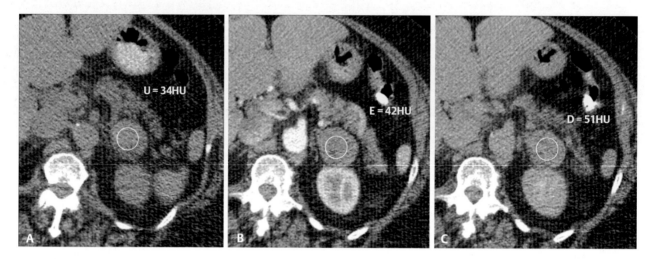

Fig. 65.1 Adrenal protocol computed tomography (CT) scans in a patient with endometrial carcinoma and an incidental left adrenal mass (*circles*). **(A)** Unenhanced scan, **(B)** portal venous phase enhanced scan, and **(C)** 10-minute delayed CT.

Radiologic Findings

- 4 cm left adrenal mass
- Unenhanced attenuation of the adrenal mass is > 10 Hounsfield units (HU).
- Progressive enhancement on adrenal protocol computed tomography (CT) (i.e., no washout)

Diagnosis

Metastatic disease to the adrenal glands

Differential Diagnosis

- Adrenal adenoma
- Adrenal cysts
- Pheochromocytoma
- Primary adrenal carcinoma
- Adrenal pseudocysts
- Lymphoma/leukemia

Discussion

Background

Adrenal metastases are quite common due to the gland's rich blood supply, with metastases found in ~27% at autopsy in patients with a primary malignancy. In patients with a known extra-adrenal primary malignancy, an adrenal mass is likely to be metastatic disease in up to 70% of cases. Common extra-adrenal carcinomas with a propensity to involve the adrenal glands include lung, breast, melanoma, renal, and gastrointestinal malignancies.

Clinical Findings

Lam and Lo (2002) reported a 30-year study of patients with adrenal metastatic disease. Out of 464 patients, 95% were asymptomatic. Mass effect resulted from the adrenal metastases or hemorrhage into the mass in symptomatic individuals. Adrenal insufficiency occurred in less than one third of symptomatic patients.

Pathology

Depends on primary tumor

Imaging Findings

COMPUTED TOMOGRAPHY

- Lipid-rich adrenal adenomas would have an unenhanced attenuation of < 10 HU and would not progressively enhance (**Fig. 65.1**).
- Adrenal cysts should have fluid attenuation (e.g., < 20 HU) and not show enhancement.
- Pheochromocytoma should present with the clinical triad of palpitations, diaphoresis, and hypertension but could present with these imaging findings.
- Primary adrenal carcinoma, chronic hemorrhagic adrenal pseudocyst, and leukemia and/or lymphoma may present similarly. Because the lesion cannot be characterized as benign in the setting of a primary malignancy, it requires biopsy or surgical excision.
- Metastatic lesions are often > 4 cm (**Fig. 65.2**).
- Metastatic lesions may enhance in a similar manner as the primary tumor of origin.
- Frequently, the metastatic lesion is hypoattenuating or poorly enhancing due to areas of necrosis (**Figs. 65.2** and **65.3**) or hemorrhage.
- Calcification is not common, but when it is present, it does not necessarily imply benign disease.

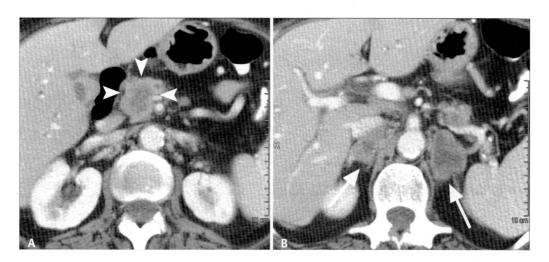

Fig. 65.2 Metastatic pancreatic cancer. **(A)** A contrast-enhanced computed tomography scan shows a low-density pancreatic head mass (*arrowheads*). **(B)** On the same scan, bilateral low-density necrotic adrenal metastases (*arrows*) measuring > 5 cm each are seen.

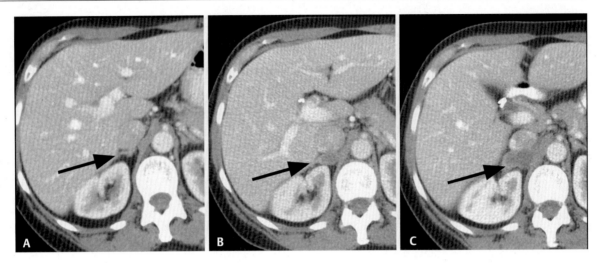

Fig. 65.3 History of lung cancer. Contrast-enhanced computed tomography (CT) scans of the right adrenal gland (*arrows*) over the span of 5 months show **(A)** a normal right adrenal gland, **(B)** developing right adrenal metastasis at 2-month follow-up CT, and **(C)** continued growth in the right adrenal metastasis at 5 months. The low density should not be confused with lipid; rather, it is a necrosis and measured > 10 HU.

- Demonstration of lesion growth on short-term follow-up indicates a high probability of a metastatic lesion (**Fig. 65.3**).

When an adrenal lesion is incidentally discovered on a routine contrast-enhanced CT (**Fig. 65.4**), relative percentage washout (RPW) is determined with a 15-minute delayed scan through the adrenal mass. RPW is calculated based on the formula [(Enhanced – Delayed)/(Enhanced)] × 100%, with a threshold of > 40% RPW yielding a sensitivity and specificity of 82 and 92%, respectively, for adenoma. *Note:* Some authors use a 10-minute delayed scan for the calculation of RPW and absolute percentage washout (APW).

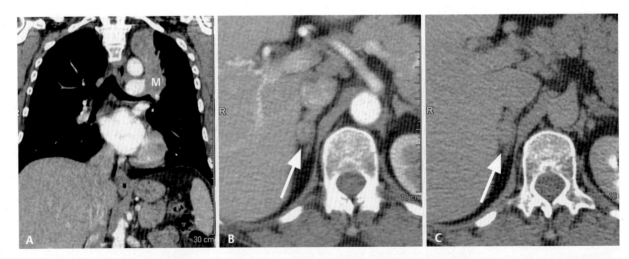

Fig. 65.4 Lung cancer. Staging contrast-enhanced computed tomography scans show **(A)** a mass (M) obstructing the left upper lobe bronchus, **(B)** a 1.5 cm mass in the right adrenal gland (*arrow*) with attenuation of 84 HU on the portal venous phase, and **(C)** a delayed scan through the right adrenal gland (*arrow*) measuring 72 HU with a calculated relative percentage washout of 15%, not consistent with an adrenal adenoma.

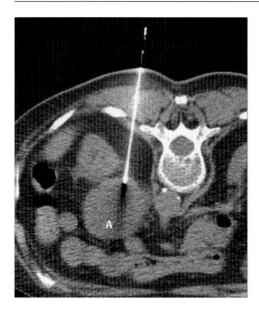

Fig. 65.5 Patient with melanoma and an adrenal mass. Noncontrast computed tomography scan with the patient prone. The biopsy needle is within the substance of the adrenal mass (A). The pathology was metastatic melanoma.

An adrenal mass is indeterminate if it is not consistent with an adrenal adenoma by density or by RPW values. It is in these patients where adrenal biopsy plays an important role.

Adrenal Biopsy

In patients with a known extra-adrenal primary malignancy and an adrenal mass that is suspected of being metastatic disease, adrenal biopsy is indicated to confirm distant metastasis (**Fig. 65.5**). In the absence of a known extra-adrenal malignancy, a biopsy of indeterminate adrenal lesions should be carefully considered. It may be difficult to differentiate adrenal cortical neoplasms from normal cortical tissue on biopsy specimens. Importantly, in the setting of an adrenal mass, exclusion of pheochromocytoma must be performed prior to any biopsy or surgery to avoid a potential hypertensive crisis.

MAGNETIC RESONANCE IMAGING

- Metastases are usually larger than adenomas (i.e., > 4 cm)
- Metastases may be hypointense on T1-weighted and hyperintense (relative to liver) on T2-weighted images but can be variable due to hemorrhage or necrosis on both T1- and T2-weighted images; may show variable enhancement
- Metastases do not have sufficient lipid to lose signal on opposed phase gradient echo (GRE) images (**Fig. 65.6**).

POSITRON EMISSION TOMOGRAPHY

- The uptake of fluorine-18 fluorodeoxyglucose (F^{18}-FDG) in positron emission tomography (PET) and PET combined with CT scans has shown sensitivity, specificity, and accuracies of 93 to 100%, 90 to 96%, and 92 to 96%, respectively, for diagnosing adrenal metastatic disease (**Fig. 65.7**).
- Small lesions (< 10 mm) and those with hemorrhage and/or necrosis may be false-negative.
- False-positives include granulomatous disease, pheochromocytoma, and brown fat in the suprarenal fossa.

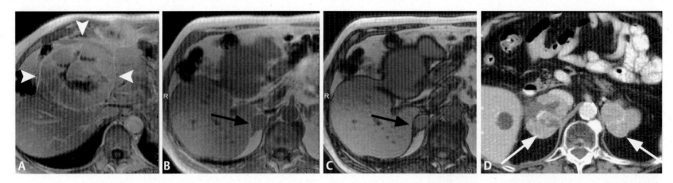

Fig. 65.6 Hepatocellular carcinoma. **(A)** A gadolinium enhanced T1 gradient echo (GRE) axial image shows an enhancing hepatic mass (*arrowheads*). An adrenal mass (*arrows*) was also seen on the **(B)** in phase and **(C)** opposed phase GRE images before intravenous contrast. On visual inspection, the adrenal lesion does not drop in signal on the opposed phase image when compared with the in phase image. The signal intensity index for the adrenal lesion, with spleen as an internal control, showed a drop of only 5% (with the criterion for adenoma being > 25% drop). Thus, this lesion is not consistent with an adrenal adenoma by magnetic resonance imaging. **(D)** A follow-up CT scan shows increasing right and new left adrenal metastases (*arrows*).

- Adrenal adenomas can also be false-positive in up to 5% of cases for unknown reasons.

Treatment

- Extra-adrenal primary malignancy with spread to the adrenal glands is consistent with diffuse metastatic disease and is generally treated as advanced disease (i.e., with palliative care).

Prognosis

- Survival rate < 10% at 5 years for all patients

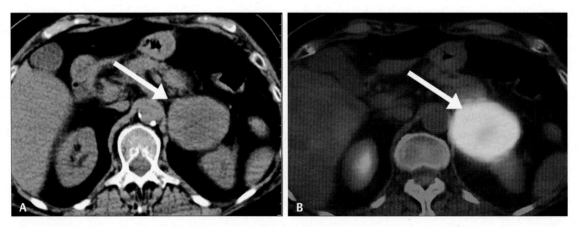

Fig. 65.7 Positron emission tomography/computed tomography (PET/CT) imaging in a patient with non-small cell lung carcinoma. **(A)** Nonenhanced CT scan reveals a large left adrenal mass (*arrow*) measuring 5.5 cm with no detectable lipid. **(B)** PET/CT image shows significant fluorodeoxyglucose metabolism in the left adrenal mass with a maximum standardized uptake value of 14.5, consistent with a malignant deposit.

- Adrenal metastases occur late in the course of a primary malignancy.
- Common finding at autopsy

PEARLS

- Some metastases actually increase in attenuation on delayed CT imaging (i.e., they progressively enhance). Thus, absolute or relative percentage washout values equal zero.

Suggested Readings

Chong S, Lee KS, Kim HY, et al. Integrated PET-CT for the characterization of adrenal gland lesions in cancer patients: diagnostic efficacy and interpretation pitfalls. Radiographics 2006;26(6):1811–1824.

Dunnick NR, Korobkin M. Imaging of adrenal incidentalomas: current status. AJR Am J Roentgenol 2002;179(3):559–568.

Hussain HK, Korobkin M. MR imaging of the adrenal glands. Magn Reson Imaging Clin N Am 2004;12(3):515–544.

Lam KY, Lo CY. Metastatic tumours of the adrenal glands: a 30-year experience in a teaching hospital. Clin Endocrinol (Oxf) 2002;56(1):95–101.

Paulsen SD, Nghiem HV, Korobkin M, Caoili EM, Higgins EJ. Changing role of imaging-guided percutaneous biopsy of adrenal masses: evaluation of 50 adrenal biopsies. AJR Am J Roentgenol 2004;182(4):1033–1037.

Welch TJ, Sheedy PF II, Stephens DH, Johnson CM, Swensen SJ. Percutaneous adrenal biopsy: review of a 10-year experience. Radiology 1994;193(2):341–344.

Yun M, Kim W, Alnafisi N, Lacorte L, Jang S, Alavi A. 18F-FDG PET in characterizing adrenal lesions detected on CT or MRI. J Nucl Med 2001;42(12):1795–1799.

CASE 66

Clinical Presentation

A 9-year-old patient with von Hippel-Lindau disease presents with possible suprarenal fossa masses.

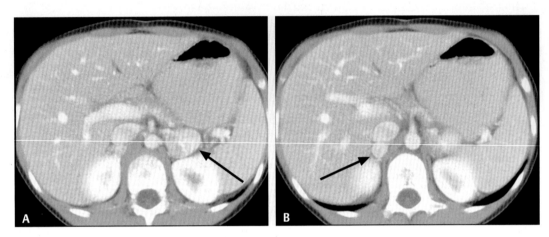

Fig. 66.1 Contrast-enhanced computed tomography scans show bilateral hyperenhancing adrenal masses (*arrows*) on the **(A)** left and **(B)** right.

Radiologic Findings

- Bilateral hyperenhancing adrenal masses in a patient with von Hippel-Lindau disease (*arrows,* **Fig. 66.1**).

Diagnosis

Bilateral pheochromocytomas

Differential Diagnosis

- Adrenal metastasis
- Wilms tumors (if inseparable from the adjacent kidney)
- Exophytic upper pole renal cell carcinomas
- Adrenal adenoma
- Adrenal cortical carcinoma

Discussion

Background

Pheochromocytomas are neuroendocrine tumors that arise from the chromaffin cells of the adrenal medulla. The rule of 10s applies to pheochromocytomas, which includes 10% bilateral, 10% malignant, 10% extra-adrenal (i.e., paragangliomas), and 10% normotensive. Previously, 10% were felt to be hereditary. However, recent research suggests that as many as one quarter of patients with spontaneous pheochromocytomas actually have some form of gene mutation predisposing to these types of tumors. Familial pheochromocytomas are autosomal dominant or are inherited in association with von Hippel-Lindau disease, multiple endocrine neoplasia (MEN) types 2A and B, Sturge-Weber syndrome, or neurofibromatosis type 1.

Clinical Findings

Pheochromocytomas secrete high levels of catecholamines, which results in paroxysms of hypertension. Ninety percent of patients have sustained or labile hypertension. At least one of the symptoms from the classic clinical triad of palpitations, diaphoresis, and headache will be seen. When symptoms suggest the diagnosis, a pheochromocytoma is confirmed with biochemical testing (resting serum cathecholamines assay and 24-hour urine norepinephrine, epinephrine, and/or vanillylmandelic acid). Imaging is then performed to localize the pheochromocytoma prior to surgical resection. A pheochromocytoma may present as an adrenal "incidentaloma" when it is clinically silent (nonfunctioning).

Pathology

Pheochromocytomas are functioning or nonfunctioning neoplasms of the adrenal medulla. Extra-adrenal pheochromocytomas are called paragangliomas and arise from the sympathetic chain from the cervical spine to the sacrum, but ~98% of pheochromocytomas are found in the abdomen. They may arise adjacent to the bladder dome or at the aortic bifurcation within the organ of Zuckerkandl.

Imaging Findings

COMPUTED TOMOGRAPHY

- Adrenal metastasis is unlikely in a child with no known malignancy.
- Coronal reconstructions would show these lesions originating from the adrenal glands, which would exclude both Wilms tumors and renal cell carcinoma.
- Adrenal adenomas may enhance intensely. In a routine setting, a 15- (or 10-) minute delayed scan would be obtained and relative percentage washout calculated. In this patient with von Hippel-Lindau disease, bilateral pheochromocytomas are likely.
- Adrenal carcinoma presents as a large tumor (> 6 cm) in one adrenal gland.
- Classically, pheochromocytomas are adrenal masses that enhance intensely following intravenous contrast administration (**Fig. 66.1**).
- Pheochromocytomas are usually well-circumscribed lesions and often > 3 cm.
- Pheochromocytomas can undergo necrosis and thus show areas of nonenhancement that may mimic a cystic lesion.
- Rarely, pheochromocytomas have been noted to contain intratumoral fat mimicking myelolipoma.
- Rarely, lipid content may be sufficient to mimic an adrenal adenoma having attenuation < 10 Hounsfield units (HU) on an unenhanced scan and washout characteristics that may approximate the criteria for adenomas.
- Calcification is occasionally seen simulating still other adrenal lesions (e.g., adrenal carcinoma, granulomatous disease, or chronic organizing adrenal hematoma).
- Due to the myriad imaging presentations, pheochromocytomas should always be considered in the differential diagnosis for an adrenal incidentaloma when a more specific diagnosis cannot be made.
- Coronal and sagittal reconstructions are useful in separating an adrenal pheochromocytoma from an upper pole renal mass.

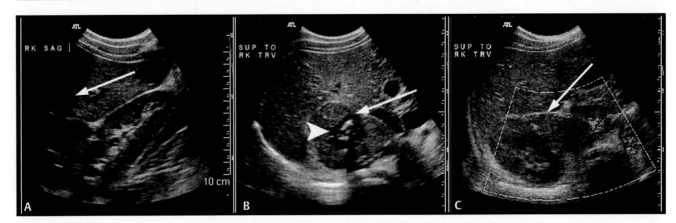

Fig. 66.2 A right upper quadrant ultrasound in a 16-year-old patient with hypertension and abdominal pain. **(A)** A sagittal image through the liver shows a mass (*arrow*) separate from the superior pole of the right kidney. **(B)** A transverse image shows calcification (*arrowhead*). **(C)** A color Doppler image shows a vascular mass (*arrow*) with a component bulging into the inferior vena cava.

ULTRASOUND

- Ultrasound findings of pheochromocytomas are nonspecific.
- Pheochromocytomas are well-marginated or encapsulated masses that range from hypoechoic to isoechoic to echogenic compared with the adjacent kidney.
- Most pheochromocytomas are solid appearing.
- Areas of hemorrhage, cystic degeneration, or necrosis give the lesion a heterogeneous appearance.
- Color flow may be detected in vascular portions of the tumor that have not undergone necrosis or cystic change (**Fig. 66.2**).

NUCLEAR MEDICINE

- I-131 metaiodobenzylguanidine (MIBG) is a guanethidine analogue that competes with norepinephrine at synaptic reuptake receptors.
- MIBG sensitivity and specificity for pheochromocytoma is 88 and 96%, respectively.

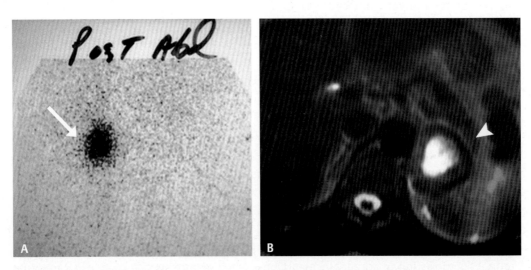

Fig. 66.3 Left adrenal pheochromocytoma. **(A)** A planar metaiodobenzylguanidine scan (posterior projection) shows intense tracer localization to the left adrenal bed (*arrow*). **(B)** T2-weighted axial magnetic resonance image shows characteristic high signal in the left adrenal gland (*arrowhead*) in the same patient. Source: Resnick, Older, Diagnosis of Genitourinary Disease, New York: Thieme, 1997: 543. Reprinted by permission.

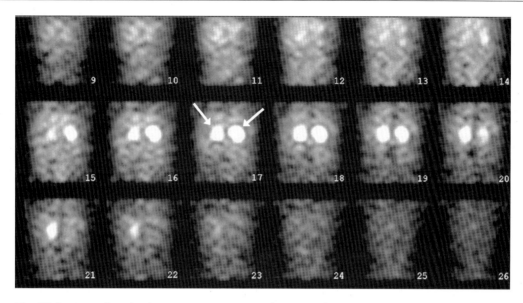

Fig. 66.4   Coronal single-photon emission computed tomography (SPECT) OctreoScan in a patient with von Hippel-Lindau disease and known bilateral pheochromocytomas. Bilateral intense uptake of the tracer is seen in the adrenal glands (*arrows*) but nowhere else in the body.

- Localized uptake on MIBG scan is indicative of pheochromocytoma (**Fig. 66.3A**). This corresponded to an abnormality that was noted on MRI (**Fig. 66.3B**).
- OctreoScan (Covidien, Hazelwood, Missouri), an indium 111-labeled somatostatin analogue, binds to somatostatin receptors on pheochromocytomas and is considered a second-line imaging agent.
- These agents are generally employed to confirm pheochromocytomas and, more importantly, to identify other foci of metastatic disease (**Fig. 66.4**).

MAGNETIC RESONANCE IMAGING

- The magnetic resonance imaging (MRI) classic appearance for pheochromocytomas is shown in **Fig. 66.5**. Pheochromocytomas are low to intermediate signal on T1-weighted imaging, intensely bright ("lightbulb bright") on T2-weighted imaging, and should show prominent enhancement on contrast-enhanced images.
- As mentioned in the CT section, these tumors can have atypical appearances, including low signal on T2-weighted imaging, high signal on T1-weighted imaging due to intratumoral fat or hemorrhage, and show little to no enhancement in regions of necrosis or cystic degeneration, as in the left adrenal gland in **Fig. 66.5E**.
- High T2 signal is not specific for pheochromocytomas, as metastases and adrenal carcinoma may have high signal.
- Calcification, if present, may not be apparent on MRI or may show magnetic susceptibility artifact.

Treatment

- Treatment is surgical resection after appropriate adrenergic blockade to prevent adverse effects of catecholamine discharge during anesthesia induction or tumor manipulation.

Prognosis

- Ten percent of pheochromocytomas are malignant. However, malignant pheochromocytomas are difficult to diagnose pathologically. Therefore, diagnosis depends on identifying distant metastases at staging and at follow-up.

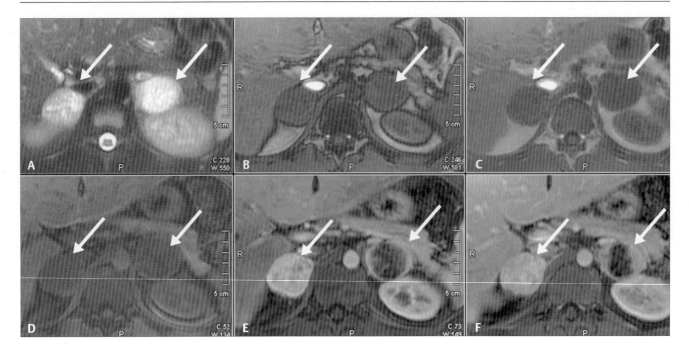

Fig. 66.5 Magnetic resonance imaging in a patient with von Hippel-Lindau disease and known pheochromocytomas. **(A)** Axial T2-weighted fat saturation show bilateral high-signal adrenal masses (*arrows*) on T2-weighted images that do not have signal drop on the opposed phase GRE. **(B)** T1 gradient echo (GRE) opposed phase, and **(C)** T1 GRE in phase images. **(D)** Axial three-dimensional GRE fat saturation and **(E)** pregadolinium and **(F)** postgadolinium images show an intensely enhancing right adrenal mass but a left adrenal mass with poorly enhancing central areas mimicking a cystic lesion owing to tumor necrosis.

PEARLS

- Pheochromocytoma should be excluded biochemically prior to percutaneous adrenal biopsy to avoid a "pheochromocytoma crisis" (i.e., a spectrum of physiologic abnormalities associated with catecholamine discharge such as hypertension, circulatory failure, and shock).
- Administration of high osmolar iodinated contrast materials should be avoided if an adrenal mass is suspected of being a pheochromocytoma because of possible instigation of a hypertensive crisis with the associated cardiovascular morbidities. Low osmolar contrast appears to be safe.
- Pheochromocytoma should be considered in the differential of any unknown adrenal mass.

Suggested Readings

Blake MA, Kalra MK, Maher MM, et al. Pheochromocytoma: an imaging chameleon. Radiographics 2004;24(Suppl 1):S87–S99.

Blake MA, Krishnamoorthy SK, Boland GW, et al. Low-density pheochromocytoma on CT: a mimicker of adrenal adenoma. AJR Am J Roentgenol 2003;181(6):1663–1668.

Klingler HC, Klingler PJ, Martin JK Jr, et al. Pheochromocytoma. Urology 2001;57(6):1025–1032.

Lee TH, Slywotzky CM, Lavelle MT, Garcia RA. Cystic pheochromocytoma. Radiographics 2002;22(4):935–940.

Manger WM. An overview of pheochromocytoma: history, current concepts, vagaries, and diagnostic challenges. Ann N Y Acad Sci 2006;1073:1–20.

Schwerk WB, Gorg C, Gorg K, Restrepo IK. Adrenal pheochromocytomas: a broad spectrum of sonographic presentation. J Ultrasound Med 1994;13(7):517–521.

Swensen SJ, Brown ML, Sheps SG, et al. Use of 131I-MIBG scintigraphy in the evaluation of suspected pheochromocytoma. Mayo Clin Proc 1985;60(5):299–304.

Welch TJ, Sheedy PF II, van Heerden JA, et al. Pheochromocytoma: value of computed tomography. Radiology 1983;148(2):501–503.

CASE 67

Clinical Presentation

A 19-year-old female presents with acute onset of right upper quadrant pain.

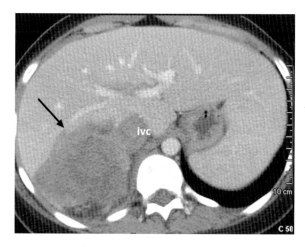

Fig. 67.1 Contrast-enhanced computed tomography scan of the abdomen in a patient with right upper quadrant pain. IVC, inferior vena cava.

Radiologic Findings

- Contrast-enhanced computed tomography (**Fig. 67.1**) shows a right upper quadrant mass cephalad to the right kidney. The mass measures 12 cm with invasion of the adjacent liver (*arrow*) and also invasion into the inferior vena cava (IVC).

Diagnosis

Primary adrenal cortical carcinoma

Differential Diagnosis

- Pheochromocytoma
- Adenoma
- Metastatic disease
- Lymphoma or leukemia

Discussion

Background

Primary adrenal cortical carcinoma is very rare (1–2:1,000,000 persons). Age distribution is bimodal, with one peak in early childhood and another in the 4th to 5th decade. Adrenal carcinomas are often quite large at diagnosis, measuring between 6 and 22 cm. Incidentally discovered adrenal lesions measuring > 6 cm are treated presumptively as adrenal carcinomas and are surgically resected after pheochromocytoma is excluded biochemically.

239

Clinical Findings

More than half of patients present with autonomous cortisol production (Cushing syndrome), but a variety of other adrenal cortical hormones may be overproduced, resulting in adrenogenital syndrome (excess sex hormones) or Conn syndrome (excess aldosterone), as well as others. The remaining patients present with pain or other symptoms referable to the mass.

Pathology

Adrenal carcinoma is diagnosed pathologically based on a combination of macroscopic features (e.g., capsule disruption, tumor weight, and presence of hemorrhage) and microscopic features (e.g., mitotic rate and nuclear atypia). The presence of fibrotic bands is a differentiating feature between benign adrenal cortical neoplasms and frank adrenal carcinoma. Pathologic analysis of percutaneous biopsy (fine needle aspiration or core needle biopsy) of adrenal carcinoma presents a challenge to pathologists, as adrenal carcinoma can appear similar to normal adrenal cortical tissue.

Imaging Findings

COMPUTED TOMOGRAPHY

- Pheochromocytoma would present with hypertension and/or the classic triad of palpitations, headache, and diaphoresis, which is not present in this case.
- Adrenal adenomas are usually < 3 cm and do not invade adjacent structures, as seen with this case (**Fig. 67.1**).
- Metastatic disease, lymphoma, and leukemia are possibilities, but there is no known extra-adrenal malignancy in this patient.
- Adrenal carcinomas characteristically present as large tumors (> 6 cm) (**Figs. 67.1** and **67.2**).
- Tumor margins are poorly defined, irregular, or frankly invasive. Invasion into adjacent structures, such as the kidney, spleen, or liver (**Fig. 67.2**), is common.
- Vascular invasion into the adrenal vein, renal vein, or IVC is common.
- The lesions are heterogeneous owing to necrosis or intratumoral hemorrhage. The lesions will enhance inhomogeneously.
- Calcification is present in ~30 to 40%.

RADIOGRAPHY

- Abdominal radiography or intravenous pyelogram (IVP) may show displacement of the kidney or other organs if the adrenal mass is large.

ULTRASOUND

- Nonspecific findings
- Adrenal carcinoma will be heterogeneous. Hypoechoic areas will be seen, representing cystic change, with viable tumor or necrotic areas being more echogenic.
- Color flow may be observed in viable tumor tissue. Vascular invasion may be easier to detect with ultrasound, but false-positives from compressive mass effect have been reported.
- A well-defined capsule is seen surrounding most or the entire tumor in half of all patients.

NUCLEAR MEDICINE

- There is probably no benefit to specialized adrenal scintigraphy (e.g., iodocholesterol imaging) over standard computed tomography (CT) or magnetic resonance imaging (MRI).

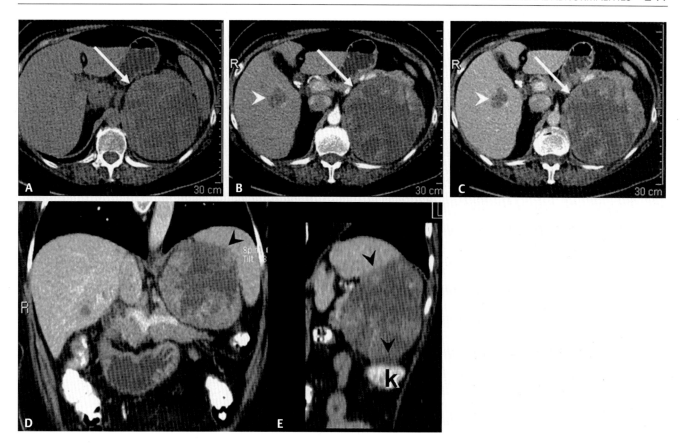

Fig. 67.2 Adrenal protocol computed tomography (CT) scans in a patient with left-sided pain and an adrenal mass on prior imaging. **(A)** Unenhanced, **(B)** enhanced, and **(C)** 10-minute delayed CT scans show a large heterogeneous left upper quadrant mass (*arrows*) with large areas of poor enhancement representing necrosis. Note the hepatic metastasis in the liver (*arrowhead*). Three-dimensional reconstruction images in the **(D)** coronal and **(E)** sagittal planes show invasion of the spleen (*black arrowheads*) by the mass and tumor invading the renal capsule (*black arrowheads*) of the inferiorly displaced left kidney (k). Both organs were invaded at surgery.

MAGNETIC RESONANCE IMAGING

- Morphologic features are similar to CT. MRI strengths include multiplanar reconstructions that allow definitive localization of the tumor within the adrenal gland. This plus vascular sequences can improve radiologists' confidence that tumor is or is not invading adjacent organs and vessels.
- Large, irregularly marginated or invasive masses will be seen with mass effect upon, or frank invasion into, adjacent organs and vascular structures (**Fig. 67.3**).
- Solid portions of tumor will show moderate to marked enhancement in a nodular pattern following gadolinium administration.
- Necrosis is common and will show a variable pattern on T1-weighted images and high intensity on T2-weighted images with areas of corresponding poor enhancement following gadolinium (**Fig. 67.3**).
- Hemorrhage is common and will show variable signal on T1- and T2-weighted images depending on the age of the blood present in the hemorrhagic mass.
- An important pitfall to note is that there can be lipid contained within the adrenal carcinoma that might mimic an adrenal cortical adenoma with a drop in signal on opposed phase gradient echo (GRE) images. Drop in signal may not be uniform due to irregular dispersion of lipid in the adrenal mass.

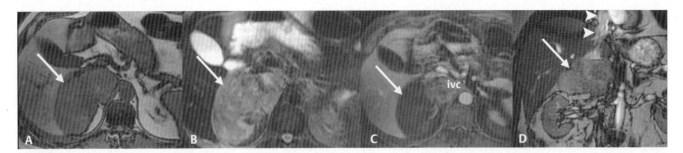

Fig. 67.3 Axial magnetic resonance imaging in a patient with right flank pain. **(A)** T1 gradient echo (GRE) shows a homogeneous right adrenal mass (*arrow*). **(B)** T2-weighted image with fat saturation shows the lesion to be heterogeneous and high signal. **(C)** Postgadolinium three-dimensional GRE shows significant portions of tumor not enhancing, representing necrosis. Only the portion invading the inferior vena cava (IVC) enhances. **(D)** Coronal magnetic resonance venogram showing tumor invasion into the IVC (*arrowheads*) just inferior to the heart.

- Calcification may not be discernible on MRI or may cause magnetic susceptibility artifact on T1 GRE images.

POSITRON EMISSION TOMOGRAPHY

- Positron emission tomography (PET) has been shown to be accurate in the differentiation of benign from malignant adrenal lesions. However, there is some contradictory literature, and the final role of PET in adrenal carcinoma has not been defined.

Treatment

- Primary surgical resection is both diagnostic and therapeutic for these lesions.
- In patients with advanced disease and distant metastases at the time of presentation, adrenal biopsy can be entertained to obtain a diagnosis prior to initiation of chemotherapy.

Prognosis

- Adrenal carcinoma has a very poor prognosis, with a mean survival time of < 18 months.
  - Although diagnosis at an earlier stage does convey some survival benefit, overall 5-year survival is still abysmal (16–38%).

PEARLS _____

- Percutaneous biopsy of an incidentally discovered adrenal mass in a patient with no known primary malignancy (the "adrenal incidentaloma") should be discouraged because cytologic analysis cannot differentiate adrenal cortical neoplasms from normal adrenal cortical tissue.
- In general, biopsy of suspected primary adrenal carcinomas should not be performed; rather, they should be referred to an adrenal surgeon for surgical removal. Biopsy needle track seeding is a possibility.
- In any patient with an incidentally discovered adrenal mass, pheochromocytoma should be excluded biochemically, especially prior to any intervention.

Suggested Readings

Allolio B, Fassnacht M. Adrenocortical carcinoma: clinical update. J Clin Endocrinol Metab 2006; 91(6):2027–2037.

Anonymous. NIH state-of-the-science statement on management of the clinically inapparent adrenal mass ("incidentaloma"). NIH Consens State Sci Statements 2002;19(2):1–25.

Elsayes KM, Mukundan G, Narra VR, et al. Adrenal masses: MR imaging features with pathologic correlation. Radiographics 2004;24(Suppl 1):S73–S86.

Fishman EK, Deutch BM, Hartman DS, et al. Primary adrenocortical carcinoma: CT evaluation with clinical correlation. AJR Am J Roentgenol 1987;148(3):531–535.

Hamper UM, Fishman EK, Hartman DS, Roberts JL, Sanders RC. Primary adrenocortical carcinoma: sonographic evaluation with clinical and pathologic correlation in 26 patients. AJR Am J Roentgenol 1987;148(5):915–919.

Lockhart ME, Smith JK, Kenney PJ. Imaging of adrenal masses. Eur J Radiol 2002;41(2):95–112.

Schlund JF, Kenney PJ, Brown ED, et al. Adrenocortical carcinoma: MR imaging appearance with current techniques. J Magn Reson Imaging 1995;5(2):171–174.

Slattery JM, Blake MA, Kalra MK, et al. Adrenocortical carcinoma: contrast washout characteristics on CT. AJR Am J Roentgenol 2006;187(1):W21–W24.

CASE 68

Clinical Presentation

Abdominal pain

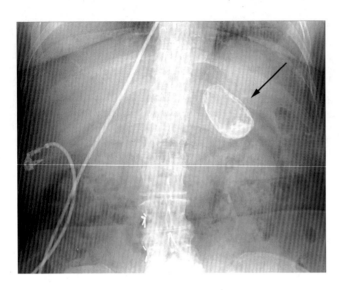

Fig. 68.1 Abdominal plain film in a patient with abdominal pain. Radiograph shows a large oval calcified mass in the left upper quadrant (*arrow*).

Radiologic Findings

- On abdominal radiograph, a large oval mass with calcified rim is seen in the left upper quadrant (**Fig. 68.1**)
- On abdominal computed tomography (CT), a large oval mass with calcified rim is seen arising from the left adrenal gland (**Fig. 68.2**)

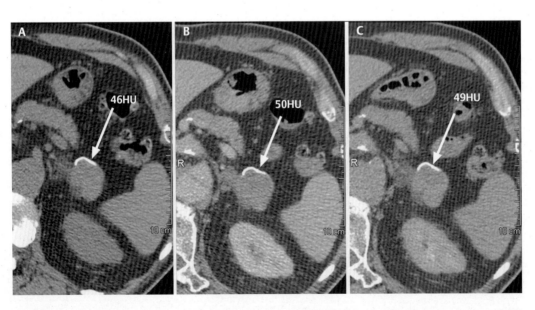

Fig. 68.2 Same patient as in **Fig. 68.1**. Adrenal protocol computed tomography with **(A)** unenhanced, **(B)** enhanced, and **(C)** 10-minute delayed images shows a calcified left upper quadrant mass (*arrows*) with no discernible enhancement.

- Baseline high attenuation may be due to proteinaceous contents or calcification.
- No significant enhancement in lesion

Diagnosis

Adrenal pseudocyst

Differential Diagnosis

- Adrenal cyst
- Adrenal adenoma
- Adrenal hemorrhage
- Cystic adrenal neoplasm, including pheochromocytoma, primary adrenal carcinoma, and cystic metastases to the adrenal gland

Discussion

Background

Adrenal cysts are rare. The most common are adrenal pseudocysts. Other cystic adrenal lesions have been previously categorized as (1) endothelial cysts, (2) epithelial cysts, and (3) parasitic (hydatid) cysts. In a 25-year review of cystic adrenal neoplasms at the Mayo Clinic (Erickson), 78% of adrenal cystic lesions were pseudocysts, 20% were endothelial lined cysts, and 2% were epithelial lined cysts. No hydatid cysts were reported in this series. Nineteen percent of adrenal pseudocysts are associated with adrenal tumors, including adrenal adenoma, adrenal cortical carcinoma, and pheochromocytoma.

Clinical Findings

In the Mayo study, most patients presented with symptoms of pain referable to the size of the cystic adrenal lesion. Gastrointestinal symptoms and a palpable mass at physical exam have also been reported.

Pathology

Pseudocysts are cystic structures with definable walls but no identifiable lining. Most pseudocysts are believed to evolve from previous adrenal hemorrhage or infection. Some are related to hemorrhage into an associated adrenal tumor. Endothelial lined cysts arise from angiomatous tissues. Epithelial lined cysts and hydatid disease are extremely uncommon.

Imaging Findings

RADIOGRAPHY

- Abdominal radiography is nonspecific for this diagnosis.
- Calcifications may be conspicuous on plain film radiography, but the true nature may be confused with calcified renal cysts, calcified cysts in the liver or spleen, or vascular calcification/aneurysms. Cross-sectional imaging is usually undertaken.

COMPUTED TOMOGRAPHY

- Adrenal cysts will be round or oval, measure simple fluid [0–20 Hounsfield units (HU)], and show no enhancement following intravenous (IV) contrast.

- Adrenal adenomas may have low attenuation in the simple fluid range, but they will show enhancement following IV contrast.
- Adrenal hemorrhage will show no enhancement but should resolve on short-term follow-up CT scans.
- Adrenal pseudocysts may be high density (i.e., > 20 HU) because of intracystic hemorrhage, infection, or calcifications.
- Granulation tissue within adrenal pseudocysts may enhance minimally.
- Cystic adrenal neoplasms, including pheochromocytoma, primary adrenal carcinoma, and metastases, can mimic adrenal pseudocysts. Biopsy or surgical excision is usually required for definitive diagnosis when there is high clinical suspicion of one of these mimics.

ULTRASOUND

- Adrenal cysts will contain anechoic simple fluid.
- With cyst hemorrhage or infection, a fluid debris level may be present.
- Chronic pseudocysts will have complex contents ± calcification.

MAGNETIC RESONANCE IMAGING

- Adrenal cysts will follow the signal intensity of simple fluid on all sequences (**Fig. 68.3A–C**) and will not enhance (**Fig. 68.3D**).
- Adrenal pseudocysts may be more complex, have varying signal on both T1- and T2-weighted images, and may show minimal enhancement.

Treatment

- For painful adrenal pseudocysts, treatment is simple surgical excision after excluding pheochromocytoma.
- Asymptomatic lesions can be followed to confirm stability, but any change or new symptom warrants surgical removal.

Prognosis

- True adrenal cysts and pseudocysts are benign.

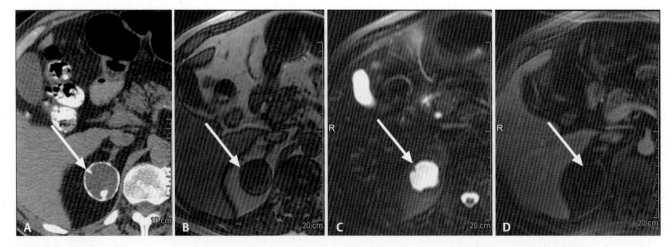

Fig. 68.3 **(A)** Noncontrast computed tomography shows a calcified mass emanating from the medial limb of the right adrenal gland (*arrow*). **(B)** T1-weighted gradient echo (GRE) axial image, **(C)** T2-weighted axial image with fat saturation, and **(D)** T1-weighted GRE axial image with gadolinium show the mass to be cystic and without enhancement (*arrows*).

PEARLS _____

- Several cystic neoplasms occur in the adrenal gland that can mimic adrenal cysts and pseudocysts. Adrenal cortical carcinomas and pheochromocytomas may calcify and/or may undergo cystic degeneration. Adrenal adenomas or myelolipomas may undergo hemorrhagic transformation that may evolve to a cystic adrenal lesion. An adrenal pseudocyst is therefore a diagnosis of exclusion.

Suggested Readings

Erickson LA, Lloyd RV, Hartman R, Thompson G. Cystic adrenal neoplasms. Cancer 2004;101(7):1537–1544.

Habra MA, Feig BW, Waguespack SG. Image in endocrinology: adrenal pseudocyst. J Clin Endocrinol Metab 2005;90(5):3067–3068.

Korobkin M, Francis IR. Imaging of adrenal masses. Urol Clin North Am 1997;24(3):603–622.

CASE 69

Clinical Presentation

Patient having work-up for hematuria

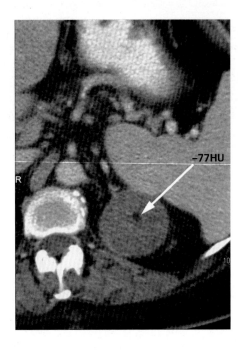

Fig. 69.1 Hematuria work-up. Contrast-enhanced computed tomography scan shows a 4 cm intermediate density left adrenal mass with a low density center (*arrow*) that measures –77 HU.

Radiologic Findings

- Incidental 4 cm left adrenal mass (**Fig. 69.1**) with a central low density (*arrow*) measuring –77 Hounsfield units (HU), which is in the range of macroscopic fat and is diagnostic of an adrenal myelolipoma

Diagnosis

Myelolipoma

Differential Diagnosis

- Adrenal adenoma
- Adrenal cyst
- Exophytic angiomyolipoma from the adjacent upper pole of the kidney
- Retroperitoneal liposarcoma

Discussion

Background

Adrenal myelolipomas are adrenal neoplasms that contain mature adipose cells and hematopoietic elements resembling bone marrow. They are uniformly benign and are easily recognized when macroscopic fat is present in an adrenal mass on computed tomography (CT) or magnetic resonance imaging (MRI). The belief is that myelolipoma results from a metaplastic process in the adrenal gland, but this theory has not been proven.

Clinical Findings

Unless there has been incidental hemorrhage in the myelolipoma resulting in pain, patients are generally asymptomatic, and the adrenal mass is detected while the patient is undergoing imaging for other reasons.

Pathology

Grossly, fatty yellow tissue is seen mixed with reddish marrow elements. Microscopically, mature fat mixed with hematopoietic tissues is diagnostic.

Imaging Findings

COMPUTED TOMOGRAPHY

- Lipid-rich adrenal adenomas measure < 10 HU on unenhanced CT scans. Density should not approach that of macroscopic fat, which is in the range of –30 to –120 HU.
- Adrenal cysts are fluid density (i.e., 0–20 HU).
- Coronal reconstructions would best show that this lesion arises from the adrenal gland and not the adjacent kidney, as would an exophytic angiomyolipoma.
- To exclude retroperitoneal sarcoma, you must be certain the lesion arises from within the adrenal gland. If the retroperitoneal lesion is outside the adrenal gland or appears to be invading the adrenal gland, sarcoma should be considered.
- Lesions should be well circumscribed and be contained within the adrenal gland (**Fig. 69.2**).
- Nearly all myelolipomas contain some areas of macroscopic fat.
- Macroscopic fat density measures between –30 and –120 HU and is grossly similar in density to subcutaneous and retroperitoneal fat (**Fig. 69.2**).
- Soft tissue density in myelolipomas is related to the hematopoietic elements. Myelolipomas composed mostly of hematopoietic elements measure higher density (**Fig. 69.1**) and can enhance, making detection of fat more difficult.
- Twenty percent of myelolipomas will contain calcifications.

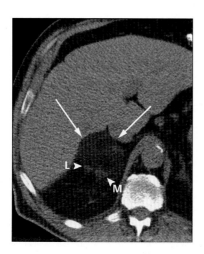

Fig. 69.2 A fatty mass arising within the right adrenal gland. Unenhanced computed tomography scan through the right adrenal gland shows a fatty mass (*arrows*) replacing the adrenal gland. The mass clearly arises from the adrenal gland because the lateral (L, *arrowhead*) and medial (M, *arrowhead*) limbs of the gland are enlarged by the presence of the fatty mass. A retroperitoneal liposarcoma is excluded because the organ of origin for this fatty mass is assuredly the adrenal gland.

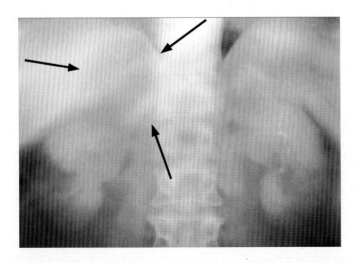

	321	322	323	324	325	326	327	328	329
	44	24	28	39	48	42	37	13	-5
	77	52	39	45	45	41	48	40	42
	17	27	9	-28	-30	15	34	48	50
	13	31	0	-55	-77	-56	-20	22	6
	13	30	-1	-39	-44	-32	11	44	40
	55	42	-12	-56	-63	-54	-17	15	14
	45	51	-17	-73	-65	-63	-29	36	44
	50	38	2	-32	-28	14	35	43	27
	-3	8	18	-6	15	15	16	24	1
	57	57	52	57	52	44	41	30	29
	41	53	56	27	13	31	31	42	44

A   B

Fig. 69.3 Pixel map. **(A)** Contrast-enhanced computed tomography scan with a region of interest (*rectangle*) drawn around the low-density component of an otherwise high-density adrenal mass. **(B)** Pixel map of the rectangular region of interest drawn in the left adrenal mass. This lesion has a focal area of macroscopic fat densities (*circle*) in the range of −30 to −120 HU on the pixel map, corresponding to the low-density component, confirming that this adrenal mass is an adrenal myelolipoma.

- If the fatty tumor is separate from the adrenal gland or if the fatty lesion appears to be invading the adrenal gland, an aggressive retroperitoneal process, such as liposarcoma, should be considered.

Pixel Map

In difficult cases where manually drawn regions of interest (ROIs) may be equivocal for fat density Hounsfield values, the radiologist may request a pixel map. The CT technologist will draw an ROI around the low-density portion of the adrenal mass (**Fig. 69.3**). A map or table of the attenuation values of all the pixels in that ROI will be displayed on the CT console. If there are values matching that of macroscopic fat, the diagnosis of adrenal myelolipoma is confirmed.

RADIOGRAPHY

- A large myelolipoma may be detectable on abdominal radiography, such as an intravenous pyelogram (IVP), as a space-occupying lesion with displacement of adjacent structures (**Fig. 69.4**), but most will be nondetectable on standard radiographs.

Fig. 69.4 Intravenous pyelogram (IVP). View coned to the kidneys from the IVP shows a right suprarenal low-density mass (*arrows*) with mass effect on the subadjacent upper pole of the right kidney. This mass was confirmed to be a fat containing myelolipoma on a subsequent computed tomography scan.

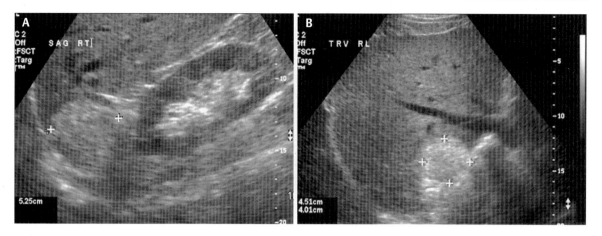

Fig. 69.5 Abdominal sonogram in the same patient as in **Fig. 69.2.** **(A)** Sagittal and **(B)** transverse images through the right suprarenal space show an echogenic mass (*calipers*) corresponding to the lesion seen in **Fig. 69.2.** On this ultrasound, it may be difficult to separate the mass from the upper pole of the right kidney. Exophytic renal cell carcinoma, angiomyolipoma, and other renal tumors need to be excluded with computed tomography or magnetic resonance imaging.

ULTRASOUND

- Ultrasound findings are not specific for myelolipoma.
- Normal adrenal glands are not ordinarily visualized in adults with sonography.
- An adrenal mass, especially on the right, can be conspicuous because the adjacent liver serves as an acoustic window to see the adjacent adrenal mass (**Fig. 69.5**).
- On ultrasound, fatty tumors such as myelolipomas are echogenic, but this is a nonspecific finding (**Fig. 69.5**).

MAGNETIC RESONANCE IMAGING

- Detection of macroscopic fat on MRI is performed with T1-weighted sequences without and with the application of fat saturation:
  - If an adrenal lesion contains areas of high signal on T1 sequences that saturates out (i.e., gets darker) on fat saturation sequences, this confirms the lesion contains macroscopic fat and is consistent with myelolipoma (**Fig. 69.6A,B**).
  - Lesions may also decrease in signal on opposed phase T1 gradient echo (GRE) sequences compared with their appearance on in phase T1 GRE sequences, but only if there are equal amounts of fat and soft tissue in the same pixel elements (required for chemical shift artifact) (*arrow*, **Fig. 69.6C,D**). Complementary CT also confirms fat density (*arrow*, **Fig. 69.6E**).

Treatment

- Myelolipomas are true leave-alone lesions because they are benign.
- Pain from necrosis or interval hemorrhage may require surgical removal or angiographic embolization for continued bleeding.
- Those lesions associated with hormonal imbalance can undergo surgical resection for normalization of endocrine function.

Prognosis

- There is no malignancy potential.

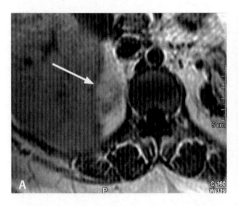
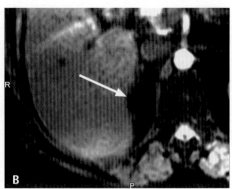
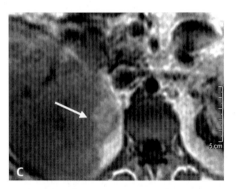
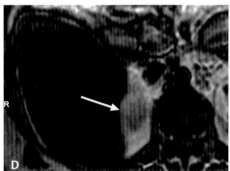
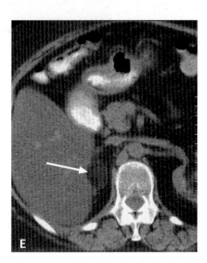

Fig. 69.6   A fatty adrenal mass (*arrow*) evaluated by magnetic resonance imaging (MRI) with comparison computed tomography (CT). Axial MRI using **(A)** T1 gradient echo (GRE) without fat saturation, **(B)** T1 GRE with fat saturation, **(C)** in phase GRE, and **(D)** opposed phase GRE. A drop of signal on fat saturation sequences **(A,B)** confirms macroscopic fat in the adrenal lesion. There is little change on chemical shift imaging (in and opposed phases) because the lesion is almost entirely fat, as confirmed on the accompanying contrast-enhanced CT scan of same patient **(E)**.

PEARLS

- When asked to biopsy an atypical myelolipoma to exclude metastatic disease, core biopsy is required to show macroscopic fat and hematopoietic elements, which are required for definitive diagnosis of myelolipoma.

Suggested Readings

Dunnick NR, Korobkin M. Imaging of adrenal incidentalomas: current status. AJR Am J Roentgenol 2002;179(3):559–568.

Han M, Burnett AL, Fishman EK, Marshall FF. The natural history and treatment of adrenal myelolipoma. J Urol 1997;157(4):1213–1216.

Rao P, Kenney PJ, Wagner BJ, Davidson AJ. Imaging and pathologic features of myelolipoma. Radiographics 1997;17(6):1373–1385.

CASE 70

Clinical Presentation

Patient presents with elevated cortisol levels and failure to adequately suppress on overnight dexamethasone suppression test. Patient has hypertension and some facial edema.

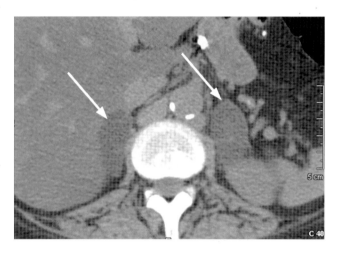

Fig. 70.1 Noncontrast computed tomography scan through the adrenal glands (*arrows*) in a patient with Cushing syndrome.

Radiologic Findings

- Bilateral. low-density [< 10 Hounsfield units (HU)] enlarged adrenal glands (*arrows,* **Fig. 70.1**) on noncontrast computed tomography (CT) scan. Adrenal glands maintain an adreniform shape, consistent with bilateral adrenal hyperplasia.

Diagnosis

Cushing syndrome due to bilateral adrenal hyperplasia (BAH)

Differential Diagnosis

- Bilateral adrenal pheochromocytomas
- Bilateral adrenal adenomas
- Bilateral adrenal metastasis
- Adrenal lymphoma

Discussion

Background

Bilateral adrenal hyperplasia (BAH) in Cushing syndrome may be primarily due to intrinsic adrenal overgrowth with excess cortisol production. However, hypercortisolism may be the result of stimulation from a pituitary adenoma resulting in adrenocorticotropic hormone (ACTH) overproduction (Cushing disease). Ectopic ACTH secretion by a primary malignancy (usually small cell lung cancer) can also occur, resulting in a paraneoplastic syndrome. More than 90% of non-ACTH-dependent Cushing syndrome cases result from a functioning adrenal adenoma or adrenal carcinoma.

Imaging Findings

COMPUTED TOMOGRAPHY

- Bilateral pheochromocytomas would be found in a patient with hypertension, possibly in association with von Hippel-Lindau disease. There is no such history in this case.
- With bilateral enlarged adrenal glands, and therefore the possibility of bilateral adrenal hyperplasia, clinical correlation regarding functional adrenal abnormalities is essential. Cushing syndrome is the most common manifestation of adrenal hyperplasia. In the absence of biochemical abnormalities, bilateral nonfunctioning adenomas, metastatic disease, and lymphoma become realistic considerations.
- Hyperplasia is recognized as smooth or nodular enlargement of both the adrenal body and the limbs.
- Size measurements can be performed, but it may be challenging to measure reproducibly, given the small size of these structures. In general, in BAH, the gland's body and limbs have a "beefy" appearance but maintain an adreniform shape. This finding, however, is not specific for hyperplasia, as adrenal adenomas may present similarly.
- The hyperplastic glands may contain high amounts of cholesterol (intracytoplasmic lipid), so the adrenal glands may measure < 10 HU on an unenhanced CT scan (**Fig. 70.1**) and drop in signal on opposed phase T1-weighted gradient echo (GRE) magnetic resonance imaging (MRI) sequences compared with in phase sequences, just as adenomas do.

Treatment

Therapy depends on the cause of hypercortisolism:

- For a pituitary tumor, surgical therapy is indicated.
- For an adrenal adenoma, adrenalectomy is indicated.
- For BAH, medical therapy is directed at ameliorating the effects of hormone overproduction. If medical therapy fails, bilateral adrenal resection may be undertaken, but the patient will require lifelong cortisol supplementation as a result.
- For ACTH-producing tumors, treatment is directed at the tumor.

Prognosis

- Depends on the etiology of the hypercortisolism

PEARLS _____

- The diagnosis of Cushing syndrome is made clinically, and the role of imaging, primarily with CT, is to determine if a functioning adrenal adenoma or adrenal carcinoma is present.

Suggested Readings

Rockall AG, Babar SA, Sohaib SA, et al. CT and MR imaging of the adrenal glands in ACTH-independent cushing syndrome. Radiographics 2004;24(2):435–452.

CASE 71

Clinical Presentation

Following a motor vehicle collision, a patient presents with an incidentally noted right adrenal mass. No other acute injury is noted on routine computed tomography (CT) scans. A follow-up CT scan was recommended.

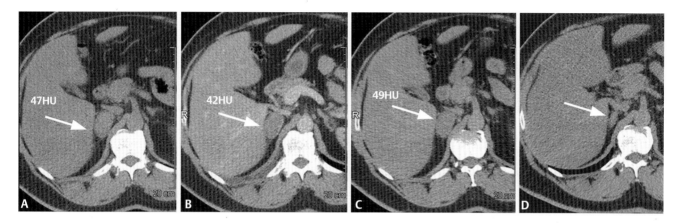

Fig. 71.1 Status post–motor vehicle collision. Follow-up adrenal protocol computed tomography (CT) with **(A)** unenhanced, **(B)** portal venous phase enhanced, and **(C)** 10-minute delayed imaging through the upper abdomen shows no enhancement within the right adrenal mass. **(D)** Unenhanced CT 5 months later shows resolution of the right adrenal mass.

Radiologic Findings

- Well-defined oval right adrenal mass (arrows, **Figs. 71.1A–C**)
- Minimal periadrenal stranding
- No significant change in attenuation from unenhanced through delayed scans, consistent with a nonenhancing lesion.
- The lesion resolved on follow-up CT (**Fig. 71.1D**), which is essential to making this diagnosis.

Diagnosis

Traumatic adrenal hemorrhage

Differential Diagnosis

- Adrenal adenoma
- Adrenal metastasis
- Adrenal cortical carcinoma
- Pheochromocytoma
- Lymphoma/leukemia

Discussion

Background

Traumatic adrenal hemorrhage is found in ~2% of trauma patients who undergo CT. Adrenal hemorrhage is seen more frequently in more severe traumas, and there is a high association with other traumatic injuries and a higher mortality. Isolated adrenal hemorrhage is rare, and a search for other injuries should be undertaken in this situation. In the absence of other traumatic injury, consider an adrenal "incidentaloma" as the diagnosis and recommend adrenal protocol CT follow-up.

Clinical Findings

In the setting of trauma, an adrenal mass is presumed to represent post-traumatic adrenal hemorrhage. Follow-up adrenal protocol CT is recommended to confirm resolution of the mass. With spontaneous adrenal hemorrhage, patients present with vague abdominal or flank pain, which may result in an abdominal CT scan, where the diagnosis is suggested and follow-up is required.

Imaging Findings

COMPUTED TOMOGRAPHY

- None of the lesions in the differential would show so little change in attenuation over the three-phase adrenal protocol CT scan.
- Short-term follow-up is the key to this diagnosis showing resolution of the adrenal hemorrhage. With follow-up imaging, most hemorrhages should resolve or at least decrease in size and also decrease in attenuation, separating adrenal hemorrhage from all of the other differential possibilities. Periadrenal stranding should resolve.
- Adrenal hemorrhage will present as a round or oval high-attenuation mass within the adrenal gland, or obscuring it, with or without periadrenal stranding.
- Adrenal hemorrhage attenuation measures ~40 to 60 Hounsfield units (HU).
- No enhancement in the adrenal hemorrhage is seen when an unenhanced CT (or delayed CT) is available for comparison.
- Adrenal hematomas range from 2 to 4 cm.
- Some hematomas become chronic and do not resolve. They display benign features (e.g., remain stable over years). They may show varying amounts of calcification (**Fig. 71.2**). Chronic hematomas may become adrenal pseudocysts.

ULTRASOUND

- Ultrasound is useful for the evaluation and follow-up of suspected adrenal hemorrhage in newborns (**Fig. 71.3**).
- Adrenal hemorrhage will present acutely as a complex heterogeneous solid-appearing mass in the suprarenal fossa. The lesion will show no blood flow on color or power Doppler unless active bleeding is present.
- The mass will gradually resolve over time, with a decrease in size and change from hyperechoic to hypoechoic centrally as the clot retracts and resorbs. Resolution excludes neuroblastoma as a possibility.
- The lesion may completely resolve, or a residual fluid collection or mass may remain in the suprarenal fossa.
- In adults, the adrenal glands are difficult to visualize with ultrasound.

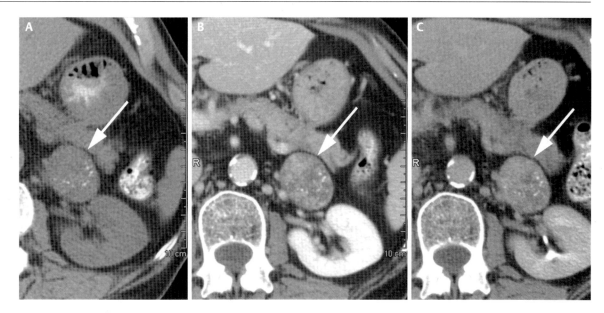

Fig. 71.2 Adrenal protocol computed tomography (CT) showing **(A)** unenhanced CT with a 4 cm left adrenal mass (*arrow*) containing stippled calcification. **(B)** Contrast-enhanced CT shows patchy areas of enhancement within the mass (*arrow*). **(C)** A 10-minute delayed CT shows little washout from the mass (*arrow*), consistent with an indeterminate lesion. Following surgical resection, pathologic analysis showed chronic hemorrhage within a degenerated adrenal adenoma.

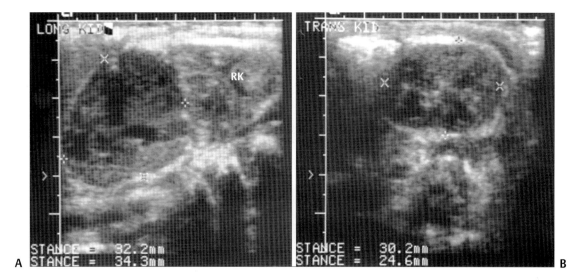

Fig. 71.3 Abdominal sonogram in a newborn with a distended abdomen and neonatal adrenal hemorrhage. **(A)** Sagittal and **(B)** transverse images of the right suprare- nal fossa show a heterogeneous soft tissue mass (*calipers*) above the right kidney (RK).

MAGNETIC RESONANCE IMAGING

- Blood and its breakdown products show various signal intensities depending on the time period after the hemorrhage when the magnetic resonance imaging is performed (**Fig. 71.4**). See **Table 71.1.**

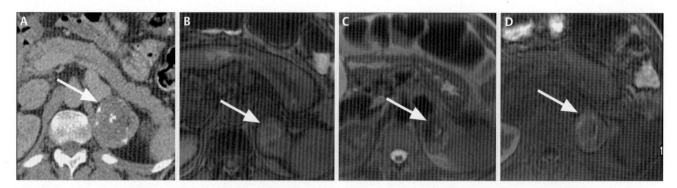

Fig. 71.4 Magnetic resonance imaging showing adrenal hemorrhage of varying ages within a chronic organizing hematoma. **(A)** Contrast-enhanced computed tomography scan shows a lesion (*arrow*). **(B)** T1-weighted gradient echo (GRE) axial image shows a predominantly high-signal left adrenal mass (*arrow*), suggesting methemoglobin. **(C)** T2-weighted axial image with fat saturation shows a heterogeneous mass (*arrow*) with high signal areas (suggesting methemoglobin) and low signal areas (suggesting hemosiderin). **(D)** Postgadolinium T1-weighted GRE axial image with fat saturation shows no significant enhancement in the mass (*arrow*, i.e., similar to **B**).

Table 71.1   Appearance of Adrenal Hematoma on Magnetic Resonance Imaging

Time Period	T1 Weighted	T2 Weighted	Enhancement	Other
< 1 week	Iso- to hypointense	Hypointense	None	Intracellular deoxyhemoglobin
1 to 7 weeks	Hyperintense	Hyperintense	None	Methemoglobin
> 7 weeks	Hypointense rim	Hypointense rim	None	Hemosiderin deposition and pseudocapsule formation

Treatment

- Adrenal hemorrhage is self-limited when not due to coagulopathy or anticoagulation.
- Treatment is directed at the underlying cause of the hemorrhage.
- In patients who develop adrenal insufficiency from adrenal hemorrhage, corticosteroid supplementation is instituted until adrenal function recovers.

Prognosis

- Depending on the cause, adrenal hemorrhage can be self-limited and benign, or it can be a part of sepsis and a cascade with an ultimately fatal conclusion (e.g., meningococcemia).

PEARLS _____

- If asymptomatic and there is strong suspicion the lesion represents hemorrhage, a short-term follow-up in 1 to 3 months can be performed, as adrenal hemorrhage resolves rapidly.

Suggested Readings

Dunnick NR, Korobkin M. Imaging of adrenal incidentalomas: current status. AJR Am J Roentgenol 2002;179(3):559–568.

Kawashima A, Sandler CM, Ernst RD, et al. Imaging of nontraumatic hemorrhage of the adrenal gland. Radiographics 1999;19(4):949–963.

Rana AI, Kenney PJ, Lockhart ME, et al. Adrenal gland hematomas in trauma patients. Radiology 2004;230(3):669–675.

Vella A, Nippoldt TB, Morris JC III. Adrenal hemorrhage: a 25-year experience at the Mayo Clinic. Mayo Clin Proc 2001;76(2):161–168.

CASE 72

Clinical Presentation

Right flank pain

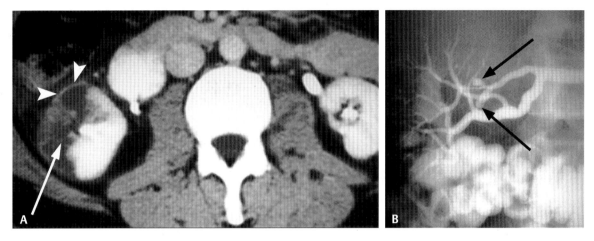

Fig. 72.1 **(A)** Enhanced computed tomography scan through the right kidney. **(B)** Right renal arteriogram.

Radiologic Findings

- Sharply demarcated absent nephrogram anteriorly and laterally, corresponding to segmental artery distribution (*arrow,* **Fig. 72.1A**)
- Rim sign laterally produced by patent capsular vessels, a sign of a renal infarct (*arrowheads,* **Fig. 72.1A**)
- Occlusion of anterosuperior segmental artery on renal angiogram (*black arrows,* **Fig. 72.1B**)

Diagnosis

Renal infarct

Differential Diagnosis

- Acute pyelonephritis
- Renal contusion
- Renal cell carcinoma
- Radiation changes

Discussion

Background

Renal infarction is most commonly an embolic event arising from a cardiac source or peripheral vascular disease. Other causes of renal infarctions include arterial emboli or thrombosis, trauma, vasculitis, renal vein thrombosis, and septic shock.

261

Clinical Findings

Depends on the etiology. A renal infarct may be entirely asymptomatic, or the patient may present with flank pain and/or hematuria.

Pathology

Important to the pathogenesis of renal infarction is the "end organ" nature of the kidney's blood supply. There is little collateral blood flow to the kidneys other than small capsular vessels. Infarcts may be solitary or multiple and bilateral. Infarcts are wedge-shaped areas of ischemic coagulative necrosis, with the apex directed toward the medulla and the base at the cortex.

Imaging Findings

COMPUTED TOMOGRAPHY

- Hypodensities associated with acute pyelonephritis could appear similar to this case, but the very sharp demarcation, distribution, and peripheral rim sign indicate infarction.
- Renal contusion could appear similar to this case, but there was no history of trauma.
- There is no mass in this case to suggest a neoplasm, only an absent nephrogram. The sharp relatively linear demarcation with the normal parenchyma also would not fit with a mass lesion.
- Radiation can produce a sharply marginated area of diminished nephrogram. No history or other findings on the images suggest prior radiation.
- Classic findings in renal infarction include
  - Sharp demarcation with normal-enhancing renal parenchyma, as seen in **Fig. 72.1A**
  - Wedge-shaped area of nonenhancing tissue
  - Persistent enhancement of the renal capsular vessels producing the so-called rim sign (*arrowheads,* **Fig. 72.1A**)

ANGIOGRAPHY

- Second-line imaging following computed tomography (CT) for diagnosis

MAGNETIC RESONANCE IMAGING

- There is no advantage of magnetic resonance imaging over CT for acute diagnosis of renal infarction unless the patient has a sensitivity to iodinated contrast materials.
- T1- and T2-weighted images show variable signal in the infarcted areas.
- On T1-weighted imaging following gadolinium, a sharp demarcation is seen between the infarcted and normal renal parenchyma.
- The cortical rim sign may not be well seen.

Treatment

- Treatment is directed towards the underlying cause (e.g., treat atrial fibrillation with anticoagulants to prevent further clot formation and embolization).

Prognosis

- Depends on the extent of renal parenchymal infarction. Limited infarction will result in atrophy and scarring of the infarcted renal segment.

- In equivocal cases between renal mass lesion and infarction, a repeat CT in 6 to 8 weeks will show that an infarct will begin to decrease in size and eventually produce renal atrophy with scarring.

Suggested Readings

Kim SH, Park JH, Han JK, et al. Infarction of the kidney: role of contrast enhanced MRI. J Comput Assist Tomogr 1992;16(6):924–928.

Kumar V, ed. Robbins and Cotran: Pathologic Basis of Disease. 7th ed. Philadelphia: Elsevier; 2005.

Saunders HS, Dyer RB, Shifrin RY, et al. The CT nephrogram: implications for evaluation of urinary tract disease. Radiographics 1995;15(5):1069–1085.

CASE 73

Clinical Presentation

A 60-year-old patient presents with uncontrolled hypertension despite multiple medications.

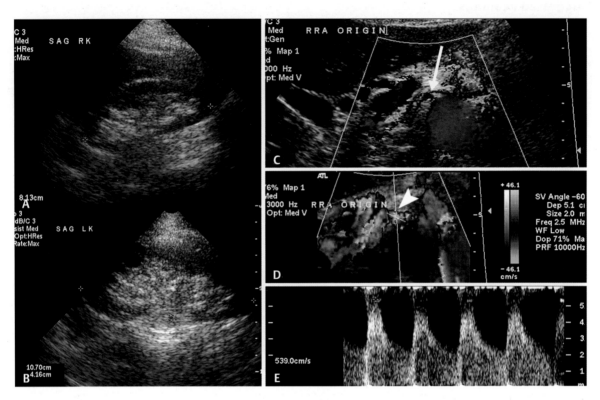

Fig. 73.1 Gray scale sonogram of both kidneys shows size discrepancy, with **(A)** the right kidney measuring 8.1 cm and **(B)** the left kidney measuring 10.7 cm. **(C)** Color flow shows aliasing at the right renal artery origin (*arrow*). **(D)** Angle-corrected sample volume is placed in the region of maximal aliasing (*arrowhead*). **(E)** Spectral analysis shows peak systolic velocity > 539 cm/sec.

Radiologic Findings

- Size discrepancy > 2 cm between the two kidneys—left > right (**Fig. 73.1A,B**)
- Small, smooth right kidney compared with the left (**Fig. 73.1A–C**)
- Aliasing at the right renal artery origin on color flow imaging (**Fig. 73.1D**)
- Spectral analysis at the area of greatest aliasing, showing elevated velocities consistent with high-grade stenosis (**Fig. 73.1E**)

Diagnosis

Renal arterial stenosis (RAS) at the right renal artery origin

Differential Diagnosis

- Renal infarction
- Chronic pyelonephritis

264

- Postobstructive atrophy
- Radiation nephritis
- Congenital hypoplasia

Discussion

Background

Most hypertension is essential. Only ~6% of hypertension is renovascular in origin. The leading form of RAS is atherosclerotic (90%), seen in older patients, with men being affected more often than women. Disease is located at the renal artery ostia. The second leading form of RAS is fibromuscular dysplasia (FMD), which is responsible for 10% of renovascular hypertension. FMD occurs in females between 15 and 50 years of age. Disease is located in the mid to distal renal artery.

Clinical Findings

Hypertension is often abrupt in onset or acutely worsens. It presents before the age of 30 or after 55 in renovascular hypertension. Often the duration of hypertension is < 1 year and may be refractory to treatment despite multiple antihypertensive medications.

Pathology

RAS results in a decrease in renal perfusion pressure that activates the renin-angiotensin-aldosterone system to increase blood pressure and thereby increase renal perfusion pressures. Although this supports perfusion to the affected kidney, it may produce intrinsic damage to the unaffected kidney.

Imaging Findings
ULTRASOUND

- Renal infarction and chronic pyelonephritis would present with a small kidney. The cortex, however, would be scarred and not smooth, as in this case.
- Postobstructive atrophy would present with a small, smooth kidney, but often with some residual calyceal dilatation, not seen in this case.
- Radiation nephritis may present similar to this case, but there is no history given of radiation or malignancy.
- Congenital hypoplasia is a possibility, except that congenitally hypoplastic kidneys are frequently > 50% smaller than the contralateral kidney.
- Significant RAS of > 60% estimated diameter reduction is diagnosed with the following criteria:
  - Absolute peak systolic velocity of 180 cm/sec in the involved renal artery
  - Renal to aortic ratio (RAR) of > 3.5
  - Sensitivity and specificity ~90% in dedicated vascular laboratories

COMPUTED TOMOGRAPHY

- A small, smooth kidney is seen with size discrepancy compared with the contralateral kidney.
- The stenosis is well depicted and quantifiable with contrast-enhanced computed tomography angiography (CTA), although poor renal function may be a contraindication to intravenous iodinated contrast administration (**Fig. 73.2**).
- In a review by Vasbinder et al (2004), CTA sensitivity and specificity for RAS were ~64 and 92%, respectively, but many other studies have had much higher sensitivities.

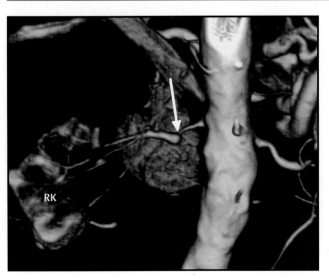

Fig. 73.2 Computed tomography angiography of the same patient as **Fig. 73.1** shows a significant stenosis in the proximal one third of the right renal artery (*arrow*). Note the atrophic-appearing right kidney (RK).

MAGNETIC RESONANCE IMAGING

- Magnetic resonance angiography (MRA) is an excellent alternative imaging strategy for RAS over CT, although in patients with decreased glomerular filtration rate (GFR, < 60 mL/min), concerns regarding nephrogenic systemic fibrosis (NFS) may prevent the use of gadolinium (see Case 10).
- Time of flight techniques (without gadolinium) and gadolinium-enhanced imaging both may quantify RAS.
- In a review by Vasbinder et al (2004), MRA sensitivity and specificity for RAS were ~62 and 84%, respectively, but many other studies have had much higher sensitivities.

ANGIOGRAPHY

- Digital subtraction angiography with angioplasty is the gold standard test for diagnosing and treating RAS.
- Clinically relevant and treatable stenosis ranges from 50 to 99% diameter reduction (**Fig. 73.3**).

NUCLEAR MEDICINE

- Captopril renogram shows characteristic poor tracer uptake and excretion by the involved kidney.
- This study lacks the anatomical information provided by other tests.

RADIOGRAPHY/INTRAVENOUS PYELOGRAM

- Because of decreased perfusion pressure with decreased uptake and excretion of contrast, the symptomatic kidney may show delayed contrast excretion as well as decreased size (i.e., small, smooth kidney).
- Intravenous pyelogram is contraindicated due to its need for iodinated contrast in patients with compromised renal function and because of the limited information obtained.

Treatment

- Medical management, including addressing atherosclerotic risk factors (e.g., cholesterol, diet)
- Angioplasty with or without stenting
- Renal vascular surgery

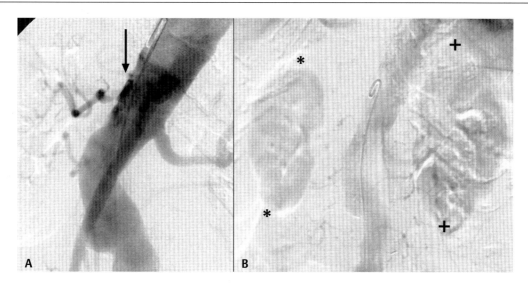

Fig. 73.3 **(A)** Diagnostic aortogram shows marked narrowing of the right renal artery ostium (*arrow*), consistent with significant renal artery stenosis. **(B)** Delayed imaging shows a small, smooth right kidney nephrogram (*asterisks*) compared with the normal contralateral kidney (*plus signs*).

Prognosis

- Fibromuscular dysplasia is also quite responsive to angioplasty.
- Bilateral RAS is most responsive to angioplasty.
- Unilateral atherosclerotic RAS is less responsive, and hypertension may in fact be essential and unrelated to the renal artery changes.
- Following revascularization, up to 55% of hypertension patients improve, but up to 30% worsen.

Suggested Readings

Safian RD, Textor SC. Renal-artery stenosis. N Engl J Med 2001;344(6):431–442.

Vasbinder GB, Nelemans PJ, Kessels AG, et al. Accuracy of computed tomographic angiography and magnetic resonance angiography for diagnosing renal artery stenosis. Ann Intern Med 2004;141(9):674–682.

Vashist A, Heller EN, Brown EJ Jr, Alhaddad IA. Renal artery stenosis: a cardiovascular perspective. Am Heart J 2002;143(4):559–564.

CASE 74

Clinical Presentation

A 67-year-old male presents with chronic right flank pain.

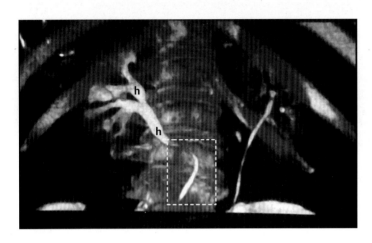

Fig. 74.1 CT-IVP three-dimensional reconstruction in the coronal plane.

Radiologic Findings

- Mild right hydronephrosis and proximal hydroureter (h, **Fig. 74.1**)
- The right ureter extends medially to the midline, crossing behind the inferior vena cava (IVC) (dashed rectangle, **Fig. 74.1**).

Diagnosis

Retrocaval ureter

Differential Diagnosis

- Ureteropelvic junction (UPJ) obstruction
- Ureteral stricture
- Congenital megaureter

Discussion

Background

As a consequence of a persisting right posterior cardinal vein, the ureter wraps around behind the vena cava and is deviated toward the midline in the L3–L4 region. Although this may be without consequence, it can result in hydronephrosis.

Clinical Findings

If hydronephrosis is present, symptoms may occur.

Pathology

Embryologically, retrocaval ureter arises as a result of persistence of the embryonic right posterior cardinal vein as the adult vena cava.

Imaging Findings

COMPUTED TOMOGRAPHY

- Mild hydronephrosis is seen with a mild UPJ obstruction, but medial deviation of the ureter would not be present.
- Ureteral stricture could be considered if it were not for the medial movement of the ureter behind the IVC.
- Megaureter would show a dilated ureter extending to the bladder, not shown in this case.
- Computed tomography (CT) is the preferred method of diagnosis. With a retrocaval ureter, CT will show
    - The right ureter moving posteriorly behind the IVC with hydronephrosis proximally
    - The right ureter emerges anterior to the IVC further distally with normal caliber

RADIOGRAPHY/INTRAVENOUS PYELOGRAM/RETROGRADE PYELOGRAM

- The classic finding for a retrocaval ureter on an intravenous pyelogram (IVP) (**Fig. 74.2**) and retrograde pyelogram (**Fig. 74.3**) is medial deviation of the midureter, resulting in hydronephrosis.

ULTRASOUND

- Hydronephrosis will be seen if present, but findings may mimic a UPJ obstruction. It would require an astute sonographer to detect the retrocaval ureter.

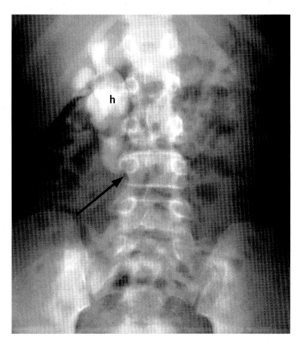

Fig. 74.2 Delayed abdominal radiograph from an intravenous pyelogram showing hydronephrosis (h), with the right ureter extending medially (*arrow*) secondary to a retrocaval ureter.

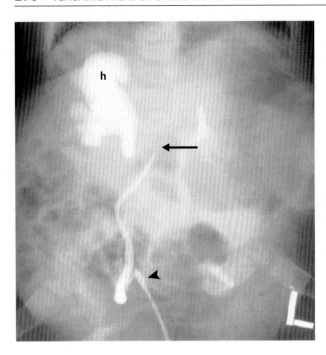

Fig. 74.3 Retrograde pyelogram in a newborn with multiple congenital anomalies, including right hydronephrosis. Classic medial deviation of the ureter (*arrow*) with hydronephrosis (h) proximally and normal caliber distally is consistent with a retrocaval ureter proven at surgery. Cannula is seen in the right ureteral orifice (*arrowhead*).

Treatment

- Open surgical repair with resection of the retrocaval ureteral component and reanastomosis of proximal and distal ureters

Prognosis

- Good

Suggested Readings

Bass JE, Redwine MD, Kramer LA, Huynh PT, Harris JH Jr. Spectrum of congenital anomalies of the inferior vena cava: cross-sectional imaging findings. Radiographics 2000;20(3):639–652.

Hsu T, Streem S, Nakada S. Management of upper urinary tract obstruction. In: Wein A, ed. Campbell-Walsh Urology. 9th ed. Philadelphia: Saunders Elsevier; 2007:1227–1271.

CASE 75

Clinical Presentation

A young black female presents with gross hematuria.

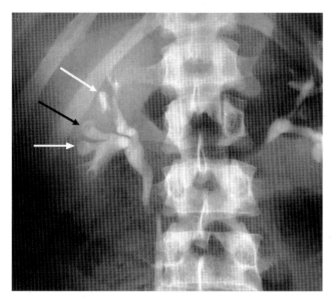

Fig. 75.1 Intravenous pyelogram, 10-minute radiograph. Scout film did not show stones.

Radiologic Findings

- Ring sign (*black arrow,* **Fig. 75.1**)
- Clubbed calyces (*white arrow,* **Fig. 75.1**)

Diagnosis

Papillary necrosis

Differential Diagnosis

- Transitional cell carcinoma
- Blood clots
- Chronic pyelonephritis
- Nonopaque stones

Discussion

Background

Papillary necrosis is well associated with several clinical entities: diabetes mellitus, analgesic abuse, renal obstruction, infection, and sickle cell disease. Women are affected more often than men, probably as a result of increased numbers of urinary tract infections (UTIs). Up to one third of patients present with more than one predisposing factor (e.g., diabetes mellitus and UTI).

271

Clinical Findings

Papillary necrosis may present with UTI or urinary tract obstruction, or it may be an incidental finding. In Eknovan et al, major presenting signs/symptoms included fever and chills in 67% of cases, flank pain and dysuria in 41%, and gross hematuria in 19%.

Pathology

Inciting events lead to vascular stasis, blockage, or thrombosis in the vasa recta, resulting in ischemic necrosis of the medullary papilla.

Imaging Findings

RADIOGRAPHY/INTRAVENOUS PYELOGRAM

- Tumor and clot may present as filling defects, but the constellation of ring sign, clubbed calyx, and patient age favors papillary necrosis.
- Chronic pyelonephritis will produce a clubbed calyx, but it also produces associated parenchymal scarring, not seen in this case; additionally, chronic pyelonephritis will not produce the ring sign.
- Nonopaque stones can produce filling defects, which could be similar to the ring sign, but the lack of stones on the scout film in conjunction with gross hematuria makes this diagnosis much less likely.
- The ring sign represents necrotic papilla still in place but separated from the medulla and therefore surrounded by contrast (*black arrow,* **Fig. 75.1**).
- Clubbed calyx represents sloughed papilla no longer in place (*white arrow,* **Fig. 75.1**).
- Early papillary necrosis will present as smaller contrast collections in the pyramids, which can produce the "golf ball on tee" appearance, as in **Fig. 75.2.**

COMPUTED TOMOGRAPHY

- On CT-IVP, contrast material fills the clefts in the necrotic medulla, revealing early changes of necrosis (*arrow,* **Fig. 75.3**).
- Clefts may be central or at the fornices, forming a "lobster claw" configuration.
- Complete necrosis with papillary sloughing will demonstrate contrast surrounding the sloughed papilla and is analogous to "ring shadows" seen on IVP.
- Blunting of the calyces will be seen following passage of the sloughed papilla into distal portions of the collecting system.

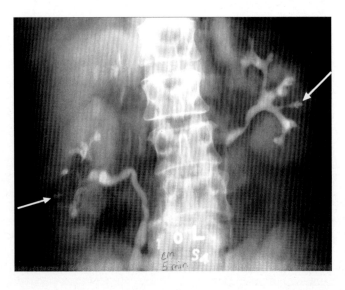

Fig. 75.2 A 5-minute intravenous pyelogram film demonstrates bilateral papillary necrosis with multiple areas of contrast in pyramids, including the classic "golf ball on tee" sign in both kidneys (*arrows*).

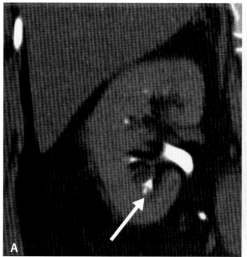
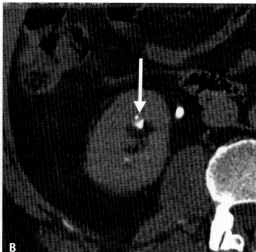

Fig. 75.3 Pyelogram phase of a CT-IVP with coronal three-dimension reconstruction **(A)** and axial image through the right kidney **(B)**. Patient had a history of right side urinary tract obstruction that was subsequently relieved. Excavation of the right midpole renal pyramid is seen, with contrast filling the cleft (*arrow*), consistent with papillary necrosis.

- If the sloughed papilla results in obstruction, hydroureteronephrosis will be seen.

Treatment

- Recognize an at-risk patient (e.g., diabetic patient with frequent UTIs or stone disease) early in the disease.
- Treat the underlying cause (e.g., treat UTI and/or obstruction and control diabetes).

Prognosis

- Depends on the cause and severity of the renal parenchymal damage

PEARLS

- A sloughed papilla may cause urinary tract obstruction and present as renal colic.
- Sloughed papillae may calcify and mimic collecting system calculi (excavated medulla will be the clue to papillary necrosis as the cause for the calcification).
- Gross hematuria in a young black individual should raise the question of sickle cell trait or disease.

Suggested Readings

Dyer RB, Chen MY, Zagoria RJ. Intravenous urography: technique and interpretation. Radiographics 2001;21(4):799–821.

Eknoyan G, Qunibi WY, Grissom RT, Tuma SN, Ayus JC. Renal papillary necrosis: an update. Medicine (Baltimore) 1982;61(2):55–73.

Griffin MD, Bergstralhn EJ, Larson TS. Renal papillary necrosis: a sixteen-year clinical experience. J Am Soc Nephrol 1995;6(2):248–256.

Jung DC, Kim SH, Jung SI, Hwang SI, Kim SH. Renal papillary necrosis: review and comparison of findings at multi-detector row CT and intravenous urography. Radiographics 2006;26(6):1827–1836.

CASE 76

Clinical Presentation

A 35-year-old female presents with cervical carcinoma.

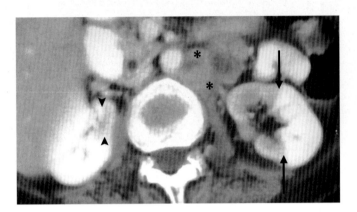

Fig. 76.1 Enhanced computed tomography scan through the kidneys.

Radiologic Findings

- Sharply defined focal decreased nephrogram in the left kidney (*arrows*, **Fig. 76.1**)
- Small area of decreased right nephrogram (*arrowheads*, **Fig. 76.1**)
- Left periaortic adenopathy (*asterisks*, **Fig. 76.1**)

Diagnosis

Radiation-induced ischemia/nephropathy

Differential Diagnosis

- Renal infarct
- Renal contusion
- Acute pyelonephritis

Discussion

Background

Radiation nephropathy can be the result of direct radiation, such as from a radiation therapy port, as in this case. However, radioactive pharmaceuticals that are metabolized or excreted in the urine can also cause renal damage. Sharply focused radiation ports in current radiation therapy limit this sort of renal damage.

Clinical Findings

The patient may be asymptomatic. Renal changes occur 6 to 12 months after the exposure and lead to chronic renal insufficiency. Proteinuria and hypertension may be observed earlier.

274

Pathology

A direct dose of up to 20 Gray can cause radiation nephropathy. Radiation-induced ischemia is secondary to a vasculitis produced by the radiation.

Imaging Findings

COMPUTED TOMOGRAPHY

- Renal infarct can appear similar, but medial distribution does not fit well with infarct. No cortical rim sign is present.
- Contusion is usually not as sharply defined, and no history of trauma was given.
- Acute pyelonephritis will produce focal hypodense areas, but not with the sharp demarcation from normal parenchyma seen in this case. No striated nephrogram is present, and there was no clinical information to suggest infection.
- The key diagnostic feature in this case is the sharp, medial distribution of the nephrographic abnormalities in both kidneys (*arrows and arrowheads,* **Fig. 76.1**). The pattern of abnormal nephrogram fits perfectly with the projected radiation field for the periaortic adenopathy.

Treatment

- None

Prognosis

- Portions of the kidney exposed to high doses of radiation will atrophy.

Suggested Readings

Cohen EP, Robbins ME. Radiation nephropathy. Semin Nephrol 2003;23(5):486–499.

Saunders HS, Dyer RB, Shifrin RY, et al. The CT nephrogram: implications for evaluation of urinary tract disease. Radiographics 1995;15(5):1069–1085, discussion 1086–1088.

CASE 77

Clinical Presentation

Right scrotal mass

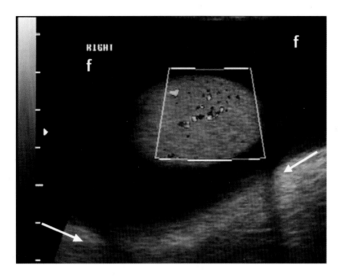

Fig. 77.1   Right scrotal sonogram utilizing power Doppler.

Radiologic Findings

- Large anechoic fluid collection surrounding the right testis (f, **Fig. 77.1**)
- Increased posterior through-transmission of sound secondary to fluid collection (*arrows,* **Fig. 77.1**)
- Normal Doppler flow to the testis

Diagnosis

Large simple hydrocele

Differential Diagnosis

- Reactive hydrocele
- Spermatocele
- Varicocele

Discussion

Background

Simple hydrocele is the most common cause of painless scrotal swelling. Causes of hydroceles include traumatic, inflammatory, and infectious etiologies, but it may be idiopathic. Tumor and torsion can present with hydrocele. In young children, a hydrocele may develop from a patent processus vaginalis that allows abdominal fluid to enter the scrotum. In adults, the cause of a hydrocele should be sought and treated.

Clinical Findings

A simple hydrocele usually presents as painless scrotal swelling. The cause will determine the symptomatology.

Pathology

A large collection of fluid between the visceral and parietal layers of the tunica vaginalis results in a hydrocele. The collection surrounds the anterior and lateral aspects of the testicle.

Imaging Findings

ULTRASOUND

- Reactive hydrocele is typically caused by infection and contains septa or debris, not seen in this case.
- Spermatocele is a well-circumscribed fluid collection within the epididymis, as opposed to a hydrocele, which is fluid within the layers of the tunica vaginalis surrounding portions of the testis.
- Varicocele represents dilated venous channels and would be filled with color flow, as opposed to the avascular fluid in this case.
- Simple hydrocele is seen as a simple fluid collection surrounding the anterior and lateral aspects of the testicle (f, **Fig. 77.1**).
- No color or power Doppler flow is observed within the hydrocele.

Treatment

- Treat the cause of the hydrocele (e.g., treat the epididymitis in a reactive hydrocele).
- Large symptomatic hydroceles can be drained.

Prognosis

- Depends on etiology; generally good

Suggested Readings

Dogra VS, Gottlieb RH, Oka M, Rubens DJ. Sonography of the scrotum. Radiology 2003;227(1):18–36.

Older RA, Watson LR. Ultrasound anatomy of the normal male reproductive tract. J Clin Ultrasound 1996;24(8):389–404.

CASE 78

Clinical Presentation

Swollen tender left hemiscrotum with fever

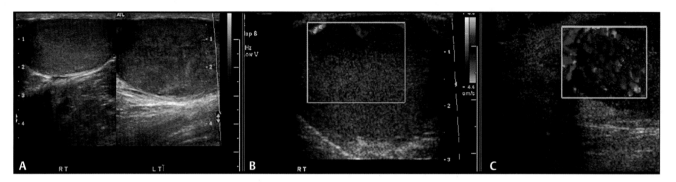

Fig. 78.1 Scrotal sonogram. **(A)** Transverse view of both testicles. Color Doppler of the **(B)** right and **(C)** left testicles.

Radiologic Findings

- Enlarged and heterogeneous symptomatic left testicle compared with the right (**Fig. 78.1A**)
- Normal color flow in the asymptomatic right testicle (**Fig. 78.1B**), compared with marked increased color flow consistent with hyperemia on the left (**Fig. 78.1C**).
- The left epididymis was also enlarged and hyperemic (not shown).

Diagnosis

Orchitis of the left testis

Differential Diagnosis

- Testicular tumor
- Metastatic disease, lymphoma, or leukemia
- Trauma

Discussion

Background

Primary orchitis is rare but can occur as a result of testicular infection (usually from mumps) or from granulomatous disease (sarcoid). Orchitis is most commonly a result of the spread of infection from the adjacent epididymitis, as in this case, resulting in epididymo-orchitis.

Clinical Findings

Painful, swollen hemiscrotum with or without fever and other constitutional symptoms

Pathology

Common infecting organisms include the same organisms that cause epididymitis (*Escherichia coli, Klebsiella, Neisseria gonorrhoeae, Chlamydia trachomatis*). Mumps orchitis and sarcoidosis can also cause an orchitis.

Imaging Findings

ULTRASOUND

- Testicular tumor could have this appearance, but no definite mass is seen. To exclude neoplasm, a follow-up ultrasound can be performed to ensure resolution of the findings.
- Metastatic disease, lymphoma, and leukemia are unlikely, given no history of a primary malignancy. Again, follow-up sonography showing resolution excludes this diagnosis.
- There is no history of trauma.
- Sonographic features for orchitis, when compared with the asymptomatic testis, include the following:
  - Enlarged testis
  - Heterogeneous appearance on gray scale
  - Hyperemia on color and power Doppler

Treatment

- Antibiotics for bacterial orchitis

Prognosis

- Resolution with appropriate antibiotic coverage

PEARLS _____

- Follow-up exam to resolution is recommended, as the sonographic appearance of orchitis is non-specific, and testicular neoplasm can present similarly.

Suggested Readings

Dogra VS, Gottlieb RH, Oka M, Rubens DJ. Sonography of the scrotum. Radiology 2003;227(1):18–36.

CASE 79

Clinical Presentation

Enlarged right testicle

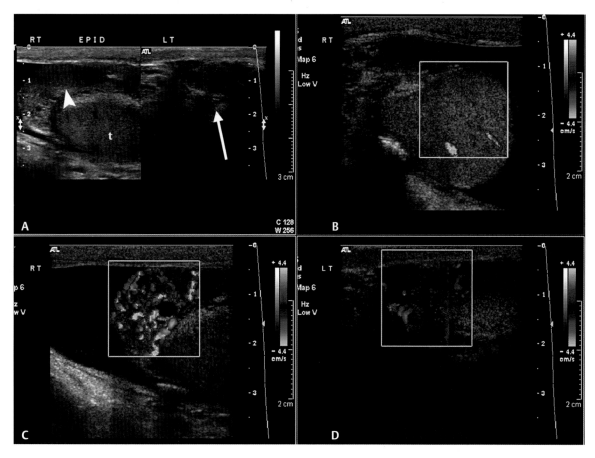

Fig. 79.1 Scrotal sonogram. **(A)** Gray scale side-by-side images of right epididymitis (*arrowhead*) and left epididymis (*arrow*). t, right testicle. Color Doppler images of the **(B)** right testicle, **(C)** right epididymis, and **(D)** left epididymis.

Radiologic Findings

- Enlarged right epididymis compared with the left (**Fig. 79.1A**)
- Normal flow in the right testicle excludes torsion (**Fig. 79.1B**).
- Hyperemic right epididymis compared with the left (**Fig. 79.1C,D**)

Diagnosis

Epididymitis

Differential Diagnosis

- Testicular torsion
- Varicocele
- Epididymal cyst

281

Discussion

Background

Epididymitis is the most common cause of painful swelling of the testis in young adult males. Urinary tract infection (UTI) is the most common cause of epididymitis in very young and older patients (i.e., prepubertal boys and men > 35 years of age). Sexually transmitted disease is the most common cause in adult men younger than 35.

Clinical Findings

Gradual onset of scrotal pain, fever, urethral discharge, and other urinary symptoms is common. The hemiscrotum may be swollen, with the epididymis being tender, enlarged, and/or indurated. Testicular torsion must be excluded in a young male with testicular pain, as 50% of epididymitis cases are clinically misdiagnosed as testicular torsion.

Pathology

In the sexually transmitted diseases age group, *Neisseria gonorrhoeae* and *Chlamydia trachomatis* are common infecting organisms. UTI secondary to *Escherichia coli* or *Proteus* spp. may be causative in other age groups.

Imaging Findings

ULTRASOUND

- Testicular torsion is excluded by the presence of intratesticular flow on the symptomatic side (**Fig. 79.1B**).
- A varicocele represents dilated veins of the pampiniform plexus usually seen superior to the testis and not within the substance of the epididymis, as in this case.
- An epididymal cyst would be fluid filled and not contain vascularity.
- Gray scale images may show a hypoechoic or heterogeneous epididymis that is enlarged, as in **Fig. 79.1A**.
- Increased color and power Doppler flow is seen in the symptomatic epididymis out of proportion to the asymptomatic side (**Fig. 79.1C,D**).
- The key differentiating feature between epididymitis and torsion is the presence of normal testicular flow on the symptomatic side with epididymitis.
- Increased flow in the adjacent testicle indicates orchitis as well as epididymitis.

Treatment

- Culture of urethral swabs is required to direct antimicrobial treatment. The patient's sexual partners should be treated if a sexually transmitted organism is identified.

Prognosis

- Excellent with appropriate treatment

PEARLS _____

- Both epididymitis and testicular torsion present with an acutely painful scrotum. Therefore, testicular torsion must always be excluded in cases of acute scrotum.

Suggested Readings

Black JA, Patel A. Sonography of the abnormal extratesticular space. AJR Am J Roentgenol 1996;167(2):507–511.

Dogra VS, Gottlieb RH, Oka M, Rubens DJ. Sonography of the scrotum. Radiology 2003;227(1):18–36.

CASE 80

Clinical Presentation

A 28-year-old male presents with a prior left orchiectomy for a testis tumor.

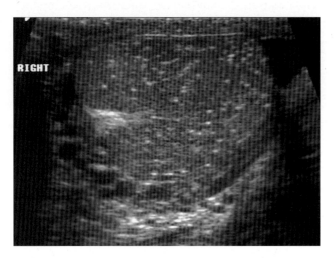

Fig. 80.1 Right testicular sonogram. Normal-sized testis with multiple tiny echogenic foci but no mass lesion present.

Radiologic Findings

- Normal-sized testis
- Multiple tiny echogenic foci (**Fig. 80.1**)
- No mass lesion present

Diagnosis

Testicular microlithiasis

Differential Diagnosis

- Testicular teratoma
- Mixed germ cell tumor
- Sertoli cell tumor

Discussion

Background

Testicular microlithiasis has about a 2 to 3% prevalence in the asymptomatic young male population. There is considerable literature documenting cases of testicular carcinoma in men with testicular microlithiasis, but no definitive association has been proven. Testicular microlithiasis may be associated with conditions that predispose to testicular carcinoma. There is controversy regarding the risk of developing a testicular tumor in a patient with testicular microlithiasis; therefore, there is controversy regarding management. No definitive guidelines exist at this time for the management of asymptomatic patients with testicular microlithiasis. A conservative approach is to follow closely with ultrasound and/or physical exam.

Clinical Findings

No signs or symptoms are specifically referable to testicular microlithiasis.

Pathology

The testicular microliths are located in the seminiferous tubules. They represent calcification of intracellular debris surrounded by concentric collagen laminations.

Imaging Findings

ULTRASOUND

- Coarse calcifications are present along with an intratesticular mass in teratoma, mixed germ cell, and Sertoli tumors. There is no associated mass in this case (**Fig. 80.1**).
- Testicular microlithiasis appears as innumerable tiny nonshadowing echogenic intratesticular foci. More than five echogenic foci without shadowing (i.e., microliths) per ultrasound field is one definition of microlithiasis.
- Ultrasound is the primary imaging modality.
- Computed tomography and magnetic resonance imaging have no role in the primary diagnosis.

Treatment

- Urology referral is appropriate.

Prognosis

- No long-term definitive prognosis has yet to be determined.

Suggested Readings

Backus ML, Mack LA, Middleton WD, et al. Testicular microlithiasis: imaging appearances and pathologic correlation. Radiology 1994;192(3):781–785.

Cast JE, Nelson WM, Early AS, et al. Testicular microlithiasis: prevalence and tumor risk in a population referred for scrotal sonography. AJR Am J Roentgenol 2000;175(6):1703–1706.

Middleton WD, Teefey SA, Santillan CS. Testicular microlithiasis: prospective analysis of prevalence and associated tumor. Radiology 2002;224(2):425–428.

Vegni-Talluri M, Bigliardi E, Vanni MG, Tota G. Testicular microliths: their origin and structure. J Urol 1980;124(1):105–107.

CASE 81

Clinical Presentation

A 33-year-old male presents with an abnormal testis on a physical exam.

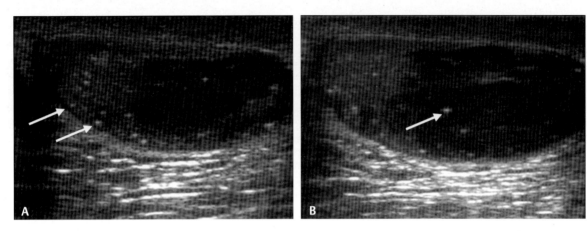

Fig. 81.1 **(A,B)** Testis sonographic images in the long axis.

Radiologic Findings

- Multiple small echogenic foci representing microlithiasis (*arrows,* **Fig. 81.1**)
- Hypoechoic, relatively homogeneous testis mass

Diagnosis

Seminoma and microlithiasis

Differential Diagnosis

Malignant testis tumors other than seminoma

Discussion

Background

The incidence of testicular cancer in the United States has increased by up to 50% over the past few decades, but it is unclear why. According to the National Cancer Institute (SEER), there were nearly 8000 cases of testicular carcinoma in 2004, with ~50% representing seminoma. Most occur in the 4th decade of life, with the peak incidence between 25 and 35 years of age. Cryptorchidism is a predisposing condition, and it is controversial if orchiopexy offers any risk prevention.

Testicular microlithiasis has a high association with malignant testis tumors, although there is considerable controversy regarding the likelihood of developing testis tumor in patients with microlithiasis and no tumor at the time that microlithiasis is detected.

Clinical Findings

Most patients present with testicular symptoms, including pain, swelling, hardness, or any combination. The minority of patients present with a painless testicular mass. Because infection may present similarly, a trial of antiobiotics is often undertaken, but if symptoms do not resolve, testicular sonography is indicated.

Pathology

Seminoma is a malignancy arising from the epithelium of the seminiferous tubules. It may be a precursor to nonseminomatous germ cell tumors (NSGCTs). Fifteen percent of men who have seminoma may relapse with NSGCT following initial treatment. Twenty percent of seminoma patients may have elevated levels of β-subunit of human chorionic gonadotropin (HCG) (up to 60% of patients with NSGCT have HCG elevation).

Imaging Findings

ULTRASOUND

- Any intratesticular mass in a young man is considered malignant until proven otherwise, but associated microlithiasis makes a benign process even less likely (**Fig. 81.1**).
- Ultrasound is the study of choice for a suspected testis mass. The key point is to separate intratesticular lesions, which are generally malignant, from extratesticular lesions, which are usually benign.
- Seminoma is generally more homogeneous than NSGCTs, but ultrasound is not reliable for differentiation.

COMPUTED TOMOGRAPHY

- Computed tomography (CT) is used for staging purposes once a testicular mass is identified. Adenopathy involves the retroperitoneal lymph nodes because the embryonic origin of the testes is retroperitoneal with descent into the scrotum during development. Thus, the lymphatic drainage of the testicles is to the retroperitoneum.

POSITRON EMISSION TOMOGRAPHY

- Positron emission tomography (PET) has been shown, in some studies, to be more sensitive and specific for staging testicular carcinoma than CT.

Treatment

- Testicular resection, along with removal of the spermatic cord and paratesticular tissues
- Postoperative pelvic radiation
- For recurrence or advanced disease, combination chemotherapy, including cisplatin

Prognosis

- Staging and prognosis are based on the extent of disease and serum tumor markers.
- Excellent prognosis when diagnosis and treatment are at an early stage (> 95% 5-year survival rate for seminoma)
- Testicular carcinoma is highly curable even in advanced cases with metastatic disease.

PEARLS _____

- Extragonadal germ cell tumors occur in the anterior mediastinum. However, in the setting of a mediastinal mass in a young male, primary testicular germ cell tumors with metastatic spread to the mediastinum should be excluded with testicular ultrasound.

Suggested Readings

Backus ML, Mack LA, Middleton WD, et al. Testicular microlithiasis: imaging appearances and pathologic correlation. Radiology 1994;192(3):781–785.

Bosl GJ, Motzer RJ. Testicular germ-cell cancer. N Engl J Med 1997;337(4):242–253.

Cast JE, Nelson WM, Early AS, et al. Testicular microlithiasis: prevalence and tumor risk in a population referred for scrotal sonography. AJR Am J Roentgenol 2000;175(6):1703–1706.

Howlett DC, Marchbank ND, Sallomi DF. Pictorial review: ultrasound of the testis. Clin Radiol 2000;55(8):595–601.

Middleton WD, Teefey SA, Santillan CS. Testicular microlithiasis: prospective analysis of prevalence and associated tumor. Radiology 2002;224(2):425–428.

National Cancer Institute. SEER Cancer Statistics Review, 1975–2005. Available at: http://seer.cancer.gov/csr/1975_2005/. Accessed July 15, 2008.

CASE 82

Clinical Presentation

Palpable mass in the right testis

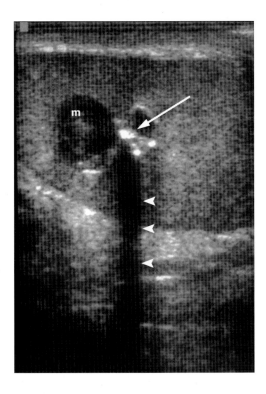

Fig. 82.1 Longitudinal sonographic view of the right testis. Source: Resnick, Older, Diagnosis of Genitourinary Disease, New York: Thieme, 1997: 105. Reprinted by permission.

Radiologic Findings

- Intratesticular mass (m, **Fig. 82.1**)
- Heterogeneous mass with cystic areas as well as calcification (*arrow,* **Fig. 82.1**) with shadowing (*arrowheads,* **Fig. 82.1**)

Diagnosis

Mixed cell-type germ cell tumor

Differential Diagnosis

- Epidermoid cyst
- Intratesticular abscess
- Seminoma

Discussion

Background

Testicular cancer incidence in the United States has increased by up to 50% over the past few decades, but it is unclear why. Fifty percent of testicular carcinomas are nonseminomatous germ cell tumors

(NSGCTs). They occur most commonly in the 3rd decade of life. Cryptorchidism is a predisposing factor. It is unclear if early orchiopexy offers any protection.

Clinical Findings

Most patients present with symptoms such as testicular mass and/or pain.

Pathology

Often testicular cancer has a mix of histologies, including embryonal carcinoma, choriocarcinoma, teratoma, and yolk sac tumor. Most tumors elaborate human chorionic gonadotropin (HCG) and/or alpha fetoprotein (AFP). Fifteen percent of men who have seminoma may relapse with NSGCT following initial treatment. Up to 60% of patients with NSGCT have HCG elevation.

Imaging Findings

ULTRASOUND

- Epidermoid cyst demonstrates the target sign produced by alternating rings of high and low echogenicity, not present in this case.
- Abscess may contain echogenic gas with dirty shadowing, but the echogenic material in this case is calcium with clean acoustic shadowing.
- Most seminomas are homogeneous and hypoechoic, unlike this case.
- Nonseminomas such as teratoma, embryonal cell, and choriocarcinoma are more likely to be cystic, heterogeneous, contain shadowing calcification, and cannot be separated from the mixed germ cell tumor in this case.
- Any intratesticular mass in a young male is considered malignant until proven otherwise.

COMPUTED TOMOGRAPHY

- Computed tomography (CT) plays a major roll in staging lymph node metastasis and distant metastasis (lung, liver, or bone).
- Lymph node metastasis occurs in the retroperitoneum first (e.g., left para-aortic region next to the left renal vein, interaortocaval, and right paracaval regions). The testes originated in the retroperitoneum and descended to the scrotum during development, but they maintained their lymphatic drainage to the retroperitoneum.

POSITRON EMISSION TOMOGRAPHY

- Positron emission tomography has been shown to be more sensitive and specific than CT for staging testicular carcinoma.

Treatment

- Orchidectomy, lymph node dissection, pelvic radiation, and chemotherapy, depending on the stage
- For recurrence or advanced disease, combination chemotherapy, including cisplatin

Prognosis

- Staging and prognosis are based on the extent of disease and serum tumor markers.
- Prognosis is not as good as seminoma, but still very good (> 90% 5-year survival rate).
- Testicular carcinoma is highly curable even in advanced cases with metastatic disease.

Suggested Readings

Bosl GJ, Motzer RJ. Testicular germ-cell cancer. N Engl J Med 1997;337(4):242–253.

Hahn NM, Sweeney CJ. Germ cell tumors: an update of recent data and review of active protocols in stage I and metastatic disease. Urol Oncol 2005;23(4):293–302.

Howlett DC, Marchbank ND, Sallomi DF. Pictorial review: ultrasound of the testis. Clin Radiol 2000; 55(8):595–601.

National Cancer Institute. SEER Cancer Statistics Review, 1975–2005. Available at: http://seer.cancer.gov/csr/1975_2005/. Accessed July 15, 2008.

Testicular tumors and tumorlike lesions. In: Hricak H, Hamm B, Kim B, eds. Imaging of the Scrotum. New York: Raven Press; 1995.

CASE 83

Clinical Presentation

A 79-year-old male presents with a scrotal mass.

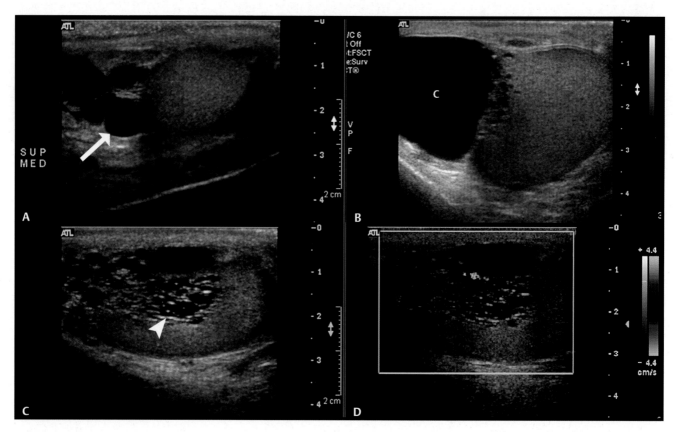

Fig. 83.1 Right testicular sonogram. **(A,B)** Sagittal through the epididymis, **(C)** sagittal through the right testicle, and **(D)** color Doppler images of the right testicular lesion.

Radiologic Findings

- Epididymal cysts (*arrow*, **Fig. 83.1A**)
- Large epididymal cyst (c, **Fig. 83.1B**)
- Tubular channels in the mediastinum of the right testis (*arrowhead*, **Fig. 83.1C**)
- No significant color flow within tubular channels (**Fig. 83.1D**)

Diagnosis

Tubular ectasia of the rete testis (TER)

Differential Diagnosis

- Testis tumor
- Lymphoma
- Intratesticular varicocele

Discussion

Background

TER is a benign condition possibly resulting from partial or complete obstruction of the efferent ducts. It occurs in older men (median age range 62–65 years) and is often bilateral. Disorders associated with efferent duct obstruction (i.e., vasectomy, spermatocele, or epididymitis) may be associated with TER.

Clinical Findings

This is an incidentally discovered finding in patients who have scrotal sonography for scrotal mass or pain.

Pathology

Dilated rete tubules

Imaging Findings

ULTRASOUND

- This pattern (**Fig. 83.1**) is an unusual finding for seminoma or nonseminomatous germ cell tumor. The pattern is classic for TER, and in the absence of a solid component, it should not be mistaken for testicular neoplasm. Also, patients are generally older than typical for testicular neoplasm.
- Lymphoma typically presents as a solid mass, commonly bilateral. Cysts are not a common finding in lymphoma.
- An intratesticular varicocele would demonstrate color flow with venous signature on spectral analysis, not seen in this case (**Fig. 83.1D**).
- It is the combination of findings that leads to the diagnosis of TER:
  - Epididymal cyst or cysts (**Fig. 83.1A,B**)
  - Dilated tubular channels adjacent to the mediastinum testes (**Fig. 83.1C**)
  - Testicular cysts
- It is important not to mistake the architectural distortion produced by the dilated tubules for a cystic testis neoplasm. The constant presence of an epididymal cyst should lead to high suspicion for rete tubular ectasia.
- Evaluation of the opposite testis is helpful, as tubular ectasia is often bilateral.
- Tubular ectasia is found in an older age group than most testis tumors.

MAGNETIC RESONANCE IMAGING

- When differentiation between benign TER and a testicular neoplasm is difficult, magnetic resonance imaging can be used in equivocal cases.
- On T1-weighted imaging, TER shows lower signal than adjacent testicular parenchyma. On T2-weighted imaging, TER shows a multilobular pattern that is difficult to distinguish from a normal testicle. With gadolinium, TER does not enhance and is identified as cystic malformations in the mediastinum.

Treatment

- None

Prognosis

- Benign, usually incidental finding

PEARLS

- Whenever there is an epididymal cyst in association with what appears to be architectural distortion within the mediastinum testis, think of tubular ectasia of the rete testis.

Suggested Readings

Burrus JK, Lockhart ME, Kenney PJ, Kolettis PN. Cystic ectasia of the rete testis: clinical and radiographic features. J Urol 2002;168(4 Pt 1):1436–1438.

Dogra VS, Gottlieb RH, Oka M, Rubens DJ. Sonography of the scrotum. Radiology 2003;227(1):18–36.

Older RA, Watson LR. Tubular ectasia of the rete testis: a benign condition with a sonographic appearance that may be misinterpreted as malignant. J Urol 1994;152(2 Pt 1):477–478.

Tartar VM, Trambert MA, Balsara ZN, Mattrey RF. Tubular ectasia of the testicle: sonographic and MR imaging appearance. AJR Am J Roentgenol 1993;160(3):539–542.

CASE 84

Clinical Presentation

Painful left testicle

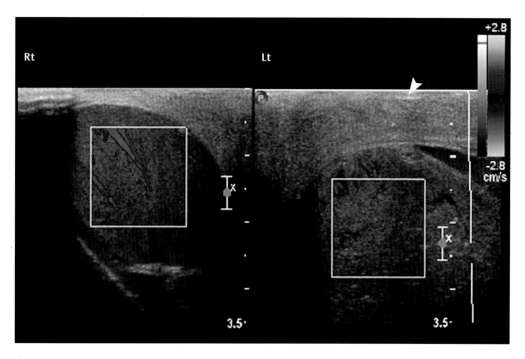

Fig. 84.1 Testicular sonogram shows color flow boxes (*rectangles*) over both the right (Rt) and left (Lt) testicles. Note the heterogeneous echotexture to the left testicle.

Radiologic Findings

- No color flow in the left testis
- Heterogeneous enlarged left testis (Lt, **Fig. 84.1**)
- Normal color flow in the right testis (Rt, **Fig. 84.1**)
- Scrotal skin thickening over the ischemic left testis (*arrowhead*, **Fig. 84.1**)

Diagnosis

Left testicular torsion with probable evolving infarction

Differential Diagnosis

- Orchitis
- Epididymitis
- Scrotal abscess

295

Discussion

Background

Testicular torsion results from twisting of the testicle on its vascular pedicle. Torsion most commonly occurs in adolescent boys. It represents a surgical emergency.

Clinical Findings

Symptoms include acute onset of testicular pain with nausea, vomiting, and low-grade fever. Swollen, inflamed, and tender hemiscrotum is found on physical exam. Epididymitis and testicular torsion present similarly. Clinical differentiation between testicular torsion and epididymitis is difficult, with a nearly 50% false-positive rate of diagnosis of torsion based on clinical findings alone. Torsion of the appendix testis or appendix epididymis may mimic the symptoms of testicular torsion.

Pathology

With testicular twisting on the vascular pedicle, venous congestion ensues, followed by arterial compromise, followed by testicular infarction. Bell clapper deformity is felt to be the main cause for testicular torsion where the tunica vaginalis completely encircles the testicle and spermatic cord. Normally, the tunica vaginalis partially encircles the testicle and fixes it to the posterolateral wall of the scrotum. The bell clapper deformity allows for free rotation of the testicle within the tunica, resulting in torsion.

Imaging Findings

ULTRASOUND

- If a diagnostic study is indicated to evaluate potential testicular torsion, sonography with color Doppler imaging is the study of choice.
- Orchitis produces increased testicular flow. In **Fig. 84.1,** the normal right testis does not show increased flow, and the left testis shows no flow.
- Epididymitis, which can be confused clinically with testicular torsion, demonstrates increased color Doppler flow and swelling in the epididymis, neither of which is shown in this case.
- Scrotal abscess would be seen as a fluid collection with variable internal echoes; no such fluid collection is present in this case.
- Color and power Doppler confirms no intratesticular flow, verifying the diagnosis of testicular torsion.
- Gray scale changes within the testicle vary with the length of ischemia, but they are not diagnostic of testicular torsion. Normal testicular echogenicity on gray scale imaging, however, suggests a viable testicle.

NUCLEAR MEDICINE

- Technetium 99-M pertechnetate testicular scintigraphy remains an option in cases where the color or power Doppler imaging is nondiagnostic.
- Scintigraphy will show a photopenic defect in the region of the torsed testicle. There may be a rim sign that represents hyperemia (increased tracer) corresponding to inflamed paratesticular tissues.

Treatment

- Detorsing of the symptomatic testicle should be performed as soon as possible after onset of pain to restore blood flow. If the testicle appears nonviable at surgery, it is removed. With viable testes, bilateral orchiopexy is performed to prevent further bouts of testicular torsion on the symptomatic side but also for the contralateral side, which is at increased risk for torsion.

Prognosis

- There is a nearly 100% testicle salvage rate when testicular torsion is diagnosed and treated within the first 6 hours after the onset of pain.

PEARLS

- With suspected torsion, the epididymal findings are not the key to diagnosis, as torsion can produce a swollen epididymis. The presence or absence of normal testicular blood flow is always the critical diagnostic finding.

Suggested Readings

Dogra VS, Gottlieb RH, Oka M, Rubens DJ. Sonography of the scrotum. Radiology 2003;227(1):18–36.

Older RA, Watson LR. Ultrasound diagnosis of testicular torsion: beware the swollen epididymis. J Urol 1997;157(4):1369–1370.

CASE 85

Clinical Presentation

Incidental finding

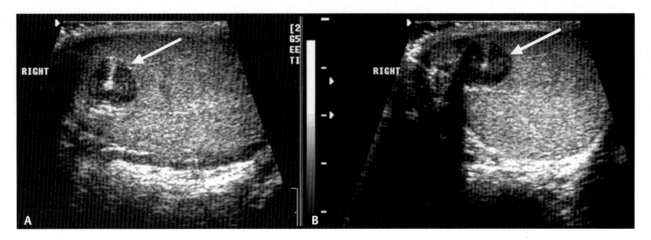

Fig. 85.1 Testicular sonogram. **(A)** Longitudinal and **(B)** transverse imaging of the right testis.

Radiologic Findings

- Intratesticular mass (*arrows,* **Fig. 85.1**)
- Target or bull's-eye sign produced by central echogenic lesion surrounded by echo-poor material

Diagnosis

Epidermoid cyst

Differential Diagnosis

- Seminoma
- Nonseminomatous germ cell tumor
- Testicular cyst

Discussion

Background

Epidermoid cysts account for ~1 to 2% of resected testicular masses. They are benign lesions without malignant potential, and surgeons may use conservative surgery if imaging strongly suggests an epidermoid cyst. This is controversial, however.

Clinical Findings

Nontender testicular mass, usually an incidental finding

Pathology

A benign, cystic lesion composed of keratin debris

Imaging Findings

ULTRASOUND

- Seminoma is typically a homogeneous hypoechoic solid lesion.
- Nonseminomatous germ cell tumors are typically heterogeneous and often contain calcium and cystic areas.
- Testicular cysts are anechoic with increased through-transmission and no internal echoes, which does not fit this case.
- Epidermoid cyst of testis presents on sonography as a well-demarcated intratesticular cystic mass.
- The target or bull's-eye sign represents the echogenic center to an otherwise hypoechoic testicular mass. The central echogenic focus is keratinized material of the epidermoid (**Fig. 85.1**).
- An "onion ring" appearance represents alternating layers within an epidermoid, including an echogenic capsule, followed by an inner hypoechoic rim with an echogenic center, not seen in this case.

MAGNETIC RESONANCE IMAGING

- Laminated appearance similar to the onion ring described by ultrasound showing alternative bands of hypo- and hyperintense signal on T1- and T2-weighted images
- Limited to no enhancement following contrast

Treatment

- With strong suspicion of a benign epidermoid cyst, enucleation of the tumor and immediate frozen-section histologic evaluation can be performed, sparing the testicle if pathology confirms an epidermoid. This, however, is a controversial issue among surgeons.

Prognosis

- Epidermoid cysts are benign.

PEARLS

- The target sign raises the possibility of a benign process and allows consideration of less radical surgery. This requires good communication between the radiologist and the referring urologist.

Suggested Readings

Langer JE, Ramchandani P, Siegelman ES, Banner MP. Epidermoid cysts of the testicle: sonographic and MR imaging features. AJR Am J Roentgenol 1999;173(5):1295–1299.

CASE 86

Clinical Presentation

An 18-year-old male with a history of treated acute lymphoblastic leukemia (ALL) presents with right scrotal swelling representing possible recurrent tumor.

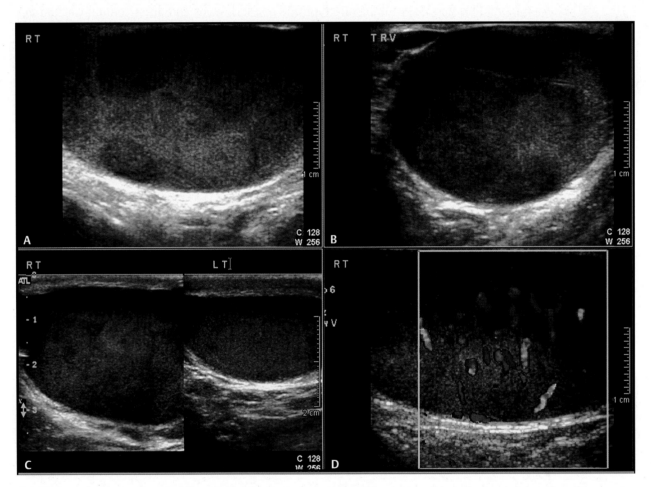

Fig. 86.1 Testicular sonogram. **(A)** Long- and **(B)** short-axis views of the right testicle show multiple hypoechoic masses nearly replacing the right testicle. **(C)** Comparison view shows the right testicle to be much larger than the left. **(D)** Significant vascularity is seen on a color flow image on the right compared with the left testicle (not shown).

Radiologic Findings

- Intratesticular mass(es) in the right testis (**Fig. 86.1A–C**)
- Increased color Doppler flow in the mass(es) (**Fig. 86.1D**)
- Significant improvement with high-dose chemotherapy (**Fig. 86.2**)

Diagnosis

Leukemic infiltration in the right testicle

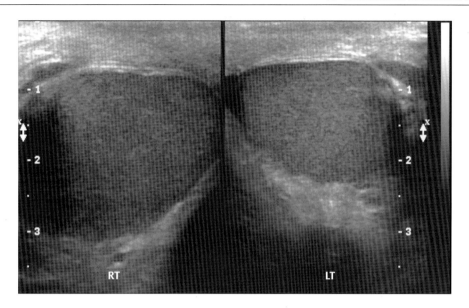

Fig. 86.2   Follow-up testicular sonogram following high-dose chemotherapy for acute lymphoblastic leukemia. Short-axis views of both testicles show resolution of right testicular masses. The right testicle is still somewhat larger than the left. No increased flow was seen on color Doppler images (not shown).

Differential Diagnosis

- Seminomatous and nonseminomatous germ cell tumor
- Intratesticular abscess

Discussion

Background

The testicle is the most common location for ALL relapse. The blood–gonad barrier prevents sufficient chemotherapeutic agent to accumulate within the testicles at initial therapy, despite complete eradication of tumor elsewhere. ALL is seen in children and young adults. Testicular lymphoma can present similarly in elderly males. Both entities commonly present with bilateral disease.

Clinical Findings

A painless, swollen testicle is the usual presenting symptom. Clinical history helps point to metastatic involvement of the testicle by the patient's primary leukemia. Improvement following high-dose chemotherapy directed at the patient's ALL confirms involvement of the testicle by ALL.

Pathology

Leukemic filtrates are found in the interstitium and seminiferous tubules of the testis.

Imaging Findings

ULTRASOUND

- Primary testis tumors could have a similar appearance, and diagnosis depends on the response to chemotherapy directed at ALL.

- Infection would present with similar imaging findings but would have different clinical findings guiding treatment. Follow-up imaging after appropriate antibiotic therapy would confirm the diagnosis and exclude testis tumor.
- As described above, leukemic or lymphomatous infiltration of the testicle would show an enlarged testicle, with increased color or power Doppler flow. The key to diagnosis is the response to high-dose or combination chemotherapy.

Treatment

- Chemotherapy directed at the patient's ALL. A blood–gonad barrier exists that can prevent accumulation of chemotherapy in the testis. Thus, the testis can harbor foci of viable tumor in leukemia and lymphoma (so-called sanctuary organ), requiring additional bouts of chemotherapy. If that fails, orchiectomy is indicated. Given the high risk of bilateral disease, the other testis should be biopsied to exclude ALL.

Prognosis

- Related to the patient's overall response to chemotherapy

PEARLS _____

- Any intratesticular mass in a young male is considered malignant until proven otherwise.

Suggested Readings

Mazzu D, Jeffrey RB Jr, Ralls PW. Lymphoma and leukemia involving the testicles: findings on gray-scale and color Doppler sonography. AJR Am J Roentgenol 1995;164(3):645–647.

CASE 87

Clinical Presentation

Blunt trauma to the scrotum suffered in a motor vehicle accident

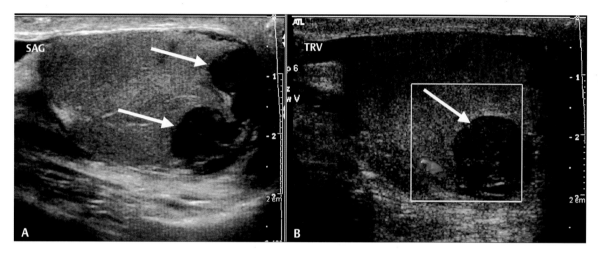

Fig. 87.1 Gray scale sonographic images of the right testicle in **(A)** sagittal view and color flow image in **(B)** transverse view.

Radiologic Findings

- Hypoechoic collection confined to the testicle (*arrows,* **Fig. 87.1A**)
- No flow seen on color or power Doppler (*arrow,* **Fig. 87.1B**)

Diagnosis

Testicular hematoma

Differential Diagnosis

- Malignant testicular neoplasms
- Testicular epidermoid

Discussion

Background

Fifty percent of scrotal injuries will show testicular hematoma. Most injuries are sports related, and fewer are the result of motor vehicle collisions. Up to 15% of testicular neoplasms may present in the setting of trauma. Therefore, follow-up is critical to confirm resolution of the intratesticular finding and exclude an underlying testicular neoplasm.

Clinical Findings

Swollen, painful scrotum. Scrotal trauma.

Pathology

Blood contained within an intact tunica albuginea represents an intratesticular hematoma.

Imaging Findings

ULTRASOUND

- The absence of flow is reassuring that this finding is not a testicular neoplasm; however, a follow-up exam is mandatory to ensure resolution.
- Nonseminomatous germ cell tumors may have cystic components; again, follow-up is mandatory.
- A testicular epidermoid would appear as a cystic structure with no flow. Internal hemorrhage may mimic the "onion skin" appearance of an epidermoid. An epidermoid would not resolve on follow-up scan.
- Testicular hematoma may have a variety of appearances depending on the age of the hematoma. It may be echogenic (acute) or hypoechoic with retracting clot (i.e., evolving hematoma).
- Testicular hematoma is confined to the tunica albuginea. If a contour abnormality is seen, suspect testicular rupture.

Treatment

- Symptomatic treatment only
- Large hematomas may become infected or may infarct, requiring orchiectomy.

Prognosis

- Depends on the severity of trauma. Most hematomas will resolve.

PEARLS _____

- Resolution on follow-up is key to the diagnosis of hematoma and exclusion of tumor.
- Any suspicion of testicular rupture requires emergent surgery.

Suggested Readings

Dogra V, Bhatt S. Acute painful scrotum. Radiol Clin North Am 2004;42(2):349–363.

CASE 88

Clinical Presentation

Asymptomatic, but palpable scrotal abnormality

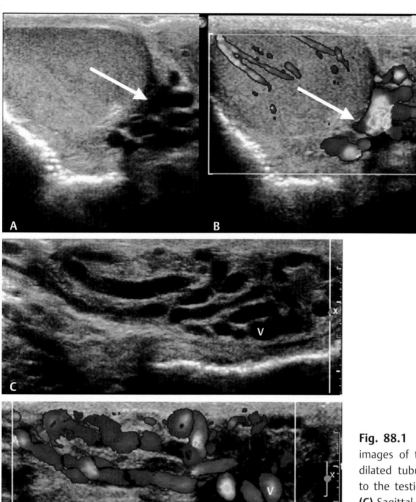

Fig. 88.1 Transverse gray scale and color images of the left hemiscrotum show **(A)** dilated tubular structures (*arrow*) adjacent to the testicle with **(B)** color Doppler flow. **(C)** Sagittal gray scale and **(D)** color Doppler images show the tubular structures represent vessels cephalad to the testicle in the spermatic cord.

Radiologic Findings

- Dilated tubular structures > 2 mm adjacent to the testicle (**Fig. 88.1A,C**)
- Color Doppler flow is present (**Fig. 88.1B,D**).

Diagnosis

Varicocele

Differential Diagnosis

None

Discussion

Background

Varicoceles represent dilated scrotal veins and are found in ~15% of adult men. This percentage increases with age and is much more common on the left. Varicoceles are seen in 40% of men presenting with infertility.

Clinical Findings

A varicocele may present as a palpable abnormality likened to a "bag of worms." It may be discovered during the work-up for infertility, or it may be an incidental finding on scrotal sonography performed for other reasons.

Pathology

Incompetent valves within the gonadal veins result in dilated scrotal veins. Venous reflux with adverse effects on testicular temperature may result in varicocele-induced infertility.

Imaging Findings

ULTRASOUND

- In addition to the above findings, spectral analysis within the varicocele will show venous waveforms.
- With the Valsalva maneuver, flow reversal may be detected within the varicocele, resulting from incompetent gonadal vein valves.

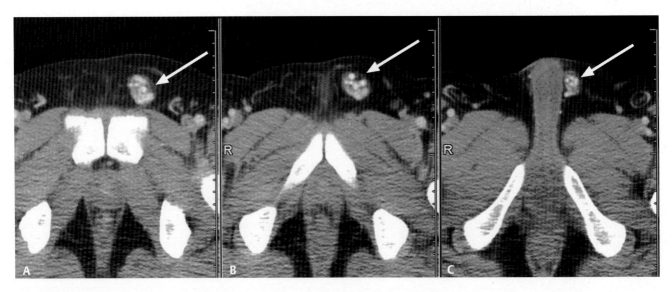

Fig. 88.2 Contrast-enhanced computed tomography through the pelvis. **(A–C)** Axial images through the left spermatic cord show a serpiginous collection of contrast-enhanced structures (*arrow*) consistent with an incidentally detected varicocele.

COMPUTED TOMOGRAPHY

- Usually incidentally detected
- Contrast-enhanced tubular structures noted in the inguinal region (**Fig. 88.2**)

Treatment

- Embolization, sclerotherapy, or surgical repair of the varicocele when infertility is a concern

Prognosis

- Up to 90% of varicoceles will resolve following the above treatments. Restoration of fertility is less certain, but the treatments are still recommended when a varicocele is found in an infertile man.

PEARLS _____

- Varicoceles may result from obstruction of the gonadal veins in the retroperitoneum (e.g., mass effect from tumor or adenopathy) or from renal cell carcinoma with involvement of the left renal vein, where the left gonadal vein drains. Urologists may obtain cross sectional imaging to exclude retroperitoneal masses as the cause for varicocele.

Suggested Readings

Bhatt S, Rubens DJ, Dogra VS. Sonography of benign intrascrotal lesions. Ultrasound Q 2006;22(2):121–136.

CASE 89

Clinical Presentation

Mass in the right groin

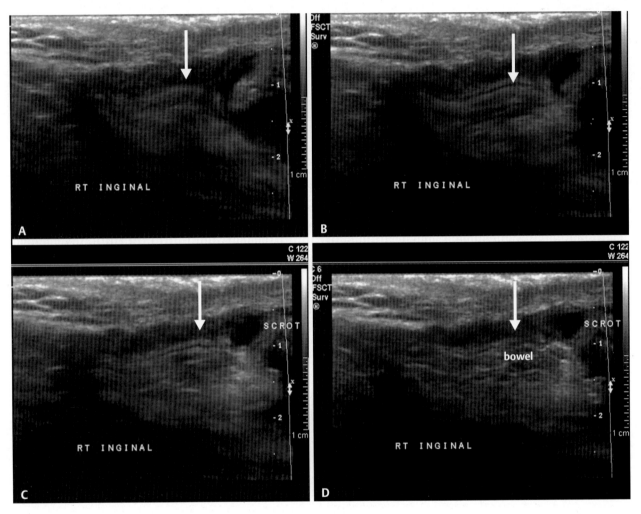

Fig. 89.1 **(A–D)** Gray scale sonogram images in the right inguinal region (*arrows*) show bowel extending down through the inguinal canal during a prolonged Valsalva maneuver.

Radiologic Findings

- No finding initially (**Fig. 89.1A**)
- Progressive Valsalva maneuver reveals the bowel moving through the inguinal canal (*arrow*, **Fig. 89.1B**) and into the right scrotum (*arrow*, **Fig. 89.1C,D**).
- Peristalsis is seen on real-time imaging within the herniating mass, confirming the bowel.

Diagnosis

Right inguinal hernia

Differential Diagnosis

- Extratesticular fluid collection (e.g., abscess, spermatocele, hydrocele, or hematocele)
- Extratesticular mass in inguinal region (e.g., lymphadenopathy)
- Testicular mass with spread to the paratesticular tissues

Discussion

Background

Inguinal hernias are quite common. Physical exam is usually sufficient for diagnosis. In equivocal cases, cross-sectional imaging may be required.

Clinical Findings

Painful right scrotum and/or right inguinal bulge

Pathology

Direct hernias (hernia through a weakness in the abdominal wall musculature at Hesselbach triangle) are medial to the inferior epigastric vessels. Indirect hernias (enter the inguinal canal through the deep inguinal ring) are lateral to the inferior epigastric vessels.

Imaging Findings

ULTRASOUND

- Observing valvulae conniventes and/or bowel peristalsis is required to exclude extratesticular fluid collections and extratesticular masses as the cause of the scrotal mass and to confirm hernia.
- The "mass" in this case was not associated with the testicle, and the testicle was otherwise normal (not shown).
- Attempt to demonstrate the defect in the abdominal wall musculature (not always apparent without provocative maneuvers).
- A small bowel hernia will appear as a heterogeneous mass, with gut signature or containing gas, surrounding normal elements of the spermatic cord but separate from the testis.
- An omental hernia will present as an echogenic mass, due to fat, separate from the testis.
- Exclude testicular pathology by the demonstration of a normal testicle.

COMPUTED TOMOGRAPHY

- Defect in the abdominal wall in the inguinal region
- Herniation of the omentum, large or small bowel, or other structures (e.g., bladder) into the canal (**Fig. 89.2**)
- Stranding around the hernia indicates inflammation, such as bowel incarceration or strangulation.

Treatment

- Symptomatic hernias are treated with repair of the abdominal wall weakness (i.e., herniorrhaphy).

Prognosis

- Excellent if no bowel strangulation

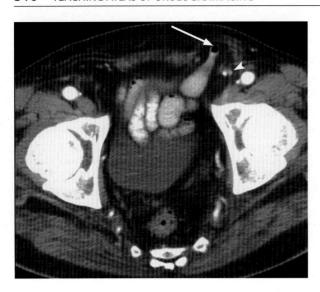

Fig. 89.2 Contrast-enhanced computed tomography shows a left inguinal hernia containing the small bowel (*arrow*) just medial to the inferior epigastric vessels (*arrowhead*), representing a direct hernia.

PEARLS

- Provocative maneuvers to demonstrate an inguinal hernia include maneuvers that raise the intra-abdominal pressure, such as a Valsalva maneuver, or performing the exam with the patient standing.

Suggested Readings

Subramanyam BR, Balthazar EJ, Raghavendra BN, Horii SC, Hilton S. Sonographic diagnosis of scrotal hernia. AJR Am J Roentgenol 1982;139(3):535–538.

CASE 90

Clinical Presentation

A 30-year-old male with history of resected testis tumor and chemotherapy

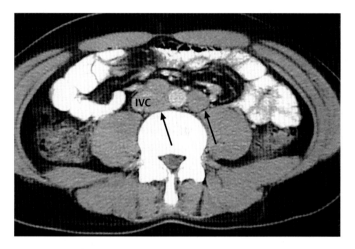

Fig. 90.1 Axial enhanced computed tomography scan through the midabdomen. IVC, inferior vena cava.

Radiologic Findings

- Left periaortic and aortocaval adenopathy (*arrows,* **Fig. 90.1**)

Diagnosis

Metastatic testis tumor to the retroperitoneal lymph nodes

Differential Diagnosis

- Retroperitoneal fibrosis
- Lymphoma

Discussion

Background

Presenting symptoms in ~10% of patients with testicular cancer may be due to metastases.

Clinical Findings

Lumbar back pain may be due to bulky retroperitoneal disease involving the psoas muscle or nerve roots. Unilateral or bilateral lower extremity swelling may be due to venous obstruction or thrombosis resulting from retroperitoneal adenopathy. A new or increasing varicocele may result from a retroperitoneal mass.

Pathology

Anatomical studies show that lymphatic drainage of the testis is primarily to the interaortocaval region for right-sided testicular tumors and to the left para-aortic and preaortic nodes for left-sided testicular tumors. Nodal masses usually occur close to the renal vein on the left and close to the insertion of the gonadal vein into the IVC on the right. Crossover may occur, especially from right to left. These anatomical studies serve as the basis for regional control with para-aortic lymph node dissection following orchiectomy.

Imaging Findings

COMPUTED TOMOGRAPHY

- The history of prior testis tumor in a young man makes any enlarged lymph nodes in the peri-aortic region highly suspect for metastatic disease even if not in a typical location.
- Retroperitoneal fibrosis (RPF) can produce abnormal soft tissue surrounding the aorta and inferior vena cava, but this is more often a conglomerate mass of tissue rather than focal round masses, representing adenopathy, as present in this case (**Fig. 90.1**).
- Lymphoma is a consideration given the adenopathy present; although lymphoma is not excluded by imaging features, it is unlikely given the history.
- Computed tomography (CT) is very sensitive for detecting lymph node enlargement.

MAGNETIC RESONANCE IMAGING

- CT and magnetic resonance imaging are equally accurate for detecting lymph node enlargement.
- RPF will appear as a plaquelike mass surrounding the aorta. T1-weighted imaging will show low signal, with variable signal on T2-weighted imaging, depending on the phase of the disease; that is, in the early (active) phase, the plaque will be high signal on T2-weighted imaging, and in the late (quiescent) phase, the plaque will be low signal. These findings are not specific for RPF, however.

POSITRON EMISSION TOMOGRAPHY

- Positron emission tomography (PET)-CT has been shown to be more sensitive and specific than CT for staging testicular carcinoma.

Treatment

- Various combinations of radiation and chemotherapy with or without retroperitoneal lymph node dissection

Prognosis

- The 5-year survival rate for seminoma with adenopathy is > 90%, 70 to 92% for nonseminomatous germ cell tumor with adenopathy (stage II disease). The greater the tumor burden and/or the presence of distant metastasis, the lower the survival rate.

PEARLS _____

- Lymph nodes measuring 1 cm in the short axis is the generally accepted definition for adenopathy in the abdomen and retroperitoneum. However, this may result in a 22 to 44% false-negative rate in detecting lymph node metastases with testicular cancer. Some authors advocate using a smaller node size (4 mm) to diagnose adenopathy (with resultant decrease in specificity) in the expected sites of lymph node metastases in testicular carcinoma (i.e., inferior to the right renal vein and adjacent to the left renal vein).

Suggested Readings

Richie J, Steele G. Neoplasms of the testis. In: Wein A, ed. Campbell-Walsh Urology. 9th ed. Philadelphia: Saunders Elsevier; 2007:893–934.

Woodward PJ, Sohaey R, O'Donoghue MJ, Green DE. From the archives of the AFIP: tumors and tumorlike lesions of the testis: radiologic-pathologic correlation. Radiographics 2002;22(1):189–216.

CASE 91

Clinical Presentation

A 50-year-old male presents with decreasing renal function.

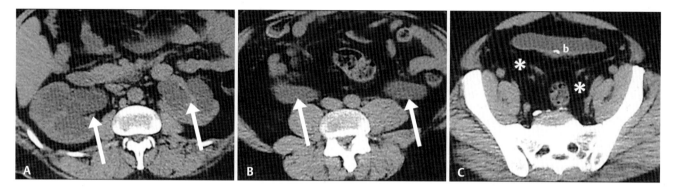

Fig. 91.1   Noncontrast computed tomography scans at the level of the **(A)** kidneys, **(B)** ureters, and **(C)** bladder.

Radiologic Findings

- Bilateral hydronephrosis and hydroureter (*arrows*, **Fig. 91.1A–C**)
- Teardrop or pear-shaped bladder (b, **Fig. 91.1C**) with incidentally noted bladder stone
- Excessive fat surrounding the bladder (*asterisks*, **Fig. 91.1C**)

Diagnosis

Pelvic lipomatosis

Differential Diagnosis

- Pelvic hematoma
- Pelvic tumor
- Lymphoma

Discussion

Background

Pelvic lipomatosis is a rare and benign condition with accumulation of fat in the pelvis with resultant mass effect. Men are significantly affected more often than women (almost 20:1). Two thirds of patients are black, and one third are white. Obesity may be associated but not uniformly causative.

Clinical Findings

Fifty percent of patients have urinary symptoms; 25% may have constipation. Occasional renal failure secondary to ureteral obstruction may occur.

315

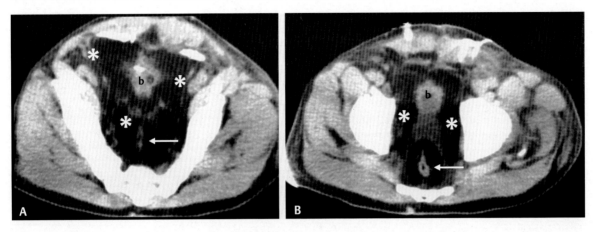

Fig. 91.2 Pelvic computed tomography imaging with intravenous contrast at two levels shows exuberant pelvic fat (*asterisks*) as the cause of elevation of the bladder (b) and mass effect on the rectum (*arrows*).

Pathology

Pelvic lipomatosis is an idiopathic accumulation of copious nonmalignant but infiltrative fat in the pelvis, which causes mass effect on the bladder and adjacent structures.

Imaging Findings

COMPUTED TOMOGRAPHY

- Both hematoma and tumor would have Hounsfield units well above the negative numbers shown for fat. Fresh blood, in fact, would be very high density.
- The bladder may be deformed by enlarged pelvic lymph nodes, but there are none present in this case, excluding lymphoma.
- Computed tomography (CT) allows a specific diagnosis to be made by showing that it is fat and not blood, tumor, or adenopathy deforming the bladder.
- Narrowing of the rectum is also apparent on CT (**Fig. 91.2**), as it would also be on a barium enema (**Fig. 91.3**).

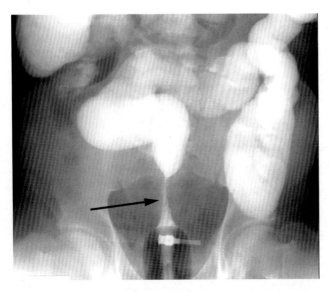

Fig. 91.3 Pelvic radiograph from contrast enema in the same patient as **Fig. 91.2** shows characteristic narrowing of the rectum in this patient with constipation due to pelvic lipomatosis.

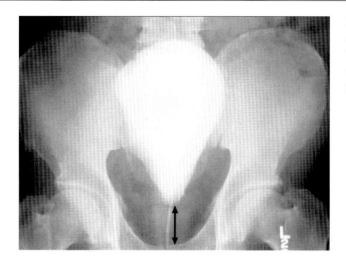

Fig. 91.4 Pelvic radiograph from a cystogram in same patient as in **Figs. 91.2** and **91.3** shows elevation of the bladder base (*double-headed arrow*) and characteristic lightbulb shape to the bladder in this patient with pelvic lipomatosis.

RADIOGRAPHY/INTRAVENOUS PYELOGRAM

- Cystography or IVP reveals a bladder that is elevated out of the pelvis and has a teardrop, pear, or lightbulb configuration (**Fig. 91.4**), which is typical of pelvic lipomatosis. This appearance, however, is not specific on intravenous pyelogram, as hematoma, tumor, or even adenopathy can produce similar findings.

Treatment

- Long-term follow-up to evaluate for ureteral obstruction is recommended.
- About 40% of patients require treatment for their ureteral obstruction with stenting versus ureteral reimplantation.

Prognosis

- Ureteral reimplantation or stenting should relieve ureteral obstruction.

PEARLS

- Pelvic lipomatosis is associated with premalignant inflammatory lesions of the bladder. Patients are therefore screened for bladder malignancy with cystoscopy.

Suggested Readings

Pais V, Strandhoy J, Assimos D. Pathophysiology of urinary tract obstruction. In: Wein A, ed. Campbell-Walsh Urology. 9th ed. Philadelphia: Saunders Elsevier; 2007:1195–1254.

CASE 92

Clinical Presentation

A 54-year-old male with 3 months of abdominal pain and testicular pain presents with renal failure.

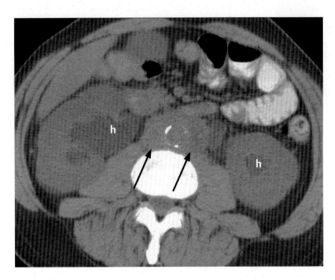

Fig. 92.1 Noncontrast computed tomography scan shows symmetric periaortic soft tissue mass (*arrows*) and bilateral hydronephrosis (h).

Radiologic Findings

- Symmetric periaortic soft tissue mass (*arrows,* **Fig. 92.1**)
- Bilateral hydronephrosis (h, **Fig. 92.1**)

Diagnosis

Retroperitoneal fibrosis (RPF)

Differential Diagnosis

- Lymphoma
- Inflammatory abdominal aortic aneurysm
- Retroperitoneal hemorrhage
- Metastatic adenopathy

Discussion

Background

RPF includes an idiopathic form (two thirds of patients) and a secondary form (one third of patients). Secondary causes include drugs (especially the ergot alkaloids, e.g., methysergide), radiation, desmoplastic reaction to retroperitoneal metastases, abdominal aortic aneurysm (AAA), and granulomatous infections, such as tuberculosis.

Clinical Findings

Poorly localized pain (abdominal, flank, or back) is the most common symptom. With involvement of the ureter(s), colicky pain may be present. Elevation of the erythrocyte sedimentation rate and C-reactive protein may be present. Men are affected 2 to 3 times more often than women. The average age of affected individuals is the 6th to 7th decade.

Pathology

The normal fatty tissue of the retroperitoneum is replaced by sclerotic collagenous or fibrotic tissue infiltrated by mononuclear cells (mostly B- and T-cell lymphocytes).

Imaging Findings

COMPUTED TOMOGRAPHY

- Lymphoma is impossible to exclude. The lack of adenopathy elsewhere may suggest an alternative diagnosis. However, biopsy is often required for definitive diagnosis.
- RPF is included in the spectrum of inflammatory periaortitis. There is no AAA in this case.
- Retroperitoneal hemorrhage would be higher attenuation in the acute setting, and hemorrhage of different ages would give a laminated appearance to the abnormal retroperitoneal tissue.
- Metastatic adenopathy is also a possibility, although no history of a known malignancy is provided.
- RPF presents as a plaquelike mass, usually in the periaortic region, which is isodense to muscle on unenhanced computed tomography (CT) without mass effect (**Fig. 92.1**). The mass is usually seen to encase the ureters, deviating them medially. Early in the inflammatory process, the plaque will enhance, but in the more chronic phases, enhancement is diminished.

RADIOGRAPHY/INTRAVENOUS PYELOGRAM

- Classic triad of medial deviation of ureters, extrinsic ureteral compression, and hydronephrosis on contrast studies of the renal collecting systems (**Fig. 92.2**).

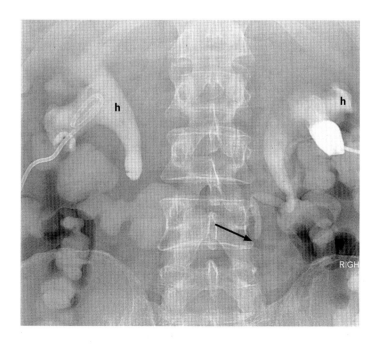

Fig. 92.2 Percutaneous nephrostomy study. Classic deviation of the left ureter medially is seen, with compression of the ureter (*arrow*) and hydronephrosis (h).

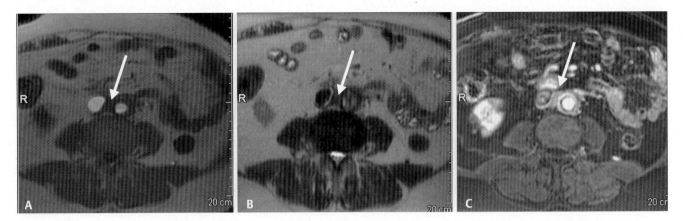

Fig. 92.3 Magnetic resonance imaging. Axial images include **(A)** T1-weighted, **(B)** T2-weighted, and **(C)** T1-weighted with fat saturation after gadolinium. A homogeneous mass (*arrows*) is seen in the periaortic space. The **(A)** T1-weighted and **(B)** T2-weighted images show low signal (likely due to a chronic lesion). The soft tissue in **C** is enhancing following gadolinium.

MAGNETIC RESONANCE IMAGING

- Magnetic resonance imaging (MRI) will show similar findings as on CT, which is that of a periaortic soft tissue mass. Tissue is low signal on T1-weighted imaging (*arrows*, **Fig. 92.3**). In the early, acute inflammatory stage of the disease, the plaque is high signal on T2-weighted imaging, but it is low signal in the chronic phase of RPF. Enhancement will be variable and usually more intense in the early phases of the process.

Treatment

- Corticosteroids to decrease the inflammatory process
- Stenting or surgery to relieve the ureteral obstruction

Prognosis

- Early diagnosis and treatment lend a favorable prognosis.
- However, the diagnosis is often made late, resulting in the complication of progressive renal failure from ureteral obstruction.

PEARLS

- Neither CT nor MRI is sufficiently specific to the diagnosis of RPF to avoid percutaneous or surgical biopsy when the diagnosis is in doubt.
- Suspected RPF requires multiple biopsies throughout the mass to ensure adequate sampling and definitive diagnosis.

Suggested Readings

Vaglio A, Salvarani C, Buzio C. Retroperitoneal fibrosis. Lancet 2006;367(9506):241–251.

Vivas I, Nicolas AI, Velazquez P, et al. Retroperitoneal fibrosis: typical and atypical manifestations. Br J Radiol 2000;73(866):214–222.

CASE 93

Clinical Presentation

Patient with human immunodeficiency virus (HIV) and acute renal failure. Both kidneys appeared similar on ultrasound.

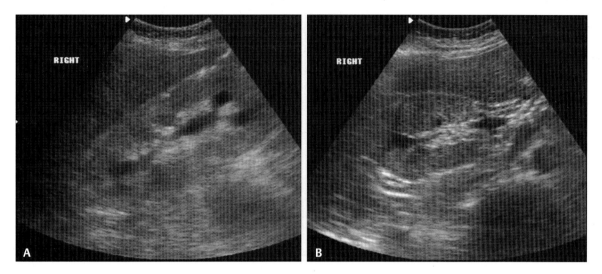

Fig. 93.1 Renal sonogram. **(A)** Longitudinal and **(B)** transverse images of the right kidney.

Radiologic Findings

- Diffusely echogenic kidney (i.e., more echogenic than adjacent liver) (**Fig. 93.1**)
- Normal-sized right kidney
- No stones and no hydronephrosis

Diagnosis

HIV nephropathy

Differential Diagnosis

- Chronic renal disease
- Medullary nephrocalcinosis
- Autosomal recessive polycystic kidney disease

Discussion

Background

Acute renal failure (ARF) etiologies are traditionally broken down into (1) prerenal causes (e.g., hypoperfusion states), (2) intrarenal (intrinsic renal disease) causes, and (3) postrenal (mechanical or functional obstruction of urine or venous blood flow) causes.

Ninety percent of intrarenal causes include ischemic nephropathy from profound or chronic ischemia to the kidneys and toxic exposures, both of which result in acute tubular necrosis (ATN). Ischemic ATN usually results from major surgery, severe trauma, burns, sepsis, or severe hypovolemia.

Nephrotoxic ATN results from toxin exposure, which has varying effects on intrarenal vasoconstriction and/or direct toxic tubular effects and/or intratubular obstruction.

The remaining 10% of intrinsic renal disease cases include large vessel disease (e.g., atheroembolic lesions), microvascular disease (e.g., vasculitis), glomerular disease (e.g., glomerulonephritis, as may be seen with HIV), and other processes of the tubulointerstitium (e.g., interstitial nephritis; infiltrative lesions, e.g., lymphoma).

Clinical Findings

Presenting features of HIV-associated nephropathy include nephrotic range proteinuria and renal failure. Black patients are affected more often than caucasian patients.

Pathology

In HIV nephropathy, focal segmental glomerulosclerosis is a prominent feature, along with diffuse mesangial hyperplasia.

Imaging Findings

ULTRASOUND

- Patients with chronic renal disease typically have echogenic kidneys, but the kidneys are small. In HIV nephropathy, however, normal-sized echogenic kidneys are seen, as in this case.
- Medullary nephrocalcinosis produces diffuse echogenicity in the medullary pyramids with occasional shadowing, but not throughout the entire kidney, as in this case.
- Autosomal recessive polycystic kidney disease produces very large echogenic kidneys in infants and children. Both the size of the kidneys (i.e., normal size) and the age of the patient exclude this diagnosis.
- Diagnostic criteria (in HIV-positive patients) for HIV nephropathy by sonography include
  - Echogenic renal cortex (i.e., greater than liver)
  - Normal-sized kidneys

Treatment

- Anti-HIV medications

Prognosis

- If treatment is begun before azotemia, the prognosis is excellent.

PEARLS _____

- Ultrasound is the primary modality of choice for imaging patients with ARF to exclude obstruction. Contrast-enhanced computed tomography and magnetic resonance imaging are contraindicated in patients with ARF.

Suggested Readings

Atta MG, Longenecker JC, Fine DM, et al. Sonography as a predictor of human immunodeficiency virus–associated nephropathy. J Ultrasound Med 2004;23(5):603–610.

Brenner B, ed. Brenner and Rector's The Kidney. 7th ed. Philadelphia: Saunders; 2004.

APPENDIX

A. MRI Glossary

Abbreviation	Full Name
GRE	• Gradient echo
T1WI	• T1-weighted image
T2WI	• T2-weighted image
VIBE	• Volume interpolated breath hold examination
FLASH	• Fast low angle shot (a T1-weighted sequence)
HASTE	• Half-Fourier acquisition single-shot turbo spin echo (a T2-weighted sequence)

B. Management of Acute Reactions in Adults*

Remember "O_2, IV, and monitor" from basic life support (BLS). These maneuvers should be performed on every patient you are called to evaluate for potential life-threatening contrast reaction until assessment shows these interventions are not needed:

- Administer oxygen (O_2) 6 to 10 L/minute via face mask.
- Maintain adequate intravenous (IV) access, preferably using an 18G antecubital angiocatheter.
- Attach a monitor for O_2 saturation, blood pressure, and heart rate.
- Ausculate breath sounds and heart.

Specific Treatments

URTICARIA

- Discontinue injection if not completed.
- No treatment is needed in most cases.
- Give H1-receptor blocker (diphenhydramine PO/intramuscular [IM]/IV 25–50 mg).
- If severe or widely disseminated: alpha agonist (arteriolar and venous constriction): epinephrine subcutaneous (SC) (1:1000) 0.1 to 0.3 mL (0.1–0.3 mg) (if no cardiac contraindications)

FACIAL OR LARYNGEAL EDEMA

- Give alpha-agonist (arteriolar and venous constriction): epinephrine SC or IM (1:1000) 0.1 to 0.3 mL (0.1–0.3 mg) or, if hypotension is evident, epinephrine (1:10,000) slowly IV 1 mL (0.1 mg). Repeat as needed up to a maximum of 1 mg.
- If the patient is not responsive to therapy or if there is obvious acute laryngeal edema, seek appropriate assistance (e.g., cardiopulmonary arrest response team).

BRONCHOSPASM

- Give beta-agonist inhalers (bronchodilators), such as metaproterenol 2 to 3 puffs; repeat p.r.n. If unresponsive to inhalers, use SC, IM, or IV epinephrine.

---

* These recommendations are taken from the American College of Radiology (ACR). Manual on Contrast Media, 5.0 edition. American College of Radiology; 1991. Reprinted with permission of the American College of Radiology. No other representation of this material is authorized without expressed, written permission from the American College of Radiology.

- Give epinephrine SC or IM (1:1000) 0.1 to 0.3 mL (0.1–0.3 mg) or, if hypotension is evident, epinephrine (1:10,000) slowly IV 1 mL (0.1 mg). Repeat as needed up to a maximum of 1 mg.
- Alternatively, give aminophylline 6 mg/kg IV in dextrose 5% in water (D5W) over 10 to 20 minutes (loading dose), then 0.4 to 1.0 mg/kg/hour, as needed (caution: may cause hypotension).
- Call for assistance (e.g., cardiopulmonary arrest response team) for severe bronchospasm or if O$_2$ saturation < 88% persists.

HYPOTENSION WITH TACHYCARDIA

- Legs should be elevated 60 degrees or more (preferred).
- Institute rapid IV administration of large volumes of isotonic Ringer lactate or normal saline.
- If poorly responsive: epinephrine (1:10,000) slowly IV 1 mL (0.1 mg) (if no cardiac contraindications). Repeat as needed up to a maximum of 1 mg.
- If still poorly responsive, seek appropriate assistance (e.g., cardiopulmonary arrest response team).

HYPOTENSION WITH BRADYCARDIA (VAGAL REACTION)

- Legs should be elevated 60 degrees or more (preferred).
- Institute rapid IV administration of large volumes of isotonic Ringer lactate or normal saline.
- Give atropine 0.6 to 1.0 mg IV slowly if patient does not respond quickly to the first two steps.
- Repeat atropine up to a total dose of 0.04 mg/kg (2–3 mg) in an adult.
- Ensure complete resolution of hypotension and bradycardia prior to discharge.

HYPERTENSION, SEVERE

- Give nitroglycerine 0.4 mg tablet, sublingual (may repeat 3×), or topical nitroglycerine 2% ointment (apply 1 inch strip).
- Transfer to the intensive care unit or emergency department.
- For pheochromocytoma, give phentolamine 5 mg IV.

SEIZURES OR CONVULSIONS

- Consider diazepam 5 mg (or more, as appropriate) or midazolam 0.5 to 1.0 mg IV.
- If longer effect is needed, obtain neurology consultation.
- Careful monitoring of vital signs is required, particularly of partial pressure of oxygen (pO$_2$), because of the risk of respiratory depression with benzodiazepine administration.
- Consider using the cardiopulmonary arrest response team for prolonged seizures or if intubation is needed.

PULMONARY EDEMA

- Elevate the torso; use rotating tourniquets (venous compression).
- Give diuretics (furosemide 20–40 mg IV, slow push).
- Consider giving morphine (1–3 mg IV).
- Transfer to the intensive care unit or emergency department.

C. Genitourinary Specific Imaging Protocols

Adrenal Protocol CT	Contrast	100 mL low osmolar contrast at 3 to 4 mL/second	
Phase	**Timing**	**Slice Thickness (mm)**	**Coverage**
Unenhanced	Precontrast	2.5	Diaphragm through midkidneys
Enhanced	70 seconds postcontrast	2.5	Diaphragm through midkidneys
Delayed	10 minutes	2.5	Diaphragm through midkidneys

Renal Mass Protocol CT	Contrast	100 cc low osmolar contrast at 3 to 4 cc/second	
Phase	**Timing**	**Slice Thickness (mm)**	**Coverage**
Unenhanced	Precontrast	3.0	Through kidneys
Enhanced	90 to 110 seconds postcontrast	3.0	Diaphragm through entire abdomen to localize kidneys
Delayed	5 minutes	3.0	Through kidneys

CT/IVP	Contrast	100 cc low osmolar contrast at 3 to 4 cc/second	
Phase	**Timing**	**Slice Thickness (mm)**	**Coverage**
Unenhanced	Precontrast	3.75	Top of kidneys to bladder base
Enhanced	90 to 110 seconds postcontrast	3.75	Diaphragm through kidneys (include pelvis in bladder cancer patients)
Delayed	8 to 13 minutes	2.50	Top of kidneys to bladder base with multiplanar reconstructions

Stone Protocol CT			
Phase	**Timing**	**Slice Thickness (mm)**	**Coverage**
Unenhanced	Precontrast	3.75	Top of kidneys to bladder base

Adrenal Protocol MRI	Contrast	0.1 mmol/kg gadolinium compound	
Sequence	**Plane(s)**	**Slice Thickness (mm)**	**Coverage**
HASTE T2 as a localizer	Coronal	3 to 5	Adrenals
T1 GRE I in phase and opposed phase	Axial	3 to 5	Adrenals
T2 with fat saturation	Axial	3 to 5	Adrenals
T1 FLASH without and with fat saturation	Axial	3 to 5	Adrenals
Postgadolinium T1 with fat saturation	Axial	3 to 5	Adrenals

Renal Mass Protocol MRI	Contrast	0.1 mmol/kg gadolinium compound	
Sequence	**Plane(s)**	**Slice Thickness (mm)**	**Coverage**
HASTE T2 as a localizer	Coronal	3 to 5	Abdomen
T1 GRE in phase and opposed phase	Axial	3 to 5	Abdomen
T2 with fat saturation	Axial and coronal	3 to 5	Abdomen
T1 FLASH without and with fat saturation	Axial	3 to 5	Abdomen
Postgadolinium Imaging			
T1 GRE 3D dynamic imaging (six acquisitions)	Axial	3 to 5	Through kidneys
Subtraction imaging performed		3 to 5	Through kidneys

MR Urogram	Contrast	0.1 mmol/kg gadolinium compound	
HASTE T2 as a localizer	Coronal	3 to 5	Abdomen/pelvis
T2 with fat saturation	Axial and coronal	3 to 5	Abdomen/pelvis
Postgadolinium Imaging			
T1 GRE 3D dynamic imaging (three acquisitions)	Coronal	3 to 5	Abdomen/pelvis
Subtraction imaging performed		3 to 5	Abdomen/pelvis

Abbreviations: CT, computed tomography; CT-IVP, computed tomography-intravenous pyelogram; FLASH, fast low angle shot; GRE, gradient echo; HASTE, half-Fourier acquisition single-shot turbo echo; MR, magnetic resonance; MRI, magnetic resonance imaging; 3D, three-dimensional.

D. Bosniak Renal Cyst Classification System

Category	Description
I	A benign simple cyst with a hairline thin wall that does not contain septa, calcifications, or solid components. It measures water density and does not enhance.
II	A benign cyst that may contain a few hairline thin septa in which "perceived"* enhancement may be present. Fine calcification or a short segment of slightly thickened calcification may be present in the wall or septa. Uniformly high-attenuation lesions < 3 cm (so-called high-density cysts) that are well marginated and do not enhance are included in this group. Cysts in this category do not require further evaluation.
IIF (follow-up)	Cysts that may contain multiple hairline thin septa or minimal smooth thickening of their wall or septa. Perceived enhancement of the septa or wall may be present. The wall or septa may contain calcification that may be thick and nodular, but no measurable contrast enhancement is present. These lesions are generally well marginated. Totally intrarenal nonenhancing high-attenuation renal lesions < 3 cm are also included in this category. These lesions require follow-up studies to prove benignity.
III	"Indeterminate" cystic masses that have thickened irregular or smooth walls or septa in which measurable enhancement is present. These are surgical lesions, although some will prove to be benign (e.g., hemorrhagic cysts, chronic infected cysts, and multiloculated cystic nephroma); some will be malignant, such as cystic renal cell carcinoma and multiloculated cystic renal cell carcinoma.
IV	These are clearly malignant cystic masses that can have all the criteria of category III, but also contain enhancing soft tissue components adjacent to, but independent of, the wall or septum. These lesions include cystic carcinomas and require surgical removal.

* Not measurable enhancement.
Source: Reprinted from *Urology*, 66(3), Israel GM, Bosniak MA, An update of the Bosniak renal cyst classification system, 484–488, 2005, with permission from Elsevier.

E. Kidney Injury Scale

Grade*	Type of Injury	Description of Injury
I	Contusion	Microscopic or gross hematuria; urologic studies normal
	Hematoma	Subcapsular, nonexpanding with parenchymal laceration
II	Hematoma	Nonexpanding perirenal hematoma confined to renal retroperitoneum
	Laceration	< 1 cm parenchymal depth of renal cortex without urinary extravasation
III	Laceration	> 1 cm parenchymal depth of renal cortex without collecting system rupture or urinary extravasation
IV	Laceration	Parenchymal laceration extending through the renal cortex, medulla, and collecting system
	Vascular	Main renal artery or vein injury with contained hemorrhage
V	Laceration	Completely shattered kidney and/or UPJ avulsion
	Vascular	Avulsion of renal hilum that devascularizes the kidney

* Advance one grade for bilateral injuries, up to grade III.
Abbreviation: UPJ, ureteropelvic junction.
Source: From Moore EE, Shackford SR, Pachter HL, et al. Organ injury scaling: spleen, liver, and kidney. J Trauma 1989;29(12):1664–1666. Reprinted with permission.

F. Bladder Injury Scale

Grade*	Type of Injury	Description of Injury
I	Hematoma	Contusion, intramural hematoma
	Laceration	Partial thickness
II	Laceration	Extraperitoneal bladder wall laceration < 2 cm
III	Laceration	Extraperitoneal (≥ 2 cm) or intraperitoneal (< 2 cm) bladder wall laceration
IV	Laceration	Intraperitoneal bladder wall laceration ≥ 2 cm
V	Laceration	Intraperitoneal or extraperitoneal bladder wall laceration extending into the bladder neck or ureteral orifice (trigone)

* Advance one grade for bilateral injuries, up to grade III.
Source: From Moore EE, Cogbill TH, Jurkovich GJ, et al. Organ injury scaling: III. Chest wall, abdominal vascular, ureter, bladder, and urethra. J Trauma 1992;33(3):337–339. Reprinted with permission.

G. Urethra Injury Scale

Grade*	Type of Injury	Description of Injury
I	Contusion	Blood at urethral meatus; urethrography normal
II	Stretch injury	Elongation of the urethra without extravasation on urethrography
III	Partial disruption	Extravasation of urethrography contrast at the injury site with visualization in the bladder
IV	Complete disruption	Extravasation of urethrography contrast at the injury site without visualization in the bladder; < 2 cm of urethra separation
V	Complete disruption	Complete transaction with ≥ 2 cm urethral separation or extension into the prostate or vagina

* Advance one grade for bilateral injuries, up to grade III.
Source: From Moore EE, Cogbill TH, Jurkovich GJ, et al. Organ injury scaling: III. Chest wall, abdominal vascular, ureter, bladder, and urethra. J Trauma 1992;33(3):337–339. Reprinted with permission.

H. Alternative Urethra Injury Scale

Type of Injury	Description of Injury
I	Posterior urethra stretched by a hematoma but intact with no extravasation on retrograde urethrogram
II	Complete or partial uretheral tear above the intact urogenital diaphragm, with extravasation only above the urogenital diaphragm on retrograde urethrogram
III	Complete or partial uretheral rupture with disruption of the urogenital diaphragm and extravasation above and below the urogenital diaphragm on retrograde urethrogram
Straddle	Injury to the bulbous urethra with local extravasation on retrograde urethrogram

Source: This article was published in J Urol, 118, Colapinto V, McCallum RW, Injury to the male posterior urethra in fractured pelvis: a new classification, 575–580. Copyright Elsevier 1977.

I. Adrenal Organ Injury Scale

Grade*	Description of Injury
I	Contusion
II	Laceration, involving only the cortex (< 2 cm)
III	Laceration, extending into the medulla (≥ 2 cm)
IV	> 50% parenchymal destruction
V	Total parenchymal destruction (including massive intraparenchymal hemorrhage) Avulsion from blood supply

* Advance one grade for bilateral injuries, up to grade III.
Source: From Moore EE, Malangoni MA, Cogbill TH, et al. Organ injury scaling: VII.: cervical vascular, peripheral vascular, adrenal, penis, testis, and scrotum. J Trauma 1996;41(3):523–524. Reprinted with permission.

Suggested Readings

Moore EE, Cogbill TH, Jurkovich GJ, et al. Organ injury scaling, III: Chest wall, abdominal vascular, ureter, bladder, and urethra. J Trauma 1992;33(3):337–339.

Moore EE, Cogbill TH, Malangoni MA, et al. Organ injury scaling. Surg Clin North Am 1995;75(2):293–303.

Moore EE, Malangoni MA, Cogbill TH, et al. Organ injury scaling, VII: Cervical vascular, peripheral vascular, adrenal, penis, testis, and scrotum. J Trauma 1996;41(3):523–524.

Moore EE, Shackford SR, Pachter HL, et al. Organ injury scaling: spleen, liver, and kidney. J Trauma 1989;29(12):1664–1666.

J. Renal Tumor Staging

Primary Tumor (T)

T_X Primary tumor cannot be assessed

T_0 No evidence of primary tumor

T_1 Tumor ≤ 7 cm in greatest dimension, limited to the kidney

    T_{1a} Tumor ≤ 4 cm in greatest dimension, limited to the kidney

    T_{1b} Tumor > 4 cm but < 7 cm in greatest dimension, limited to the kidney

    T_2 Tumor > 7 cm in greatest dimension, limited to the kidney

T_3 Tumor extends into major veins or invades the adrenal gland or perinephric tissues but not beyond Gerota fascia

    T_{3a} Tumor directly invades the adrenal gland or perirenal and/or renal sinus fat but not beyond the Gerota fascia

    T_{3b} Tumor grossly extends into the renal vein or its segmental (muscle-containing) branches, or the vena cava is below the diaphragm

    T_{3c} Tumor grossly extends into the vena cava above the diaphragm or invades the wall of the vena cava

T_4 Tumor invades beyond the Gerota fascia

Regional Lymph Nodes (N)

Laterality does not affect the N classification.

    N_X Regional lymph nodes cannot be assessed

    N_0 No regional lymph node metastases

    N_1 Metastasis in a single regional lymph node

    N_2 Metastasis in more than one regional lymph node

Distant Metastasis (M)

    M_X Distant metastasis cannot be assessed

    M_0 No distant metastasis

    M_1 Distant metastasis

Stage Grouping

Stage	T	N	M
Stage I	T_1	N_0	M_0
Stage II	T_2	N_0	M_0
Stage III	T_1	N_1	M_0
	T_2	N_1	M_0
	T_3	N_0	M_0
	T_3	N_1	M_0
	T_{3a}	N_0	M_0
	T_{3a}	N_1	M_0
	T_{3b}	N_0	M_0
	T_{3b}	N_1	M_0
	T_{3c}	N_0	M_0
	T_{3c}	N_1	M_0
Stage IV	T_4	N_0	M_0
	T_4	N_1	M_0
	Any T	N_2	M_0
	Any T	Any N	M_1

Source: From Greene F.L., Page D.L., Fleming, I.D., et al., AJCC Cancer Staging Manual, Sixth Edition. New York: Springer Science and Business Media LLC, 2002: 323–325. www.springerlink.com. Used with the permission of the American Joint Committee on Cancer (AJCC), Chicago, Illinois.

K. Bladder Tumor Staging

Primary Tumor (T)

T_X Primary tumor cannot be assessed

T_0 No evidence of primary tumor

T_a Noninvasive papillary carcinoma

T_{is} Carcinoma in situ ("flat tumor")

T_1 Tumor invades subepithelial connective tissue

T_2 Tumor invades muscularis

$\quad$ T_{2a} Tumor invades superficial muscle (inner half)

$\quad$ T_{2b} Tumor invades deep muscle (outer half)

T_3 Tumor invades perivesical tissue

$\quad$ T_{3a} Microscopically

$\quad$ T_{3b} Macroscopically (extravesical mass)

T_4 Tumor invades any of the following: prostate, uterus, vagina, pelvic wall, abdominal wall

$\quad$ T_{4a} Tumor invades any of the following: prostate, uterus, vagina

$\quad$ T_{4b} Tumor invades any of the following: pelvic wall, abdominal wall

Regional Lymph Nodes (N)

Regional lymph nodes are those within the true pelvis; all others are distant lymph nodes.

N_X Regional lymph nodes cannot be assessed

N_0 No regional lymph node metastases

N_1 Metastases in a single lymph node, $\leq$ 2 cm in greatest dimension

N_2 Metastases in a single lymph node, > 2 cm but not > 5 cm in greatest dimension; none > 5 cm in greatest dimension

N_3 Metastases in a lymph node, > 5 cm in greatest dimension

Distant Metastasis (M)

M_X Distant metastasis cannot be assessed

M_0 No distant metastasis

M_1 Distant metastasis

Stage Grouping

Stage 0_a	T_a	N_0	M_0
Stage 0_{is}	T_{is}	N_0	M_0
Stage I	T_1	N_0	M_0
Stage II	T_{2a}	N_0	M_0
	T_{2b}	N_0	M_0
Stage III	T_{3a}	N_0	M_0
	T_{3b}	N_0	M_0
Stage IV	T_{4a}	N_0	M_0
	T_{4b}	N_0	M_0
	Any T	N_1	M_0
	Any T	N_2	M_0
	Any T	N_3	M_0
	Any T	Any N	M_1

Source: From Greene F.L., Page D.L., Fleming, I.D., et al., AJCC Cancer Staging Manual, Sixth Edition. New York: Springer Science and Business Media LLC, 2002: 335–338. www.springerlink.com. Used with the permission of the American Joint Committee on Cancer (AJCC), Chicago, Illinois.

L. Adrenal Tumor Staging

Primary Tumor (T)

T_X Primary tumor cannot be assessed

T_0 No evidence of primary tumor

T_1 Tumor ≤ 5 cm in greatest dimension, confined to the adrenal gland

T_2 Tumor > 5 cm in greatest dimension, limited to the adrenal gland

T_3 Tumor extends beyond the adrenal gland but does not invade adjacent organs

T_4 Tumor invades adjacent organs

Regional Lymph Nodes (N)

N_X Regional lymph nodes cannot be assessed

N_0 No regional lymph node metastases

N_1 Metastases into regional lymph nodes

Distant Metastasis (M)

M_X Distant metastasis cannot be assessed

M_0 No distant metastasis

M_1 Distant metastasis

Stage Grouping

Stage	T	N	M
Stage I	T_1	N_0	M_0
Stage II	T_2	N_0	M_0
Stage III	T_1	N_1	M_0
	T_2	N_1	M_0
	T_3	N_0	M_0
Stage IV	T_3	N_1	M_0
	T_4	N_1	M_0
	Any T	Any N	M_1

Source: J. Healy, R Reznek, J Husband. Primary Retroperitoneal Tumours (Chapter 19). In: Imaging in Oncology. Janet E. S. Husband and Rodney H. Reznek (eds) Isis Medical Media 1998, pp. 329–350. Copyright 1998 by Taylor & Francis Informa UK Ltd - Journals. Reproduced with permission of Taylor & Francis Informa UK Ltd - Journals in the format Textbook via Copyright Clearance Center.

M. Renal Pelvis and Ureter Tumor Staging

Primary Tumor (T)

T_X Primary tumor cannot be assessed

T_0 No evidence of primary tumor

T_a Noninvasive papillary carcinoma

T_{is} Carcinoma in situ

T_1 Tumor invades subepithelial connective tissue

T_2 Tumor invades musclaris

T_3

   (for renal pelvis only) Tumor invades beyond the muscularis into the peripelvic fat of the renal parenchyma

   (for ureter only) Tumor invades beyond the muscularis into the periureteral fat of the renal parenchyma below the diaphragm

T_4 Tumor invades adjacent organs or through the kidney into the perinephric fat

Regional Lymph Nodes (N)

N_X Regional lymph nodes cannot be assessed

N_0 No regional lymph node metastases

N_1 Metastases in a single lymph node, $\leq$ 2 cm in greatest dimension

N_2 Metastases in a single lymph node, > 2 cm but not > 5 cm in greatest dimension; none > 5 cm in greatest dimension

N_3 Metastases in a lymph node, > 5 cm in greatest dimension

Distant Metastasis (M)

M_X Distant metastasis cannot be assessed

M_0 No distant metastasis

M_1 Distant metastasis

Stage Grouping

Stage 0_a	T_a	N_0	M_0
Stage 0_{is}	T_{is}	N_0	M_0
Stage I	T_1	N_0	M_0
Stage II	T_2	N_0	M_0
Stage III	T_3	N_0	M_0
Stage IV	T_4	N_0	M_0
	Any T	N_1	M_0
	Any T	N_2	M_0
	Any T	N_3	M_0
	Any T	Any N	M_1

Source: From Greene F.L., Page D.L., Fleming, I.D., et al., AJCC Cancer Staging Manual, Sixth Edition. New York: Springer Science and Business Media LLC, 2002: 329–331. www.springerlink.com. Used with the permission of the American Joint Committee on Cancer (AJCC), Chicago, Illinois.

N. Testicular Tumor Staging

Primary Tumor (T)

The extent of primary tumor is usually classified after radical orchiectomy; for this reason, a pathologic stage is assigned.

pT_{X^*} Primary tumor cannot be assessed

pT_0 No evidence of primary tumor (e.g., histologic scar in testis)

pT_{is} Intratubular germ cell neoplasia (carcinoma in situ)

pT_1 Tumor limited to the testis and epididymis without vascular/lymphatic invasion; tumor may invade into the tunica albuginea but not the tunica vaginalis

pT_2 Tumor limited to the testis and epididymis with vascular/lymphatic invasion or tumor extending through the tunica albuginea with involvement of the tunica vaginalis

pT_3 Tumor invades the spermatic cord with or without vascular/lymphatic invasion

pT_4 Tumor invades the scrotum with or without vascular/lymphatic involvement

Regional Lymph Nodes (N)

N_X Regional lymph nodes cannot be assessed

N_0 No regional lymph node metastases

N_1 Metastases with a lymph node mass $\leq$ 2 cm in greatest dimension; or multiple lymph nodes, none > 2 cm in greatest dimension

N_2 Metastases with a lymph node mass > 2 cm but not > 5 cm in greatest dimension; or multiple lymph nodes, any one mass > 2 cm but not > 5 cm in greatest dimension

N_3 Metastases in a lymph node > 5 cm in greatest dimension

Regional Lymph Nodes

Interaortocaval	Preaortic
Para-aortic	Precaval
(Periaortic)	Retroaortic
Paracaval	Retrocaval

Distant Metastasis (M)

M_X Distant metastasis cannot be assessed

M_0 No distant metastasis

M_1 Distant metastasis

M_{1a} Nonregional nodal or pulmonary metastasis

M_{1b} Distant metastasis other than to nonregional lymph nodes and lungs

Serum Tumor Markers (S)

S_X Marker studies not available or not performed

S_0 Marker study levels within normal limits

S_1 LDH < 1.5 $\times$ N* *and*

Human chorionic gonadotropin (hCG) (MIU/mL) < 5000 *and*

Alpha-fetoprotein (AFP) (ng/mL) < 1000

S_2 LDH < 1.5 to 10 $\times$ N* *or*

hCg (MIU/mL) 5000 to 50,000 *or*

AFP (ng/mL) 1000 to 10,000

S_3 LDH < 10 $\times$ N* *or*

hCg (MIU/mL) > 50,000 *or*

AFP (ng/mL) > 10,000

* N indicates the upper limit of normal for the lactate dehydrogenase (LDH) assay

Stage Grouping

Stage 0	pT_{is}	N_0	M_0	S_0
Stage I	pT_{1-4}	N_0	M_0	S_x
Stage IA	pT_1	N_0	M_0	S_0
Stage IB	pT_2	N_0	M_0	S_0
	pT_3	N_0	M_0	S_0
	pT_4	N_0	M_0	S_0
Stage IS	Any pT/T_x	N_0	M_0	S_{1-3}
Stage II	Any pT/T_x	N_{1-3}	M_0	S_x
Stage IIA	Any pT/T_x	N_1	M_0	S_0
	Any pT/T_x	N_1	M_0	S_1
Stage IIB	Any pT/T_x	N_2	M_0	S_0
	Any pT/T_x	N_2	M_0	S_1
Stage IIC	Any pT/T_x	N_3	M_0	S_0
	Any pT/T_x	N_3	M_0	S_1
Stage III	Any pT/T_x	Any N	M_1	S_x
Stage IIIA	Any pT/T_x	Any N	M_{1a}	S_0
	Any pT/T_x	Any N	M_{1a}	S_1
Stage IIIB	Any pT/T_x	N_{1-3}	M_0	S_2
	Any pT/T_x	Any N	M_{1a}	S_2
Stage IIIC	Any pT/T_x	N_{1-3}	M_0	S_3
	Any pT/T_x	Any N	M_{1a}	S_3
	Any pT/T_x	Any N	M_{1b}	Any S

Source: From Greene F.L., Page D.L., Fleming, I.D., et al., AJCC Cancer Staging Manual, Sixth Edition. New York: Springer Science and Business Media LLC, 2002: 317–320. www.springerlink.com. Used with the permission of the American Joint Committee on Cancer (AJCC), Chicago, Illinois.

O. Prostate Tumor Staging

Primary Tumor (T)

T_X Primary tumor cannot be assessed

T_0 No evidence of primary tumor

T_1 Clinically inapparent tumor neither palpable nor visible by imaging

T_{1a} Tumor incidental histologic finding in ≤ 5% of tissue resected

T_{1b} Tumor incidental histologic finding in > 5% of tissue resected

T_{1c} Tumor identified by needle biopsy (e.g., because of elevated prostate-specific antigen [PSA]) (Whitmore-Jewett A1 and A2)

T_2 Palpable tumor confined within prostate

T_{2a} Tumor involves one half of one lobe or less

T_{2b} Tumor involves more than one half of one lobe but not both lobes

T_{2c} Tumor involves both lobes (Whitmore-Jewett B1 and B2)

T_3 Tumor extends through the prostate capsule

T_{3a} Extracapsular extension (unilateral or bilateral)

T_{3b} Tumor invades seminal vesicle(s) (Whitmore-Jewett C1 and C2)

T_4 Tumor is fixed or invades adjacent structures other than seminal vesicles: bladder neck, external sphincter, rectum, levator muscles, and/or pelvic wall (Whitmore-Jewett D1 and D2)

Regional Lymph Nodes (N)

N_X Regional lymph nodes cannot be assessed

N_0 No regional lymph node metastasis

N_1 Metastasis in regional lymph node(s)

Distant Metastasis* (M)

M_X Distant metastasis cannot be assessed (not evaluated by any modality)

M_0 No distant metastasis

M_1 Distant metastasis

M_{1a} Nonregional lymph node(s)

M_{1b} Bone(s)

M_{1c} Other site(s) with or without bone disease

* When more than one site of metastasis is present, the most advanced category is used. pM1c is most advanced.

Stage Grouping

Stage I	T_{1a}	N_0	M_0
Stage II	T_{1a}	N_0	M_0
	T_{1b}	N_0	M_0
	T_{1c}	N_0	M_0
	T_1	N_0	M_0
	T_2	N_0	M_0
Stage III	T_3	N_0	M_0
Stage IV	T_4	N_0	M_0
	Any T	N_1	M_0
	Any T	Any N	M_1

Source: From Greene F.L., Page D.L., Fleming, I.D., et al., AJCC Cancer Staging Manual, Sixth Edition. New York: Springer Science and Business Media LLC, 2002: 309–316. www.springerlink.com. Used with the permission of the American Joint Committee on Cancer (AJCC), Chicago, Illinois.

Index

Page numbers followed by *f* or *t* indicate material in figures or tables, respectively.